Kia C

BRAIN BODY DIET

ALSO BY SARA GOTTFRIED

The Hormone Cure
The Hormone Reset Diet
Younger

BRAIN BODY DIET

40 DAYS TO A LEAN, CALM, ENERGIZED, AND HAPPY SELF

SARA GOTTFRIED, MD

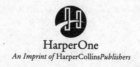

HarperOne
An Imprint of HarperCollinsPublishers

HarperOne

This book contains advice and information relating to health care. It should be used to supplement rather than replace the advice of your doctor or another trained health professional. If you know or suspect you have a health problem, it is recommended that you seek your physician's advice before embarking on any medical program or treatment. All efforts have been made to assure the accuracy of the information contained in this book as of the date of publication. This publisher and the author disclaim liability for any medical outcomes that may occur as a result of applying the methods suggested in this book.

FIRST HARPERCOLLINS PAPERBACK EDITION PUBLISHED IN 2020

Designed by Terry McGrath
Illustrations by Sara Gottfried, MD; Kevin Plottner; and Lisette Picasso

Library of Congress Cataloging-in-Publication Data is available upon request.

ISBN 978-0-06-265596-7

20 21 22 23 24 LSC 10 9 8 7 6 5 4 3 2 1

Dedicated to my daughters,
who inspire me to transform medicine
and make the world a better place

Contents

Foreword

One of the most exciting developments in the area of health and wellness over the past decade has been the recognition that gaining an understanding of a person's uniqueness opens the door to far more effective strategies for management of disease risk and treatment as well as health preservation and enhancement.

This empowering perspective has been termed *personalized medicine*, and it incorporates a vast array of information sets including genetics, standard laboratory assessments, and even information gleaned from studies of a person's gut bacteria to ultimately tailor a dedicated and specific program for the individual.

There's no doubt that this evolving approach holds great promise toward the goals of more efficient and effective health care. And moving forward, the value of incorporating a more personalized approach to the practice of medicine will gain more widespread recognition and implementation.

Standing in contrast to personalized medicine is the "one size fits all" theme that almost fully underlies the practice of medicine in the Western world. This approach values "understanding the disease a person gets" far more than "understanding the person who gets the disease."

It is a system that doesn't fully differentiate diagnostic and therapeutic techniques that represent "standard of care," for example, when comparing men and women. Children, as seen in this paradigm, are merely "small adults."

To be sure, "women's health" as a medical specialty has clearly become well, if not somewhat narrowly, defined. Typically, the term embraces those issues unique to women and overwhelmingly focuses on the reproductive process. More recently, there has been recognition that while rates for conditions like cardiovascular disease, cancer, and lung disease are similar between men and women, the disease course and response to treatment may vary considerably. These observations have helped to broaden the understanding of the uniqueness of women's health well beyond reproduction and sexuality.

Clearly, however, there remains a paucity of acceptance that significant differences exist when comparing the brains of men and women in terms of function, disease risk, and response to treatment. Why this lack of recognition and its acceptance remain pervasive is beyond the scope of this foreword, but it's certainly *not* a consequence of inadequate scientific support. Decades of research clearly demonstrate that females are at less risk for a variety of brain disorders including autism, attention deficit/hyperactivity disorder (ADHD), Tourette syndrome, and dyslexia, but have higher risk for multiple sclerosis, depression, anxiety disorder, and anorexia nervosa. Indeed, a woman's risk for Alzheimer's disease, a disease for which there exists no meaningful treatment whatsoever, is *double* that of a man's, a statistic that receives precious little mention in the media.

There are a multitude of factors at play that contribute to the brain's gender differences, many of which are influential during development. These include fundamental female/male genetic differences as well as variability in terms of how hormonal and environmental influences are operant depending on gender. Hormonal and environmental influences have a direct bearing on brain development as well as secondary effects through the mechanism of altering gene expression.

These and other mechanisms, and their unique gender-related manifestations, persist throughout our lifetimes and impart measurable differences in the brains of women in comparison to men in terms of structure as measured by sophisticated imaging technology. How these physical differences influence physiology, function, and behavior is central to an emerging body of research.

But despite a full understanding of these mechanisms, many important brain-related issues that challenge women are remarkably responsive to modification of lifestyle choices.

In the pages that follow, Dr. Sara Gottfried unpacks the science that clearly supports the heretofore politically incorrect notion that men's and women's brains are different. She deftly explores how these differences manifest in many of the pervasive issues that plague modern women including forgetfulness, weight gain, addiction, depression, anxiety, and exhaustion, and how fundamental the brain/body connection is to overall health and well-being. This connection between brain and body is further explored in the context of conditions like digestive disorders, fluid retention, and chemical sensitivity.

But the true blessing of this work is the actionable plan that builds on this science and paves the way for recovering optimal health. The Brain Body Protocol that Gottfried has created provides a powerful, user-friendly program allowing readers the opportunity to leverage the knowledge Dr. Gottfried presents to bring about a long-awaited, positive change in health destiny—for all women.

David Perlmutter, MD, FACN, ABIHM
May 2018
Naples, Florida

Introduction

Most of us don't really pay attention to our bodies. We exist solely from our heads, ignoring the rest. That's the way "smart women" are taught to survive, but this way of living isn't healthy long-term. Despite my training as a medical doctor, I had to learn that the hard way. When I was forced to confront my own health crisis, I discovered that what we know about improving and changing our bodies is incomplete. Now I'm here to teach you how to make the crucial connection between your body and your brain that will help you thrive. I'll explain how your vague lack of well-being is linked to a weak brain/body bond—and how it can be fixed, starting first with food.

Your brain controls every aspect of your body, health, daily functions, and relationships. When one of these areas breaks down, your brain does, too—and vice versa. If you're one of the hundred million women who suffer from foggy thinking, anxiety, depression, addiction, forgetfulness, overwhelm, exhaustion, and other seemingly brain-related problems, then this book is for you. If you're one of the half billion women with an inflammatory issue that puts you at risk for one of these conditions—and stubborn weight gain—then this book is for you, too. If you have a sister, mother, child, wife, or friend with any of these symptoms, they need the help described in this book. Left unaddressed, these nagging symptoms can ravage your brain and start cognitive and physical decline in your body prematurely. However, all of these symptoms have their root not merely in the brain, but also in the body.

So why isn't everyone talking about this crucial connection between the brain and body that impacts all we do? The reason is that we believe the brain is in charge—that the body blindly follows the commands of the brain, as if the instruction moves in one direction only, brain to body. But I discovered that's not true. The instruction is bidirectional.

My research has unlocked a vital missing piece of information that holds tremendous value for women: The brain is the ultimate output center for all efforts of the body, but you can't have a healthy brain if your body is out of whack, and you can't have a healthy body if your brain is out of whack. It's the ultimate interdependent relationship that is essential to long-term health and balance. The connection between brain and body is both mutually dependent and mutually supporting. I coined a new term to reflect this fundamental interconnection: *brain body*.

It's important to highlight that the female brain body is different from the male brain body. What works for men cannot be assumed to work for women, because we are not merely smaller versions of men. Toxins push the brain and body apart, and women are often more vulnerable to toxins. Similarly, the brain body breaks down in different ways for women compared with men. No wonder our rates of anxiety, depression, insomnia, and Alzheimer's are double the rates in men! I developed the Brain Body Diet to help women repair that bond, because the relationship between the body and brain is an essential foundation for us to function at our best today and protect our bodies and minds into the future.

In *Brain Body Diet*, food and lifestyle are our main "drugs" of choice. Unlike quick-fix pharmaceuticals targeting specific insurance-approved symptoms, changes in daily lifestyle are healing and restorative for the majority of people because they activate your body's innate ability to restore and maintain balance. Let's face it: pharmaceutical drugs that are prescribed for brain/body problems carry health risks, provide limited success, and most importantly, can disrupt the body's delicate healing mechanisms. Instead, I'll show you how to reverse or prevent brain/

SYMPTOMS OF BRAIN/BODY BREAKDOWN

- Feeling over-obligated and stressed, like you're churning and not making progress
- Weight gain, thicker waistline, difficulty losing weight
- Fluid retention, feeling puffy all over, dull skin color, sensitivity to chemicals
- Brain fog, sluggishness, trouble concentrating or thinking clearly, slow mental processing speed
- Complacency, less empathy, social isolation or feeling the need to dominate or control
- Leaky gut, which may appear as gas, abdominal bloating and discomfort, acid reflux, constipation, loose stool
- Overwhelm, restlessness, or anxiety
- Difficulty sleeping restfully through the night
- Burnout, depression, impulsivity, aggression
- Sugar, alcohol, or dairy cravings that you just can't ditch
- Addictive tendencies for food, alcohol, exercise, shopping, social media, or your smartphone
- "Resting bitch face"
- Feeling a lack of sovereignty, freedom, or security about your health or future
- Feeling that your short-term memory is slipping

body breakdown with evidence-based supportive nutrients from delicious food, easy-to-implement lifestyle redesign, specific exercise and mind-body practices, high-quality supplements, and, occasionally, low doses of hormones. In ancient Greece, a prescription like this was called a *diet*, or *diaita*—a prescribed way of living, of regular, daily work, not simply a restricted eating regimen that's a short-term means to an end. I consider the "prescribed way of living" to be a personalized lifestyle medicine protocol. Allow me to invite you into my medical office, to learn about the brain body and how we can knit yours back together for your greatest health and well-being. Buckle up—we're starting now!

Certain symptoms reflect a brain body out of balance. These are sacred messages, not diseases to be medicated into submission. When left unaddressed, these conditions don't simply mellow out; they tax your brain and body to the point of creating more serious conditions that are hard to reverse as those symptoms slowly establish stronger and stronger neural pathways in the brain, like a river carving a canyon. It's tough to create a new river, or pathway, but the Brain Body Diet gives you the tools you need to start digging.

Foundation of a Healthy Brain Body

Far too many of us take the brain for granted. Consider this: the brain represents only 2 to 3 percent of total body weight but consumes 25 percent of total body glucose, 20 percent of total body oxygen, and 20 percent of cardiac output. So one quarter of your fuel goes to the brain, along with one fifth of your oxygen and blood. That means the brain plays the biggest role of any organ in your body when it comes to metabolism—that is, sucking up the fuel you put inside your body. So if there's a problem with metabolism in the brain, the problem will be felt throughout the body.

The food you consume has the potential to help or hurt the gut first, then the brain, and, finally, the rest of the body. Food is information not only for the DNA of your cells but also for the DNA of the microbes in your gut, known as your microbiome (think of it as your second genome). The food on your fork determines gene expression, hormone levels, immune activity—even stress levels in your gut, your brain, and the rest of your body. Not only that, but a change in the food you eat alters the activity of the gut microbiota rapidly—within one to four days, and in some genes within six hours.[1] That's fast. And when your gut microbiota change, so does your brain. That's why nutrients matter.

In personalized lifestyle medicine, when you don't feel completely

---

[1] A tremendous amount of research fills the pages that follow. In an effort to save paper but make certain that the documentation and sources are available to everyone, I have taken the liberty of putting all of the notes on my website. Please visit at www.brainbodydiet.com.

healthy, we start first with the gut/brain connection, beginning with food. (Mainstream medicine starts with drugs.) A "food first" philosophy is the foundation of a robustly healthy brain body. If you ignore your symptoms, you raise your risk of serious cognitive decline and other brain/body problems that could be in your future sooner than you'd expect if you don't take care of your brain body now.

How do I know? Take estrogen. *Estrogen is the fundamental regulator of the female brain body.* In the brain, estrogen polices key biological functions like glucose transport, metabolism, and mitochondrial function—the way you produce energy. In the body, estrogen protects you from weight gain, ravenous appetite, insulin resistance, diabetes, and cancer. In sum, estrogen has hundreds of jobs beyond the usual female tasks that come to mind, like growing breasts and hips. When estrogen levels start to decline after age forty in perimenopause, a sequence of events unfold that lead to a woman's greater risk of insomnia, anxiety, depression, stroke, dementia, and Alzheimer's disease.[2] What's unique to women is this sudden loss of estrogen and how it makes the brain body's metabolism falter and then dramatically decline, putting women at grave risk of future disease.[3] Metabolism is further compromised by the change in crosstalk between estrogen and other chemical messengers in the body, like leptin (the hormone that tells you to put down the fork), ghrelin (the hormone that tells you to pick up the fork), adiponectin (the hormone that tells your body to burn fat), and sex hormone–binding globulin (the sponge that soaks up free levels of other sex hormones, including estrogen). Some women compensate well for the loss of estrogen that begins in their forties; most do not. If you're over forty and have been unhappy with how your body is changing, you may have brain/body dysfunction and need the help of this book.

This is what you need to understand about the brain/body connection: it's the key to health *wherever* you are in your life or healing journey. This connection holds the key to reversing many chronic symptoms that you may have felt you simply have had to live with. If you are struggling to lose weight, sleep at night, find more energy, access more joy, or simply want to maximize your health and longevity, *Brain Body Diet* is the answer you have been waiting for.

On a more macro level, women have an urgent biological imperative to pay attention to their brain body, to manage their estrogen, and to "tend and befriend" in response to stress of all kinds. Tending and befriending first oneself and then others provides something essential and profound: mental, physical, and brain immunity against all sorts of insults: toxins, unnecessary inflammation, and—more urgently— the runaway train of stress. This immunity is the downstream benefit when your brain and body are allies. When women don't heed this fundamental biological need, the result is more toxin accumulation, excess inflammation, aggression, impulsiveness, and the warning signs listed in the box on page 3.[4] Think of inflammation as an ugly low-level burn that's quietly robbing you of brain cells and the connections between them, making you fat, tired, and dim.

How I Stumbled on the Brain/Body Axis

In 2015, I hit upon a breakthrough about the brain body, and what I discovered is that the connection is not obvious. I learned this the hard way: I fainted, crashed, and smacked my head.

You'd think I was the quintessential "smart woman": a medical doctor educated at top schools with a successful career practicing medicine for more than twenty-five years—and the author of multiple *New York Times* bestselling books.

But if you looked at the biochemistry inside my cells and tissues, you'd see a civil war. You wouldn't know it at the time of my fall, but my belly was covered in itchy hives and eczema from a combination of leaky gut, rogue and imbalanced gut microbes, and inflammation (and the tight shapewear under my dress didn't help).

Back then, when there was something about my body I didn't like, my method was to make a decision about a change in behavior and just do it, like a dictator, top down. Looking back, I see it as fear-based—fear of ending up fat, divorced, alienated from my children, alone, homeless, destitute . . . other wild ideas. Fear actually works to get you started—to lose a few pounds, to work less, to be more patient with the kids. But for me, after the fear wore off, I'd fall back into my bad habits and Band-Aid solutions. For me, the Band-Aids were eating too much cheesecake in hopes of changing my emotional state, shutting down in my marriage, bingeing on drama, and, generally, working and pushing harder. I'd try to manage my disappointment and frustration by taking myself out for a manicure/pedicure, which merely added more toxins to the mix and made my brain/body problems worse.

I realize that you might approach your own life problems differently. I tend to be on the restrictive side of the spectrum. When I wanted to lose weight, I'd follow strict rules. I've worked with plenty of women who are on the permissive side of the spectrum, so when they feel put out, stressed, frustrated, or fat, they say, "Well, I deserve this chocolate." Or, "Time for that glass of wine."

I get it. My point is that while we as women may react in different ways, we've all got our Band-Aids. Our workarounds. Mine were more rules, burying myself in my work, and withdrawing from my husband— yours may be French fries or a decadent vacation.

But then I fell and hit my head and it opened a whole new world for me. I was at a cozy evening with friends. And—as I see now—I had ignored the messages my body was sending all day long, telling me it was dehydrated. Pushed too hard. Hadn't eaten and blood sugar low. Too stressed. Sleep deprived.

I set myself up for a fall.

I was standing in the kitchen, and I fainted—passed out cold. My brain did what it has evolved to do in a crisis: it shut down. Like an operating system that suddenly freezes, I lost cerebral blood flow and consciousness. I struck a cold tile floor, hitting the back of my head so hard that I had what looked like seizures due to the trauma.

When I hit my head, I was diagnosed with a severe concussion, a form of traumatic brain injury. At first I felt hopeless because I fell into a mysterious gap that most physicians are unaware of and cannot solve. As a result, I was sent home from the emergency room and doctors' offices with the typical recommendations of a health care system that didn't know what to do with me: *rest in bed in a dark room, reduce your stress, try to stay calm, give it time.* Meanwhile, my symptoms worsened. I knew something was wrong, so I set out to understand the biological imperatives that were at work behind the scenes of my symptoms. It was terrifying—until I figured out the root cause . . . and then the solution.

Yes, my fall was traumatic and terrifying, but it was also life-changing. Before I fainted, I knew little about the importance of the brain in repairing the body. I had the textbook medical knowledge, but that was only a partial view of a much more complex issue. Not only did I damage my left brain hemisphere as I fell to the ground, I emerged from the traumatic brain injury a different person. I went from being a board-certified doctor who thought she understood the importance of the brain to being humbled and full of awe about our neurological powers. Thus began my quest to be more than just a capable gynecologist and functional medicine doctor. It became essential that I understand the central role of the brain in healing the body.

These are the lessons I'm bringing to you, dear reader, in *Brain Body Diet*.

I certainly didn't know that I needed brain/body rehab until I hit my head. I'd rarely, if ever, thought about the connection. My collapse triggered an epiphany. At age forty-seven, I was in good shape hormonally due to my work as described previously in my first book, *The Hormone Cure*. My key hormones—estrogen, progesterone, thyroid, testosterone—even cortisol—were in balance. Still, even though I was no longer a hormonal nightmare, I didn't honor the biological needs of a female brain. I was more of a bulldozer than a woman. As a result, I lost the system of checks and balances in my brain and needed to re-create homeostasis—a state of physical, mental, and spiritual equilibrium. You will read about addressing all of these states in these pages.

What I discovered radically altered my understanding of how to heal the human body. It turns out that *when you take care of your brain body, you're actually taking care of all the systems in your body:* body weight set point, anxiety, depression, addictive tendencies, sex drive, heart and circulation, gastrointestinal and immune systems, and of course, the endocrine system, from your thyroid to your sex organs. Repairing the brain resolves so many small and big health issues, from the mundane and annoying to the memory-robbing and life-threatening. Mending the brain addresses the root of many of the irritating bodily symptoms that you may have, and this process you'll learn could be the most important tool in your arsenal.

The definition of a healthy brain body is that your brain and body are in sync. Healing conversations are occurring. That is, your gut is having a healing conversation back and forth with your brain, and your heart is telling your brain's overactive stress-response system that it can calm down. In short, having a healthy brain body means you are clear of the inflammation that causes brain/body breakdown. This inflammation arises as a result of the stresses and environmental toxins of modern life. Like me, you are probably unaware of your own inflammation or even brain/body symptoms. Frankly, I had built a wall between my brain and body, like the separation between church and state. Maybe you've done the same.

Typically, most of us maintain separation between our brain and our body—this is a façade, of course. For instance, when my husband's shoulder hurts after golfing, the pain and inflammation emanating from his shoulder is telling him to ice it. His brain overrides the pain with a dismissive, "I'm too busy to ice. I'll just take an ibuprofen." Yet the road to total health requires that we recognize the symbiotic connection between brain and body, which is what I teach you to do in this book. Once you understand the wall between brain and body, it will be easier to dismantle it and achieve a healthy relationship between the two once again and create lasting health.

I spent a few months being a total mess—lying in a dark room most of the time, nauseated, unable to drive for some time, exquisitely sensitive to noise, unable to work, unable to exercise because of my poor balance, unable to walk. I spent more time sitting still than ever before because I was forced to; I didn't have a choice. But some beneficial things happened as well.

I began to listen to the subtle moments of guidance that came from my heart, even though my brain was offline. At first, the softness and quiet were there because I couldn't really do much of anything. I stopped doing all the "shoulds"—I *should* exercise, I *should* work tonight. I just physically couldn't. Initially, that felt like a failure. But since I couldn't follow my inner dictator and bury myself in my work—or do the Band-Aids, the coverups, the workarounds that I performed to make myself feel better in the moment—I was stripped down to just *me*, a new version of me. I couldn't even distance myself from my husband because I was more dependent on him than ever before.

And you know what?

He loved it. He asked if I could hit my head more often. No more sitting in bed, late at night, typing aggressively on the laptop. Over time there was more laughing, sex, and stillness. Hit your head, improve your marriage!

Over time, that softness spilled out not only to my relationship with myself, or my husband, but also to how I related to my kids, sisters, parents, friends, and patients.

In the past, when my kids would come to me with something that wasn't right at school, the "smart woman" in me had immediate ideas about how to solve it. But as I lay in bed recovering from my fall, all I could do was invite them in under the covers with me. Instead of telling them the answers, I would ask them what their heart was asking for, or whispering to them.

My brain can't do this, could never do this, and won't ever be able to do this *on its own*. Instead of just being *smart*, I became *whole*. I learned that the heart can discern different and more important things than the brain. The brain is not the control center for the female body; the heart is, when you are quiet enough to listen and strong enough to surrender.

I'm here to teach you a better way to this wholeness, so you don't have to undergo the trauma that I did. It doesn't have to take you months to learn these lessons. I'm asking for forty days.

What I Was Shocked to Learn

I learned many astonishing things while healing from my brain/body injury. First, nerve cells (neurons) are quite delicate, much less hardy than I assumed. They're easy to break and damage with inflammation.

Second, I was chock-full of brain/body toxins. Even though I was living "clean" and had a hunch that detoxing once per quarter would keep me safe, there was still more to do when it came to the toxic load in my brain body—that is, there were key steps to take beyond the foundational work described in my first three books. Toxins of all sorts are linked to vague brain symptoms related to memory, focus, impulse control, resilience, libido, weight gain, and mood. They wreak havoc by disrupting normal balance in the brain and body.

Third, I had prediabetes, and this led to my fall. Prediabetes is a brain/body failure state that sent my blood sugar into wild fluctuations, changed blood flow to the brain, made my gut and then my brain leaky, damaged my mitochondria, and drove my adrenals into the ground. The root cause of my blood sugar problems—insulin block and intractable stress—became a major trigger for brain/body breakdown. I want to teach you how to manage those problems.

Your brain uses the same enzyme, called *insulin-degrading enzyme,* for a dual purpose: to process insulin after it's used, and to clear a potential toxin called amyloid beta that's associated with Alzheimer's disease. This discovery that insulin and amyloid beta share the same breakdown enzyme is a breakthrough in our understanding of the brain/body connection.[5]

Furthermore, the enzyme can't do both jobs at once. If the enzyme is busy breaking down insulin because your blood sugar is too high (like mine used to be)—thereby cranking out the insulin to try to drive the blood glucose into cells—your insulin-degrading enzyme won't be free to break down amyloid beta. As a result of reduced clearance, sticky amyloid beta can accumulate excessively in toxic seeds, then deposits, and ultimately plaques, a hallmark of Alzheimer's disease.[6] When amyloid beta builds up beyond a certain point, it becomes toxic to nerve cells, destroys synapses (the connections between nerve cells), and promotes brain inflammation, which then promotes more toxic amyloid beta accumulation. High blood sugar and amyloid beta accumulation become a vicious cycle you want to avoid—unless you prefer to lose your marbles as you age! (While the main point of this book isn't to prevent or reverse Alzheimer's, my strategies are aimed at reversing insulin block, which will also help you prevent some cases of Alzheimer's disease, including early manifestations like forgetfulness and mood changes.)

Finally, I realized that I may have never recovered my full brain function post-pregnancy, and my last pregnancy was well over a decade ago! As I flailed about, wondering why mothering was so much work—and harder compared with my career in medicine—I discovered that restoring brain function makes a huge difference in how I feel day to day.

The more I learned, the more I wanted to know why doctors and other health experts weren't talking about brain/body health. It's almost pointless—or at the very least, incomplete and counterintuitive—to address other health problems if we don't first address what's going on with the operating system of the body, the brain.

Remember: *the brain is the ultimate output center for all the efforts of the body.* If we don't eat properly, don't exercise right, and don't sleep, the primary impact is on the brain. There is not one without the other. Permit me to repeat that you can't have a healthy brain if your body is broken, and you can't have a healthy body if your brain is broken: full of toxins, inflamed, hypervigilant, and shrinking. Until we better understand the brain/body axis, we will continue to suffer from countless issues that will plague us every day and potentially shorten our lives. It's time to turn that around. You will learn how to make a dramatic difference in the way you feel, possibly even immediately, if you stick to the forty-day protocol.

How Mainstream Medicine Fails Us

To put it mildly, mainstream medicine let me down. At first, I was stung by the way my symptoms were not taken seriously. Then I got angry, because I don't want mainstream medicine to fail you, too.

Women tell me in my office: "I don't feel well. It's like I'm in a race I can never win. None of my other doctors are helping, let alone listening. I've been dismissed. You're my last hope." They feel unwell: foggier, hungrier, plumper, more forgetful, more anxious, and unhappier than ever before. Epidemiology confirms this—I break down more statistics below.

When they trot out these symptoms to their doctors, women are offered prescriptions for insomnia or anxiety or depression, perhaps issued with arrogance and impatience (or with a gentle suggestion to "go see a therapist," as if their problem were purely psychological), and it seems that the common symptoms of a woman over forty are undeserving of doctors' attention and problem-solving abilities. Those prescriptions barely work, are sometimes worse than placebos, can be addictive, and tend to numb you rather than address the root causes of your symptoms. I know it's tempting to look for the solution in a pill, but let's be honest here: when's the last time a pill really fixed your problems? Don't get me started on the side effects: more weight gain, sexual dysfunction (including difficulty achieving orgasm), and possibly dementia!

At the same time, a recent large study from Harvard of 52,135 middle-aged women, followed for twenty-two years, showed that only 13 percent of women can be classified as "healthy agers," defined as having no impairment of memory, physical fitness, or mental health, and being free of eleven major chronic diseases.[7] *Thirteen percent!* A similar study of a large group of health professionals (92,837 women and 25,303 men) showed that moderate weight gain in adulthood from age twenty-one to age fifty-five of 2.5 to 10 kilograms (5.5 to 22 pounds) is associated with significantly increased risk of major chronic diseases and decreased odds of healthy aging.[8] No surprise: weight gain is a brain/body problem that puts you at substantial risk of other chronic diseases like high blood pressure, heart disease, diabetes, and obesity-related cancer.

Brain stressors may fly below the radar for most women and physicians, but not for your body's sense of homeostasis. Over time, the sheer volume leads to toxic overload. We haven't had time to develop immunity, physical or mental. Take the rampant use of the internet and cell phones for the past decade: during that time, a parallel rise in the broken brain/body connection has occurred, especially among the "constant checkers," marked by symptoms like greater stress, anxiety, social isolation, depression, obesity, and poor quality of life.[9] It's no wonder that I'm obsessed with the brain body. Few other doctors are! And it's messing with our heads.

To summarize: Women intuitively know there's a serious epidemic of a broken-down brain body, as do scientists who measure disease rates. Doctors, by and large, do not.

Doctors may tell you, as they told me, that anxiety, depression, and having trouble finding the word on the tip of your tongue are an inevitable part of getting older. Weight gain? Doctors shrug and tell us to eat less and exercise more, even though almost none of these strategies work. You're just an unlucky person in the scheme of things.

Really? So one in three women over the age of forty is unlucky and in need of a potentially dangerous prescription? I don't think so.

That's when women end up in the offices of alternative therapists, hoping that a medical medium or crystal healer—or even voluntary bee stings—might solve their irksome complaints. The alternative approaches may help for a few hours, but they are not necessarily supported by the best evidence, such as randomized, controlled clinical trials. (Personally, I swear by acupuncture, which has centuries of effective practice behind it, combined with rigorous and proven functional medicine protocols.) Yet women are desperate (I was, too), which leads to a largely uncritical acceptance of sometimes unproven therapies that may worsen your symptoms in the long run.

Honestly, I am reluctant to criticize mainstream doctors. Instead, I want to build bridges and together figure out the best, most evidence-based approach for our patients. I was educated along with mainstream doctors at Harvard Medical School and then the University of California at San Francisco, and I used to be one, myself. I am surrounded by conventional doctors in my professional and social circles. They are not to blame; rather, they work within a broken health care system that rushes to make a quick diagnosis in seven minutes flat.

Doctors point out the progress made with diseases such as colon cancer and hip fractures,[10] yet brain-related conditions, including one's ability to focus and pay attention, lose weight, feel free of worry and depressive thoughts, and avoid Alzheimer's disease, are worsening. The uptick in these brain problems coincides with mounting exposures to toxins from food, longstanding stress, and the environment. Women are experiencing something very important: their bodies are responding normally to an abnormal set of stressors, but they have no idea that this is the case. Our work as doctors and enlightened citizens is only beginning if we want to turn this around. And you, by following the protocol in this book, are on the road to discovering the truly healthy and balanced way you can live as part of a larger ecosystem of challenges that include dysfunctional eating habits, lack of sufficient exercise, a toxic environment, inflammation in the brain body, and health that often suffers as a result.

Behind every brain-related condition is a problem present first in the body. Most physicians and their female patients have no clue that the lead in their lipstick is slowing down their thoughts, or that the typical American diet leads to dementia, or that stress on the brain turns into pain in the neck. This is a bit like yelling at your kids for asking, "What's for dinner?" when you're really pissed that your boss just added three new assignments to your already staggering workload. It's important to look further upstream instead of simply at the most immediate symptom.

Meanwhile, women feel like they're in the rat race and need to persevere despite the symptoms. They go to bed fearing that their brain function is getting worse, that their health is deteriorating, and nothing can be done. They feel stuck with the same old patterns: weight that won't budge, exercise for which they cannot find time, worries about their job or family, feeling too tired to make a change. Or they reassure themselves that maybe it's not that bad, probably because they can't see all the ways their brain/body connection isn't working. I know because not only have I lived it, I've heard about it from thousands of women in my office.

For women, problem drinking is up. So is chronic pain. Mental acuity and happiness are down. Without enough neurotransmitters—the chemical messengers that communicate information between the brain and body—to go around, there's no pause before making the next bad choice about food or other lifestyle factors that could help. The net result? You're mired in a body you don't want or need. I understand: women are too busy, tired, and stressed to prioritize future health over short-term relief.

It's a case of self-preservation gone wrong. Self-preservation keeps you stuck in your fight-flight-freeze response. The old wiring is based on survival but doesn't serve your current need for more nuanced behavior, like a resourceful response to your partner or boss. Instead, we end up with maladaptive thought patterns that create entrenched neural pathways in the brain, leading to anxiety, pain, depression, even addiction. And then your brain isn't able to serve you when you need it. Thought patterns don't change unless we change the *physiology* behind them with *physical* solutions—fresh nutrients, sufficient blood flow, and toxin-free thoughts, buttressed by an intentional practice to be more gentle and supportive with ourselves. You'll gain tools in this book that you likely are not getting at your doctor's office.

Brain/Body Breakdown by the Numbers

After my fall, I rewrote my brain destiny, and with it the destiny of my entire body. As I recovered, I was forced to reconcile a sad state of affairs when it comes to our health, a silent epidemic of brain/body disconnection, leading to brain/body failure. Here are just a few of the dire statistics:

- One in three Americans are plagued by anxiety or depression. Women are affected twice as often as men.
- One in four women over the age of forty take an antidepressant—prescriptions have tripled in the past decade despite evidence that antidepressants are often worse than placebos.
- Eighty percent of women are unhappy with their bodies, and no wonder: body weight set point keeps rising, a major sign of brain/body breakdown. Here in the United States, we just keep getting fatter.[11]
- Twenty percent of Americans, predominantly women, suffer with food addiction.[12]
- Stress levels in the United States continue to rise, with two-thirds of Americans experiencing significant stress about their future.
- More than ninety Americans are dying every day after overdosing on opioids—including prescription pain relievers, heroin, and fentanyl.
- At least twenty-four million people in the United States behave addictively with alcohol and drugs. Ten percent of US adults abuse alcohol, and women are the fastest-growing demographic.
- Traumatic brain injury is on the rise, and women fare worse than men: women sustain more concussions in sports and report more traumatic brain injury symptoms (and the symptoms they experience are more severe, and they take longer to recover).
- Internet addiction is a growing issue, affecting up to 17 percent of teenagers, and plays a role in the exponential rise of adolescent anxiety, depression, and even obesity.[13]

- Strokes are the third-leading cause of death for women, and fifth-leading cause of death for men. Women have worse outcomes than men after stroke and higher rates of recurrence.

- One in eight baby boomers complain of memory loss, which represents 13 percent of people over the age of sixty.

- In 2015, dementia was diagnosed in more than 47 million people worldwide, and the number is expected to triple by 2050.

- Alzheimer's disease is diagnosed every sixty-six seconds and currently affects 5.5 million people, but that number will quadruple by 2050.

As you can see, brain/body breakdown occurs in all stages of life, from adolescence to old age and everywhere in between. It occurs in men and women, although as a board-certified gynecologist, my focus is how to help women recover, reset, and emerge better than ever. Depending on how your specific genes interact with your environment, brain/body disconnection shows up in different ways—but what I want you to know is that these various symptoms and conditions have a similar root cause: inflammation of the brain leading to loss of physiological balance (homeostasis). The worst part is that conventional medicine usually drops the ball, because nearly all of these conditions of brain/body breakdown are preventable and reversible. Let me repeat this: I can show you how we can avoid these symptoms completely and reverse existing conditions so that you can lose weight and feel at home in your brain body again.

The root cause of your symptoms involves toxic exposures, from the toxic stress of too many obligations to getting pummeled with endocrine disruptors like obesogens (sneaky toxins that rob you of a healthy weight) and dementogens (toxins that rob you of cognitive function). When you understand how toxins can ramp up inflammation in the body and brain, causing disruption of normal activity, you will then understand the best scenarios for relieving your symptoms and resolving the real brain/body problem. I will teach you how to develop physical and mental immunity from our constant bombardment of poisons, which will help you lose weight, clear the brain fog, step away from addictive patterns, calm down, cheer up, and remember that word on the tip of your tongue.

Is this a case of unwarranted chemophobia and fearmongering about toxins? No. I believe in a science-based approach to health, and that we need to make it less complicated. We all know the key features of a healthy lifestyle: eat more vegetables, drink less alcohol, exercise more, get enough sleep, foster good relationships, and connect to purpose and meaning. Yet I know from working in the trenches that common knowledge is rarely common practice. We all need help fitting these key features—plus whatever additional strategies science has thrown our way—into our lives in a sane, productive way. Furthermore, I've noticed in my years of taking care of women that many lack the proper genes that remove toxins and reverse inflammation. Sometimes we need extra help with these complications so that we can feel our best.

When it comes to the brain/body breakdown, *Brain Body Diet* teaches you the evidence-based practices that work and clarifies what doesn't work, so you can avoid wasting your time, money, and resources. You'll feel better—fabulously *well*, in fact—as you get your brain body and your life back.

Success with the Brain Body Diet

Maybe you need to upgrade your memory, burn off brain fog, or heal a problem like an expanding waistline, depression, shopping addiction, or headaches. It may be a tendency toward moodiness, worrying, forgetfulness, or toxic overload that you no longer can tolerate. Perhaps you'll discover that your lack of impulse control stems from a dopamine deficiency, or maybe you're like me and your main goal is to stave off aging-related cognitive decline, create equanimity, and keep growing and deepening relationships. It takes the natural, innate power of the brain body to rebalance the brain and get to the root of body problems that may seem intractable.

Briefly, here are several success stories with the Brain Body Diet that you will read about in the following chapters.

Tamara, age thirty-eight, came to see me for fatigue and weight gain. We discovered she had Hashimoto's thyroiditis and that her body contained toxic levels of mercury. Testing revealed that her detoxification genes were underperforming, so we found a way to work around them. After completing the protocol, her mercury levels dropped along with her weight, for a total loss of twenty-five pounds. Tamara shows no further signs of autoimmune thyroiditis (her antibody tests are normal) and maintains a healthy weight.

Ruthie struggled with an eating disorder and food addiction that got worse after pregnancy. We traced her problem to a classic imbalance of low levels of the "pleasure" brain chemical—called dopamine—and eating too much highly palatable food like nachos and pastries. Pregnancy and sugar were literally shrinking her brain, making her less resourceful and able to override her cravings. Now, at age fifty-two, she has recovered after performing the Brain Body Diet.

Karen, age forty-five, healed her worry and anxiety with a few small but consistent changes to her food plan, altering her microbiome, swimming more regularly, and taking a natural chill pill as outlined in the protocol.

What to Expect

Brain Body Diet will show you how to address the symptoms of an imbalanced brain body. Specifically, I will provide you with tools to do the following:

- Remove toxins, including those *obesogens* and *dementogens* that I mentioned earlier. They change your mind, generate negative habits and obsessions, make you hungrier and fatigued, and increase your risk of cognitive impairment and memory loss—generally making you not feel like yourself.

- Change the body weight set point in the brain that makes it so difficult to lose weight.

- Recover the gray matter (brain cells responsible for processing and cognition) lost during pregnancy and/or through excess alcohol consumption.

- Improve strength (particularly leg strength, which is the best predictor of cognitive function years later).

- Regain and stabilize mental health and prevent burnout, depression, and anxiety.

- Add years to your life by restoring health to mitochondria that may have been damaged from the combination of too much sugar and fat, oxidative damage, heavy metals, and xenobiotics.

- Deepen sleep, enhance the glymphatic system, and clear more amyloid beta—the potential toxin that contributes to Alzheimer's disease.

- Reclaim the balance in your gut flora that prevents inflammation, autoimmunity, hormone problems, and weight gain.

- Prevent or reverse brain-related neuroinflammation and degenerative disease, such as memory loss, Alzheimer's, and multiple sclerosis.

- Create a greater sense of integrated wholeness—what I like to think of as *neurospirituality*.

I will share with you the exact principles that I researched and discovered to recover my brain/body homeostasis—and then successfully implemented with hundreds of patients.

Regardless of what you're after, change starts first in the brain and then radiates out to the body. The brain is boss—although if it overworks your body, your body can rebel and shut down the brain. Before change can occur, we need to identify patterns in the brain/body connection that are no longer working for you. Once you become aware of the unmanageable brain patterns ("But I *like* this rice that might contain arsenic!" or "My husband cheated, so I deserve my favorite dessert" or "A water filter sounds like a good idea, but I'm too busy right now"), you can take the critical action to revise and release them.

Brain health is the gateway to the best health. It must be gently triggered by faith with sensitivity, specificity, and nuance. Harsh, aggressive, bulldozing programs usually don't work over the long term, but kind and nurturing inquiry about what's true for you does. Through the Brain Body Diet, you and I working as a team for just forty days will rewire your brain with the most important tools in the lifestyle medicine arsenal: healthy unprocessed food, best times to eat, exercise, yoga, meditation, short pulses of supplements, bioidentical hormones, relationships, social support, and purpose.

Brain Body Diet will help you induce and maintain the key processes that lead to stronger nerve cells, synapses, and support cells (glial cells). The forty-day Brain Body Diet is a multistep, proven, and highly choreographed process that will lead to long-lasting changes in the molecular dance within your gut, brain, and body. You'll find individual protocols for the symptoms that bother you most, led by a questionnaire to assess if you need that particular protocol. You will reclaim your brain/body health so that you are no longer prey to overwhelming feelings of anxiety or depression. You will quell inflammation by clearing toxins, healing your brain/body connections especially between the gut and brain. You will lower your dose of toxic stress and get your needs met when it comes to sleep, sunshine, movement, emotional connection, healthy relationships, and spiritual development. You will reset the diverse hormones affecting your brain that control everything from hunger to memory. If you are overweight, you will lower your body weight set point, which is controlled by brain/body interactions. You'll reverse brain shrinkage that occurs from pregnancy, eating sugar and drinking alcohol, and lack of the types of exercise that specifically prevent brain inflammation and aging. I'll help you get off sticky prescription medications that aren't serving you. You will feel back at home in your body again with mental sharpness, able to roll with the punches and to fit into your favorite jeans, glowing from within and happy in your body. You'll have total health with brain and body back in alliance, and it doesn't have to be complicated or require expensive procedures or creams.

When you complete the Brain Body Diet, you'll feel deeply calm, energized, centered, clearheaded, lean, and smart. Your body will function more easily. You'll resolve your deepest ailments and finally feel a sense of peace. You'll make smarter decisions. You'll love better.

At this point, you are beginning to understand the relationship between brain and body and how it becomes dysfunctional. Next, we want to work together to change your daily choices and actions so that they are aligned with the best expression of your unique brain body. Learning to live in a new way with your brain body demands time and

patience. With the protocol in this book, I'm asking for just forty days
to discover this place of health and harmony. I've done it, and so have
many others. Now it's your turn. Together, we've got this covered.

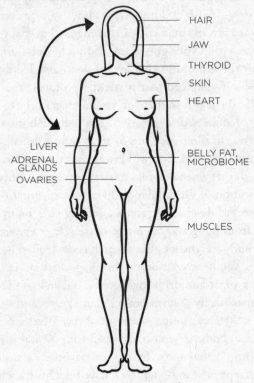

HAIR

JAW

THYROID

SKIN

HEART

LIVER
ADRENAL
GLANDS
OVARIES

BELLY FAT,
MICROBIOME

MUSCLES

Brain/Body Connections

1

The Most Precious Connection

Like me, you probably never think about the soft pink mass containing 100 billion neurons inside your skull and how it interacts with your body, yet this connection desperately needs your attention. Prior to my injury, I took my brain for granted. I toiled diligently to keep work in progress, hormones in balance, stress in perspective, gene expression optimized, and family healthy, but I didn't feel old enough to care about my brain. The possibility of Alzheimer's disease—or worse, drooling in a nursing home—felt remote, more than fifty years away. It turns out that the brain may start to decline in the thirties and forties—*decades* prior to a serious diagnosis of cognitive decline, memory problems, poor reaction time, or even Alzheimer's. Brain deterioration begins first in the body. It's up to us to do something about it, to approach the brain and body differently, to realize they are like best friends that suffer when disconnected.

What I learned is that you're not stuck with the brain you have. In fact, your brain can get better with time, even in middle and older age. Unfortunately, mainstream medicine isn't much help—it can only go so far. Mainstream doctors don't tell you, for instance, that when you become pregnant your gray matter shrinks for up to two years after birth.[1]

(Even more strange, the more it shrinks, the more you bond with your baby!) They don't tell you that of every seven depressed people they treat with a selective serotonin reuptake inhibitor, only one gets well.[2] They don't tell you that a moderate to severe concussion (a trauma-induced disturbance of brain function) in contact sports or from a fall increases your risk of dementia in the future by 90 percent, especially if the brain injury occurs in your forties, like mine.[3] Blows to the head cause microglia (a type of brain cell) to secrete mysterious microparticles that migrate across the brain, spreading inflammation far beyond the site of injury.[4] Isn't that something you would want to know before it's too late, before the brain shrinkage, anxiety diagnosis, or cancer? On the other hand, when you're armed with tools from this book, you can activate your brain to take the lead in healing your body and make your brain body stronger and sharper, starting now. You can leap out of your brain/body rut. Follow the Brain Body Diet and see the results for yourself (or put this book down, plop down in front of a television show, and take your chances!).

It took me about one year to fully recover from my concussion. During that time, I was saddled with balance issues, persistent nausea, poor memory, and extreme noise sensitivity. All of my symptoms resolved with brain/body rehab. I learned in a more personal way how the brain constantly edits itself through the building and pruning of connections between neurons, otherwise known as synapses. I've distilled the results of my brain/body dysfunction and countless hours of research so you can heal more quickly—in a research-based but easy-to-follow protocol—and certainly without hitting your head!

Here's the problem as I see it: the most important organ in your body is being ignored and overlooked as you and your doctors address what seem to be unrelated health problems. It's as if you have a world-class Olympic athlete at your disposal to train you for greatness, but you instead turn to outdated fitness fads like sauna suits and eight-minute abs. You consider the brain and think, *Yeah, it's working just fine,* and then you blow off the amazing opportunity, only to wonder why you can't remember a word midsentence or move your neck without tightness and pain.

Ultimately, we humans, especially women, are adaptation machines.

If you feed your brain body sugar, flour, alcohol, processed food, excess carbs, and high stress, then blow off exercise and perseverate on petty worries, you will adapt to be fat and demented and finally die young. If instead you feed your brain body the needed nutrients, including plenty of rainbow-colored vegetables, kundalini yoga, love, connection, purpose, HIIT exercise, and resistance training, it will get stronger as you age. The brain *can* get better with age, and a healthy brain body is the foundation.

Even though we hear so little about the brain/body connection, it's the key to just about everything related to our health. Many would agree that the brain is the seat of human identity, but most people simply aren't concerned about their brain, don't wonder if it could be working better, don't consider its secret conversation with the body, and don't think about how to fix it. Or maybe they are simply unaware of their brain body until there's a problem, but even then, they are clueless that brain health or trauma or toxins may have anything to do with their symptoms. They don't know that brain/body function is mutable. Maybe that's because we can't see brain/body changes like wrinkles on the face or feel them like a lump in the breast. Yet brain/body breakdown has more serious consequences that you should not wait to discover. Why? Because at some point, it becomes too late to change the genetic, cellular, and regulatory switches of your brain body.

I'm here to tell you: the brain controls everything you do. And if you don't take care of the brain, your body will stage a coup at some point. In fact, mutiny may be in the works right now. I want to help you become aware of your brain before there's a problem and allow it to work *for* you before it starts working *against* you. The goal is to know when and how the exposures and stresses of daily life become so severe that they seriously threaten the brain body. By understanding the specific manner in which the brain and the body interact we can heal both, reverse chronic issues, and live longer, healthier lives. This is not simply another brain book. This book is about unlocking the brain/body connection and discovering how you overcome the "broken seven," the brain problems you thought you simply "had" to live with: **toxic overload,** rising **body weight, brain fog** (postpartum, perimenopausal, and menopausal), predisposition toward **addiction, anxiety, depression,** and **memory problems.**

What Your Brain Does Well

To better understand the brain/body connection, we must first understand the brain: what it does well and what can cause it to decline.

- As a child, you create 1.8 million brain connections per second. As an adult, you're a bit slower, but by now you already have trillions of connections, or synapses, between nerve cells. You are constantly making new connections (a process called *synaptogenesis*) and occasionally pruning unused connections as needed, like a great arborist. You are aware of none of it.

- Neurologists estimate that we have sixty to seventy thousand thoughts per day, mostly the same and mostly negative.[5]

- Your brain is able to process multiple activities at once: you can eat popcorn and watch a movie at the same time, or juggle work demands on your cell phone while riding a stationary bike.

- Your brain expands your lungs, coordinates the beat of your heart, and directs your gut to digest food.

- Intelligence is tied to the supply of blood flow to the brain, which has grown 600 percent over the past three million years of hominin evolution, while brain size has grown 350 percent during the same time.[6] In other words, intelligence is related more to the brain's blood flow than to its size. Both blood flow and brain size are important, but blood flow matters more, and that means blood pressure and toxin circulation may strongly affect your brain health.

- Your brain triggers you to duck when an object is thrown at you before you have time to make sense of what's happening.

- Your brain constantly upregulates and downregulates genes and proteins (including brain chemicals and hormones) in response to cues from your environment. Feel like your kids or spouse drive you more crazy some days compared with others? It's not you; it's your brain regulation. For example, my steaming cup of green tea in the morning *upregulates* dopamine receptors in my brain, making dopamine levels rise, and I'm exquisitely sensitive to the rush of dopamine. The result is improved focus, joy, and a spring in my step. After an exhausting weekend of socializing, without some brain/body botanical like my green tea, I'm more inclined to react to my kids harping on me. Otherwise, I'm too tired, desensitized, and *downregulated*.

- Your brain turns on and off the healing response, mostly through calm body awareness.

- When you learn a new language or skill, your brain gets a reset. In response to novel experiences and learning, your brain reorganizes, remaps, repatterns, and rewires.

If you do the right things, you can make your brain smarter and stronger—and forty days on the Brain Body Diet will do just that. But we also need to know what hinders brain function. Here are some of the situations that make your brain function decline, leading to the broken seven. You can mend each of the broken seven—or all of them—with my protocol.

- A lack of gut microbes can cause anxiety, and probiotics can reverse it.

- Past emotional trauma may have shrunk your hippocampus, the part of your brain that creates memory and helps you manage emotions, leading you to now be emotionally triggered by otherwise harmless cues in your environment.

- A faulty gene may mean you have trouble making a B vitamin called methylfolate, so you feel mildly depressed. Another gene variation may cause you to accumulate too much estrogen, which can lead to "something suspicious" showing up on your mammogram.

- Toxins, such as lead in your tap water or chocolate, can start converting your low-potency stress hormones into high-potency stress hormones that may make you feel chronically overwhelmed.

- After forty, the barrier between your blood and brain, called the blood-brain barrier (BBB), gets thinner, so alcohol hits harder and hangovers linger longer.

- Your mitochondria, the powerhouses inside your cells, can slow down due to the foods you eat and the toxins you breathe, so you don't wake up feeling refreshed. Exercise in turn is depleting, so you rarely do it. You feel the mitochondrial dysfunction particularly in your brain as "brain fog."

- If you were born underweight and slightly starving, then fed formula sweetened with sugar, it may have lit up your nucleus accumbens, the reward center in your brain, like a Christmas tree. You may now need sugar to feel soothed.

- Relationship strife and lack of loving physical touch can cause your oxytocin to be too low, so you feel disconnected from others, stressed, and lonely.

- You may have inherited the gene for poor serotonin trafficking, so you run around with anxiety and mild (to you, anyway) post-traumatic stress disorder (PTSD).

- Many people use their heads while ignoring their hearts, adding unnecessary stress to the brain. The heart, like the brain, generates a powerful electromagnetic field. In fact, the electrical field of the heart (as measured in an electrocardiogram, ECG) is sixty times greater than the electrical field in an electroencephalogram (EEG) of the brain. The heart can tell you different—even more important—things than your brain.

- Eating a standard American diet, high in inflammatory carbohydrates, causes low blood flow to the "focus" part of your brain.

- A lack of emotion-management tools can cause physical distress and pain during adversity. Worry and fear activate the same neural pathways as pain, so they amplify pain sensations.

Once you identify the obstacles to your best brain function, then you can create a road map to course correct the broken seven.

When Betty, a fifty-eight-year-old woman, first came to see me, she was exasperated from months of low energy, brain fog, and sluggish memory. "I feel helpless and dumb," she confided, "and this is not how I envisioned this stage of my life." We ran a few tests and discovered she was toxic in cadmium and lead, which impair memory and cause brain breakdown (neurodegeneration). The only cadmium exposure we could find was from her daily consumption of cereal grains and rice. Her liver and her detoxification genes weren't doing their jobs well enough to keep up, and she didn't make enough glutathione, which protects your brain from toxic metals. In the forty days of the Brain Body Diet, we detoxified the heavy metals out of her system by removing grains and replacing them with tubers (sweet potatoes, potatoes, yams) and cutting out sugar and alcohol (which wreak havoc on the liver). We boosted her glutathione levels with allium vegetables (onions, garlic, leeks) and crucifers (broccoli, Brussels sprouts, cabbage, cauliflower, kale, radishes). At the end of forty days, Betty felt back to herself again and her tests confirmed normal levels of heavy metals. Starting in the next chapter, you will learn exactly what was included in her forty-day protocol so that you can try it yourself to reverse brain/body breakdown, even brain/body failure. (Or if you're like my friend Jo, you'll stop cycling through every name in the household including the dog's before calling her daughter to the dinner table.)

Road Map of the Brain

Bear with me while I go into the science of the brain to help you understand how it runs the show moment by moment in your everyday life.

On a basic level, the brain is made up of *gray matter,* consisting of the nerve cell bodies where most of the action takes place, and *white matter,* consisting of bundles of nerve cell projections, like cables, insulated by white-colored myelin for greatest transmission speed. Gray matter is gray in color, makes up the cortex of the brain, and provides processing and cognition. White matter connects different areas of gray matter to one another, like an efficient subway system. You need both to be in good form to think and behave properly.

The average brain weighs three pounds, small in size but dominant in function. The main cell types are neurons (nerve cells) and glia (includ-

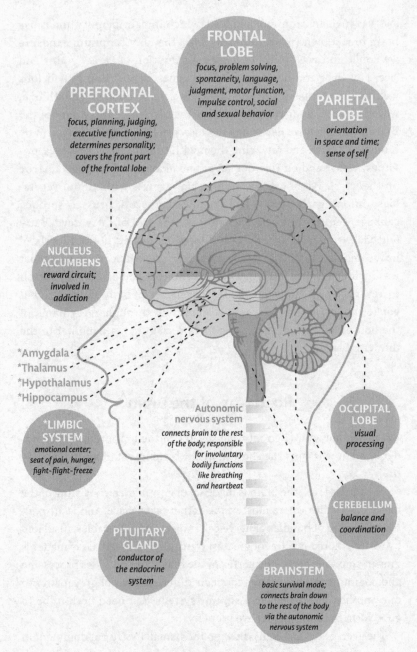

FRONTAL LOBE
focus, problem solving, spontaneity, language, judgment, motor function, impulse control, social and sexual behavior

PREFRONTAL CORTEX
focus, planning, judging, executive functioning; determines personality; covers the front part of the frontal lobe

PARIETAL LOBE
orientation in space and time; sense of self

NUCLEUS ACCUMBENS
reward circuit; involved in addiction

*Amygdala
*Thalamus
*Hypothalamus
*Hippocampus

*LIMBIC SYSTEM
emotional center; seat of pain, hunger, fight-flight-freeze

Autonomic nervous system
connects brain to the rest of the body; responsible for involuntary bodily functions like breathing and heartbeat

OCCIPITAL LOBE
visual processing

CEREBELLUM
balance and coordination

PITUITARY GLAND
conductor of the endocrine system

BRAINSTEM
basic survival mode; connects brain down to the rest of the body via the autonomic nervous system

Key Parts of the Brain

ing astrocytes, oligodendrocytes, and microglia). Nerve cells are the workhorse cells of the brain, designed to transmit information to other nerve, muscle, or glandular cells. Neurons have a cell body, an axon, and dendrites. Glial cells provide support: they surround neurons to hold them in place, supply nutrients and oxygen, and insulate one neuron from another. For the key parts of the brain to know about in order to get the most out of this book, please see the graphic on page 30.

The following key parts are the ones you want to befriend:

Limbic system: The center of emotion, survival instincts, and memory, it is the seat of pain, hunger, and the fight-flight-freeze response. It benefits from unconditional love, relationship stability, and personal safety—particularly in childhood.

- Thalamus = gathers and interprets sensory data
- Hypothalamus = master controller of the brain, in charge of autonomic nervous system
- Hippocampus = operates memory consolidation and emotional regulation (and is part of the management system for your hormones, called the hypothalamic-pituitary-adrenal [HPA] axis)
- Amygdala = the integrative center for emotions, emotional behavior, and motivation (ideally the size of an almond—one on each side of the brain—but if you're anxious, can grow to the size of a walnut)
- Basal ganglia = controls voluntary movements plus habits like teeth grinding, as well as action selection (what to do and when, at a given time). Contains the nucleus accumbens, or reward circuit, which is involved in obsession, compulsion, and addiction
- Cingulate gyrus = a bulge in the brain involved in bonding (such as between mother and child), speech production and language expression, decision-making, communication, emotional responses to pain, and behavior regulation

Pituitary: The conductor of the endocrine system, where the hormones of your thyroid, adrenal glands, ovaries (or testicles), and pineal gland are controlled.

Autonomic nervous system: Connects the brain to the rest of your body via the brainstem, and is responsible for involuntary bodily functions, like breathing and heartbeat.

Prefrontal cortex (PFC): Involved in focus, planning, judging, executive functioning, it determines personality and covers the front part of the frontal lobe.

Here's my analysis about the brain parts I injured after hitting my head back in 2015.

- **Cerebellum:** I lost my sense of balance and coordination. Two weeks after my injury, I learned the hard way that I couldn't stand on my right leg in barre class and toppled to my side.

- **Parietal lobe:** While lying on the floor having tonic/clonic convulsions, I lost my sense of orientation in space and time.

- **Brainstem:** This is the home to the nausea center; I was nauseated for approximately eight weeks after my injury. Additionally, the brainstem can keep you stuck in survival mode, as happened to me when I was coming in and out of consciousness.

- **Cervical ganglion:** This is the part of the autonomic nervous system that's in charge of maintaining homeostasis in the body. I had diminished capacity for equilibrium in my response to life because of an ongoing "brain/body failure state."

- **HPA axis** (i.e., the control system for your hormones): When this goes into overdrive, it's very hard to keep your hormones in balance, from cortisol to estrogen and insulin. The irony is that before my injury, my HPA was overactive. After the injury, it calmed down. But there are healthier, safer ways to treat trouble in the brain! Stick with me, and I'll show you how.

The New Science of the Brain in Balance

Just as your bones lose density and structural integrity over time, so does your brain. It's like age-related downsizing, but in your bones and brain, it's optional. What matters is modifying environmental cues to tell your brain to keep growing and not to shrink. Depending on your internal and external prompts, you can keep growing new nerve cell extensions (called axons) and making new connections between nerve cells.

PRINCIPLES OF NEUROGENESIS

You want neurogenesis—and lots of it. *Neurogenesis* is the ongoing growth and development of new nerve cells (neurons), which contribute to functions like learning, emotional regulation, and memory.[7] Think of neurogenesis as a sports coach who is constantly developing his or her athletes and growing the team with new recruits. So it is with your brain. As your brain continues to grow and develop, the coach keeps recruiting new support cells while taking care of the regular cells. The coach keeps an ongoing supply of precursor cells at the ready, and once they enter the matrix of the brain as new nerve cells, the coach improves the connections between them (synaptogenesis). Go, team!

Neurogenesis occurs throughout life, even in adulthood, but it can slow down, leading to declining brain function and cognition, like a team that sat on their butts over the holidays.[8] Our focus will be on how to promote more neurogenesis as an adult.

You can make as many as one thousand new nerve cells in your hippocampus each day. You want to maintain growth, density, and plasticity of these cells as you age, which means you need to keep building new connections (or teamwork) between the new cells to improve blood flow to the brain. One crucial component of ongoing healthy synaptogenesis is the "pruning shears," which come out to trim the inappropriate neural connections (the ones that are no longer useful) and make more room for the appropriate ones. This is why you don't remember every single calculus equation learned in school: your brain needed to make room for your work projects, your kid's activities, your social agenda—whatever information you need on a daily basis.

The most aggressive and healthy pruning occurs in adolescence (probably to help with learning) and again in pregnancy and postpartum (most likely to promote bonding with your baby). If you have more growth than pruning, it's better for your memory and learning. The net result is more remembering and less forgetting, as I described in my previous book *Younger*. After a certain age, too much pruning may cause memory issues, Alzheimer's disease, and schizophrenia.

Unfortunately, neurogenesis and synaptogenesis are vulnerable to brain "insults," including poor diet, chronic stress, disrupted sleep, inflammation, and toxins.[9] Microglia—the guardians of the brain—can rapidly sense changes in the brain/body balance that result from lifestyle factors.

Toxins can be created inside your body or introduced from external sources. Internal toxins like long-term stress and inflammation shrink the hippocampus by harming the microglia. An external toxin like bisphenol A (commonly known as BPA and found in the plastic coating of store receipts and canned food) negates synaptogenesis by 70 to 100 percent.[10] Heavy metals like lead can diminish neurogenesis and synaptogenesis—and you may be getting exposed through plumbing, tap water, dishware, or house dust.[11] No need to freak out your microglia (or slow down your neurogenesis) over these facts—I've got you covered in the next chapter in the kickoff for the protocol portion of *Brain Body Diet*. As you will soon discover, you can compensate for reduced neurogenesis with the right detoxifying foods, targeted exercise, and stress-relieving activities so that you can reinstate neurogenesis and keep it going as you age.[12] Together these lifestyle factors—the foundation of personalized lifestyle medicine—create more brain resilience.[13]

THE BRAIN/BODY FAILURE STATE

While there are a few notable exceptions, in my years of medical practice I've found that many of my patients are in a failure state and experiencing symptoms from one or more of the broken seven.[14] You may be, too. You may feel bone tired: too tired to socialize, too tired to go out at night, too tired to get on the floor and play with the kids, too tired to exercise. You may feel it as being overwhelmed, having trouble losing weight, being irritated with people you love, and having an appetite without end. That's a failure state in progress, a corrupted operating system. The usual mechanisms that keep you in balance are depleted. Your method of responding to stressors is overtaxed: homeostasis is elusive because the stress load is too great.

A brain/body failure state shows up differently person to person. For me at age fifty-two, it shows up as high cortisol, high blood sugar, food addiction, and the feeling that I cannot handle One. More. Thing.

Mine was a state of failure of the HPA axis—or, more technically, the hypothalamic-pituitary-adrenal-thyroid-gonadal axis. (Note that this is the management system for many of the hormones in your body, from cortisol to estrogen, progesterone, testosterone, and thyroid.) Because cortisol literally destroys brain cells (it's called a "wear and tear" hormone because it wears down body cells and tears up brain cells), my high cortisol gave me a feeling of overwhelm that was nearly constant, as was my elevated fasting blood sugar in the morning (around 105 to 110 mg/dL). My HPA was like a hormonal freeway that ground to a halt because of gridlock.

For my fifty-eight-year-old athletic husband, brain/body failure shows up as belly fat, crankiness, lack of focus, muscle fatigue, early morning awakenings, and sports injuries. For my sixty-three-year-old patient Jane, a lack of homeostasis shows up as high blood pressure in her body and lack of blood flow to her brain, which affects her memory and causes brain fog. For many of my patients, the brain body starts to fail simply because toxins clog the body and mind.

Signs of Early Brain/Body Failure

When you have brain/body failure symptoms—or even before they occur—we need to intervene to keep the brain body working properly. Brain/body failure has five root causes that lead to the broken seven. Do you recognize yourself in any of the states below? They are signs that your brain body isn't working properly, many of which may overlap.

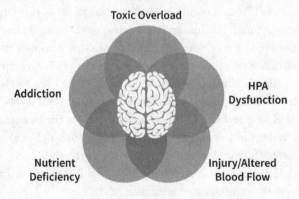

The Five States of Brain/Body Failure

Toxic Overload. Our environmental exposures are so common that we've become inured to the problem. But you deserve to know we're quite literally losing our minds to toxins (more on this in chapter 2). It's worth breaking through the apathy to understand that at least twelve everyday chemicals—found in clothing, food, and furniture—are harming our brains.

- **What goes wrong:** Toxins cause inflammation, which may lead to too much or too little pruning of synapses, a problem we addressed earlier. Toxins can also increase oxidative stress (which throws off your antioxidant defenses) as well as the daily stress that you feel. Lead converts weak and mild stress hormones into stronger stress hormones, which then tax the brain and the body.

- **Symptoms:** Nausea and balance issues (which indicate inflammation) arise from consumption of cadmium and/or arsenic. We can also experience increased symptoms of fight-flight-freeze (the default survival mode) and difficulty recovering from stressful events and toxic exposure. Toxins can also cause compromised digestion: gas, bloating, constipation, and pain near the liver. You may also experience difficulty learning new tasks or skills (i.e., difficulty rewiring the brain), memory issues, or declining intelligence or executive functioning, such as managing time or maintaining focus. I could write a book on toxins, but chapter 2 will suffice.

Hormone (Hypothalamus-Pituitary-Adrenal axis, or HPA) Dysfunction. The HPA axis regulates your mood, sex drive, immunity, digestion, energy, metabolism, and stress response (fight-flight-freeze). Think of the HPA axis as being in charge of whether your nice or bitchy side comes out. Normally, when you're stressed, the HPA ramps up to meet the challenge. Then, when you recover, the HPA becomes less sensitive to the feedback signals and calms down to normal levels, reaching its goal of homeostasis. Chronic stress signals to the hypothalamus cause the system to become overactivated and ultimately burned out (underactivated), stopping the normal HPA regulatory cycle. A dysfunctional HPA fails to re-create homeostasis, leading to irritability, excessive worry, depression, or just feeling flat.

- **What goes wrong:** There are many ways to mess up the HPA:

more stress than you can handle, poor sleep or sleep deprivation, and inflammation are the main culprits, and all lead to excessive load. Chronic stress (discussed in chapters 2 and 3) can keep your HPA in a jacked-up, overactivated state that is hard to regulate. If unaddressed, you may develop an underactivated, underresponsive HPA. Both are brain/body failure states.

- **Symptoms:** Increasing weight, brain fog, and anxiety. Anxiety is not necessarily a psychiatric diagnosis, but rather a general focus on what is wrong with life, what may be wrong, what has been wrong, or what is going to be wrong in the future. Or you may feel this sign of brain breakdown as excessive worry about something you cannot control. News flash: most things in life are beyond our control!

Addiction. Think of this as "the pleasure trap" because we are hard-wired to seek reward.[15] Addiction (covered in chapter 5) is a brain/body failure state that develops over time from seeking reward to the point of imbalance. It starts with a problem in the brain with reward feedback, leading to impulsiveness that then leads to compulsion and ultimately to uncontrollable craving, pleasure seeking, and abuse.

- **What goes wrong:** Addictive behavior changes the brain structure and function through reinforcing memory connections in certain circuits, especially the reward pathway. Eventually, problems arise with both brain biology and behavior.
- **Symptoms:** Wanting "more" of things you like to the point of harm, such as cravings for unhealthy or harmful quantities of food, exercise, alcohol, drugs, or sex; increasing weight; and anxiety. You may even begin to mistrust your instincts.

Injury/Altered Blood Flow. This root cause is the easiest to understand because we hear so much in the news and sports about head trauma. Problems with blood flow can occur from small issues that accumulate over time or a sudden insult. Examples of small injuries that can aggregate are high blood sugar, which can change blood flow to the brain and alter the body's regulation of blood pressure;[16] obesity;[17] and high blood pressure, which damages blood vessels in the brain and is the top risk factor for stroke.[18] Sudden insults include falls (perhaps from fainting or tripping), blows, concussions, motor vehicle accidents, and violence. Trauma occurs when an external force injures the brain and results in physical, social, emotional, cognitive, and behavioral symptoms. Sudden changes in blood flow can lead to fainting, stroke, and excess blood pressure. Whenever blood flow changes significantly, it can cause damage to the delicate brain tissue. Your brain is vulnerable—but resilient.

- **What goes wrong:** Small accumulated injuries result from body problems like excess carbohydrate intake and resulting blood sugar problems, high blood pressure causing damage to the brain's blood vessels, inflammation, and weight gain. When trauma occurs, the external force is the primary problem, but secondary effects may result from altered blood flow, or additional injury caused by increased pressure. Fainting is usually due to oxygen starvation, low blood pressure, low blood sugar, overheating, dehydration, heavy sweating, or exhaustion. Other causes include a blocked artery (ischemic stroke) or a burst blood vessel (hemorrhagic stroke), which interrupts or reduces blood flow and causes brain cells to die. Lack of blood flow for even a few minutes induces a low oxygen state (hypoxia), which in turn causes oxidative damage and kills brain cells. Add on top of hypoxia the lack of energy from being cut off from glucose in the blood, and you get ischemia (restriction in blood supply, causing a shortage of oxygen, glucose, and removal of metabolic wastes). *Decreased* cerebral blood flow may cause brain fog, memory loss, fatigue, anxiety, depression, low libido, hormone imbalance, and neurodegenerative disease. *Excess* blood flow can cause an increase in intracranial pressure, stroke, and brain damage. General anesthesia—such as sevoflurane, which I received for a recent surgery—is a known neurotoxin that increases intracranial pressure.

- **Symptoms:** Brain fog, moodiness, anxiety, depression, addiction, memory loss, and difficulty with multitasking: "Mommy" brain. You may or may not be diagnosed with major depression, but you feel stuck in a negative point of view about your life and/or future. You experience a loss of heart and joy. You may feel like your brain is downsizing, or what author and *New York Times* political and cultural commentator David Brooks calls becoming "hippocampally challenged."

Nutrient Deficiency. For the brain, the most important nutrients include B vitamins (B_1, B_2, B_3, B_5, B_6, B_9, B_{12}); vitamins C, D, E; DHA and EPA; the minerals calcium, magnesium, potassium, selenium, and zinc; plant phytochemicals; and hormones such as estrogen, progesterone, and oxytocin. When you lack nutrients, your brain may suffer.

- **What goes wrong:** Several brain-specific nutrients can be knocked out by chronic stress or aging, while others are imbalanced by nutritional deficiencies (i.e., eating only two or three colors of the rainbow, not all of them), and still others by toxins.
- **Symptoms:** Changes in mood, including irritability, depression, anxiety, and premenstrual syndrome; confusion, fatigue or weakness, muscle pains or tightness; vision loss; heart palpitations and shortness of breath; pale skin, anemia; digestive symptoms such as constipation, diarrhea, or gas; nerve problems like tingling or numbness; hot flashes or night sweats; "senior moments"; and disconnection and social isolation.

When was the last time someone told you to beware of these brain insults, toxins (aka *dementogens*) that rob you of your highest self? These nefarious factors are likely affecting your brain *and* your quality of life—making you feel ill-tempered, overwhelmed, unkind, and burned out. The following chapters will lead you through the steps that will heal your brain and, by extension, heal your body. You will feel whole again.

Brain to Self: Take Out the Trash

We all want to circumvent brain/body failure. A failure state shows up in daily symptoms, some of them chronic. Failure creates brain trash— early brain damage—which may be occurring for years, even decades, before you receive a diagnosis. The most common reasons I see for high levels of brain trash are:

- Weak DNA-repairing genes and habits (e.g., drinking too much alcohol)
- Marginal stress-coping habits
- Poor toxin-coping habits

Why are toxins so bad for the brain? They are substances that essentially work in direct opposition to natural healing. They either create a

---

ERIN, UNFORTUNATE MEMBER OF THE BRAIN/BODY FAILURE CLUB

Sometimes brain toxins come in the form of prescription medications that your body can't abide. Erin was a thirty-three-year-old woman who came to see me after experiencing a stroke at age twenty-nine while taking the birth control pill. After the stroke, she learned that she carries the gene mutation for a greatly increased risk of blood clot, called Factor V Leiden.[19] Taking the pill—for her and any other woman with the Factor V Leiden mutation—increased the risk of a blood clot by three- to thirteen-fold, and Erin was one of the unlucky people who learned the hard way. (Note that all women have double the risk of stroke when taking an oral contraceptive.[20]) A clot blocked an artery in her brain and cut off blood flow. Now that she's off the pill, we focused first on which of the seven parts of the Brain Body Diet she should put into her program. We investigated ways to optimize blood flow throughout her body and brain, including the use of a baby aspirin, omega-3 fats, and grounding, to keep her blood more slippery and less viscous. Note that taking a baby aspirin carries risks—discuss first with your trusted physician. She now checks her blood pressure at home and learned she has white-coat hypertension, meaning her blood pressure is more consistent when measured at home but can spike when she's anxious.

Strokes are on the rise among millennials. According to the Centers for Disease Control, strokes among women aged eighteen to thirty-four have soared 32 percent from 2003 to 2012 (and 15 percent in men), according to an analysis of 784,154 hospitalizations.[21] The problem is worse in urban areas of the West Coast and Midwest. Is it something in the air? The authors surmise that it could be the fallout of younger people getting fatter, developing diabetes, or decreasing their physical activity. We don't yet know.

negative and potentially life-altering pattern or worsen a negative pattern in the brain body. They don't respect the laws of nature. They tell your brain to stop healing the body. They can make you jittery, reactive, and mean. They cost us hundreds of billions of dollars in preventable health care costs.[22] We carry toxins in our fat tissues, and release them with fat loss. Most of us carry the most common toxins around in our bones, and every day we take in a little more lead, mercury, cadmium, and arsenic. Then, after age thirty-five, you slowly release these toxins into your bloodstream as you start to break down bone. From this internal storehouse of toxins as well as new exposures, our brain bodies become a little more poisoned each day with the food we eat (especially foods with pesticides, herbicides, genetically engineered ingredients, hormones, or mold—like grains and coffee), the water we drink, the products we use, and the air we breathe. The brain body is desperate for a wise adult, like you, to take out the trash and let it heal.

Toxins affect everyone. We live on a planet that has become increasingly toxic, especially to the brain. On freeways and at gas stations, we inhale benzene generated by fossil fuels. We drink lead-contaminated dust in our water supply. Unwittingly, we expose ourselves to chemicals in beauty products, food cans, electronics, cleaning supplies, and other household goods. It's no longer a luxury to detoxify; it's a requirement of healthy living. Consider this sad statistic: three common environmental pollutants alone are responsible for 41 million lost IQ points, as estimated by Harvard professor David Bellinger.[23] Toxins impact food choice, fears, and your sense of self. They can block your purpose, mission, and maybe even your connection to divinity.

Most of my patients have no idea about their brain's toxic load, and toxins further complicate the situation by decreasing your self-awareness. Depressing, I know! The good news is that as dire as the toxin situation may seem, I will give you the tools to minimize their impact. Moreover, what you do to remove toxins from the brain will help you with detoxification elsewhere in the body, because what is good for the brain is generally good for the entire body. You'll learn how to address these different problems based on the toxins you're harboring and your symptoms.

UNRECOGNIZED TOXIC OVERLOAD AND LEAKY BRAIN

The brain is more protected and compartmentalized than other organs because it is behind the blood-brain barrier (BBB). Think of the barrier like a firewall that keeps internet viruses from invading your computer: it's supposed to protect your brain from the entry of toxins and immune cells that can create neuroinflammation. Your BBB is like a filter, a highly selective semipermeable membrane separating circulating blood in the rest of the body from brain fluid.

However, when the tight junctions get loosened from different assaults, the BBB can become leaky, and then certain toxins *can* get into your brain. Eating a high-fat diet—of the wrong kinds of fats—can make the brain more leaky, and it's associated with negative changes to the digestive tract (including your microbiome) and depression.[24] Alcohol can alter your brain's firewall, too, by changing the normal function of your tight junctions.[25] A leaky blood-brain barrier is linked to multiple brain/body problems, such as memory issues, multiple sclerosis, stroke, and Alzheimer's disease.[26]

What's more, when specific toxins get to the brain, they can get trapped, where they then require different detoxification methods than other parts of the body. Plus, brain matter is 60 percent fat, and fat is where toxins hide. Toxins get easily stuck in the brain and stay there unless you actively do something about them.

Certain parts of the brain are particularly vulnerable to toxins. Nerve cells in a location called the locus coeruleus are highly exposed to blood circulation. If you're wondering why you should care about the locus coeruleus, here's the skinny: it's housed in the brainstem, which is the link between your brain and the rest of the body. Its main function is regulating how to respond to stress and vigilance, mobilizing the brain and body for action. Think of it as the panic button of your brain, and it can get fritzy as a result of toxin exposure.

Brain Health: Paradigm Shift

In the last few decades, research in health keeps overturning what we thought was good for us. Processed bread is out. Certain fats, such as avocado and macadamia nuts, are good. Likewise, the idea that your brain peaks in your twenties and starts heading downhill after twenty-six is now outdated. Now we know better: if you set your intention on neurogenesis and prevent or reverse neurodegeneration, you can keep enhancing your brain regardless of age.

When I was twenty-six years old, I was an intern in the Obstetrics and Gynecology residency at the University of California, San Francisco. Medical school had ramped up my left-brain wiring, and working more hours—about 120 per week—rewired me even further. I was trained to be a pattern-recognizing, linear, and analytical machine in order to keep my pregnant patients safe while in labor and to save the lives of women who came to the emergency room with a ruptured ectopic pregnancy or some other internal hemorrhage. So when I reflect on how I became so left-brain dominant, I point to medical school and residency training. It's as if I internalized a high-intensity but unsustainable thrum for how to get work done and be good at my job—and so began the process of ignoring the warning signs of a brain body out of balance. But it took hitting my head to learn that this type of negative wiring didn't serve me well or make me happy. It was an unsustainable set point that my brain body couldn't endure.

For many women, the brain and body are no longer allies; rather, they are on the brink of separation, even divorce. We're meant to have an enlivening, broad, and deep conversation between brain and body in order to feel and look our best. The relationship has dwindled, and at times it's hostile as we've become left-brain dominant, judgmental, analytical, and hurried. When we're too left-brained, we use thoughts, beliefs, feelings, and actions to try and externally manage our sense of uncertainty, scarcity, doom, or wondering when the other shoe will drop. I was no exception.

My traumatic brain injury got me to reevaluate the choices I was making that kept reinforcing the left-brain domination. I realized early on in my brain recovery that I just couldn't push myself past my limits anymore, to ignore the messages from the brain body calling for balance. A repatterning occurred—perhaps activation of the right brain, or quieting of the traumatized left brain, or both—that changed my attitude, made me more mellow, caused me to be a better listener, and stopped me from yelling at the kids.

My hope is to make neurogenesis—for both hemispheres of your brain—part of your overall health program many years, perhaps decades, before you face any symptoms of the broken seven and brain decline. Even better, let's set the intention that you're like my great-grandmother, who died at the age of ninety-seven with a keen mind and a supple body, and never faced symptoms of brain deterioration. Ever. Science proves that when you eat, think, move, and feel in novel ways, you can alter not just the function, but also the structure and blood flow of your brain. While our sociocultural conditioning limits our expectations for the aging brain, I've learned that the unfathomable sometimes becomes possible. It's the unfathomable that I wish for you and me.

The biggest secret of the type of medicine that I practice is that you have more power than any doctor to heal your body, but *healing starts with your brain*. The tricky part is that you must change the way you interact with your environment in order to change what's inside your head.

But *neuroplasticity*, the ability of mature neurons to adapt, reorganize, and recover from insults like insomnia, injury, or even dementia, is a built-in feature of your brain. Once you learn how to work with your brain to promote neuroplasticity, then you can create lasting improvement to the brain body.

Reset the Brain in Forty Days

Small actions done consistently and strategically over time lead to the most profound change. Your brain contains one hundred billion nerve cells, and each neuron links to other neurons to create many trillions of connections. That's a lot to maintain. We're going to bolster and optimize those connections with the Brain Body Diet.

We will help you to rewire your brain—to lay down new thought tracks and grooves that are clean, pure, and free of distortion—create new habits, restore the brain/body connections, and take your own self-care to a higher level.

The recommended duration of the Brain Body Diet is forty days. That said, in the first few days you'll feel an immediate payoff as symptoms like low energy, overwhelm, and brain fog start to fade immediately. Lifestyle medicine can significantly lower toxic load and improve thirty-seven different types of symptoms within the first seven days.[27] So if you were my patient, I'd advise you to jump in. Don't hesitate. Feeling better in the first week or two will be like the wind at your back, softly generating the power that you need to get through all forty days. Some people may need more time, depending on how long they've had neuroinflammation and other underlying signs of brain/body breakdown. Similar to the way hormones like estrogen and thyroid may take six weeks to reset, the length of the Brain Body Diet allows for adjustments and small changes to reconnect your brain and body. You also may be so thrilled with your results that you'll want to adopt some of these daily choices and actions permanently, and they become healthy new habits that serve your brain body into the future. Think of the forty days as a sacred container—a time of honest inquiry, committed change, and a focused time to alter old patterns and integrate new ones—a predetermined, consecutive number of days. In traditional Chinese medicine, this period of time could be considered the length of a *gong,* a Chinese word that translates as "cultivation" or "work."

I encourage you to commit to the full forty days. Why? You'll see the most profound changes. As a physician guiding women and some men through lasting health transformations, I've found that forty days is the most effective amount of time to notice the way you use your brain and then more effectively restore your brain/body connection.

You need the full forty days to detox your brain and improve all the symptoms you are experiencing in the body. You can mix and match the various parts of the protocol, depending on your issues and the results of your questionnaires at the beginning of each chapter, from chapters 2 through 8. That will allow you to personalize a forty-day protocol that serves you best. Aim to spend a few days to a week becoming familiar with the steps of each protocol, and scheduling thirty to sixty minutes each day for the actions of *Brain Body Diet* for forty days in a row. Begin with the Basic Protocol in the chapters for which you qualify based on the number of your symptoms. Take more time when available, and add the Advanced Protocol as time, resources, and energy allow.

Take your Brain Body Diet on holidays and vacations; it's important not to miss a single day if you want to heal your brain/body connection. As you make your way through the Brain Body Diet over the next forty days, your new practices will become as natural as brushing your teeth or walking the dog.

Here's a quick overview of how we will fix the broken seven:

Protocol 1: Removing Toxins

Protocol 2: Lowering the Body Weight Set Point

Protocol 3: Clearing Brain Fog

Protocol 4: Healing Reward Deficiency Syndrome and Addiction

Protocol 5: Calming Down Anxiety

Protocol 6: Emerging from Depression

Protocol 7: Restoring Memory

Each protocol is prefaced by the scientific explanations I've uncovered for each of the broken seven's roots, with discussions on the delicate balances within the greater brain body. I then finish each chapter with the Brain Body Protocol steps for you to adopt over the next forty days.

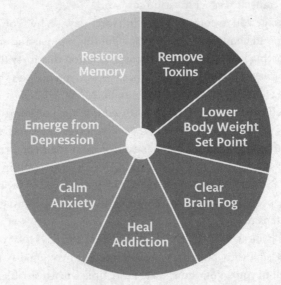

The Brain Body Protocol

Last Word

The most important lesson I've learned about brain/body rehab is that the brain can detox and then help the body heal. The brain is not just an isolated organ sitting on top of your neck but a vastly interdependent system that's connected with your body at every level. *Brain Body Diet* addresses the common everyday issues that need answers, answers that conventional medicine doesn't offer. It's never too late to repair the brain/body connection, although if you're already in a brain/body failure state—that is, you feel beset by brain fog, obesity, addiction, worry, moodiness, forgetfulness, or toxic overload—it may take longer to reactivate neuroplasticity and neurogenesis. Still, the effort is worth it. Your well-being depends on it.

What you'll find in these pages is not unvalidated opinion but scientifically proven strategies to heal the brain body—and an entertaining read that's not bogged down in scientific jargon. (The complexities of the scientific proof have been relegated to the Notes section, which is available online at brainbodydiet.com/notes.)

I'll show you how to get healthy even in an unhealthy environment and how to activate growth and repair of your nerve cells at all times. You'll learn new ways to cope with the inevitable stressors that tend to hijack most of us. You will restore homeostasis, get your brain to listen once more to your heart—as nature intended—and heal physically, mentally, and emotionally. Who doesn't want that? Following this protocol will help you not only to stay on the right side of the balance between growth and pruning, but also to inwardly reorganize your life for the better. The Brain Body Diet worked for me, and thousands of my patients, and it can work for you.

2

Toxins

Reversing the Damage to Improve Your Mood, Turn On Your Mitochondria, and Boost Energy

Tamara had developed brain fog and had gained weight over the past few years before coming to see me as a patient. She was a smart woman but couldn't figure out why she had these symptoms. Despite a grueling work schedule as a thirty-eight-year-old management consultant, she exercised regularly and ate well, so those lifestyle factors weren't to blame. Her bowel function was slower, occurring every other day instead of daily, her previous norm. Tamara felt cold most of the time, wore socks to bed, and could no longer stand to ski in the winter. She would intermittently feel low in energy, like she was moving in slow motion. When I questioned her about other symptoms, Tamara added that she was retaining fluid and her skin and hair were drier than normal.

Tamara had several abnormalities appear in her lab tests. Her thyroid function was borderline: her blood work showed elevated thyroid antibodies and a suboptimal Thyroid Stimulating Hormone (TSH) that made me concerned about the potential for an autoimmune disease (see Notes for details on Tamara's laboratory values).[1] Her mercury level was significantly high, probably because of mercury dental fillings she had received as a child, even though she had them replaced in her thirties. Tamara's blood sugar level revealed that glucose was building up in her blood instead of entering the body's cells to be used as energy—and making her body and brain inflamed. The problem was that toxins were robbing Tamara of normal thyroid function and metabolism.

Your thyroid is a major endocrine gland in the front of your neck, and its main job is to produce and store hormones that regulate weight, energy, and metabolism (the rate at which you burn calories), like the drummer in a band. If your drummer doesn't set the right pace for your cell's metabolic activity, you may feel slow—physically and cognitively—and gain weight. People with low thyroid function (hypothyroidism) may experience blood sugar problems and inflammation.[2]

Furthermore, many of the same toxins that squeeze the life out of the thyroid affect other systems in the body—weight control, blood sugar balance, even proper brain/body function. These toxins, mostly endocrine disruptors, appear in hundreds of cosmetics, plastic bottles, metal cans, toys, and the pesticides on food that isn't organic. They interfere with production, release, transportation, activity, and elimination of natural hormones, such as thyroid, insulin, estrogen, and testosterone—and as a result may cause a wide range of problems with the brain and body.

For instance, insulin is a hormone secreted by the pancreas that helps muscle and fat cells remove glucose from the blood. When your cells stop responding to insulin because you become out of balance, you have insulin resistance, which means glucose builds up in the blood, signaling the pancreas to produce even more insulin. When insulin resistance becomes severe enough, the rising blood sugar can have a toxic effect on the brain body by clumping proteins, damaging blood vessels to vital organs—increasing the risk of heart disease, kidney problems, decreasing blood flow to the brain, stroke, visual changes, and harm to nerve cells—and creating excess inflammation, putting a person at greater risk of dementia and Alzheimer's disease.

I hypothesized that if we cleared Tamara's body of the mercury and other sources of toxic inflammation, her brain fog, weight gain, and sluggish thyroid may clear up. In fact, the problems with her thyroid and blood sugar may be linked, because as TSH rises, it acts directly on insulin-making islet cells in the pancreas, causing insulin to rise along with blood glucose, indicating insulin resistance.[3] Not good. Thyroid treatment, even in subclinical hypothyroidism, lowers insulin and glucose.[4]

Some toxins are linked to both problems—slow thyroid and higher blood sugar—especially in women.[5] So we began the Brain Body Diet for Tamara. We emphasized detoxification, adding back important minerals in the appropriate ratios while removing her toxins. With my help, she used lifestyle medicine to reset insulin and rebalanced her blood sugar. She stopped using hand sanitizer or toothpaste containing triclosan because of its role as a neurotoxin and thyroid disruptor.[6] We cut out diet soda, linked to a greater risk of imbalanced gut microbes, blood sugar problems, obesity, diabetes, high blood pressure, stroke, and dementia, including Alzheimer's.[7] (Yes, soda is *that* bad. Stop immediately!) Forty days later, Tamara's blood work was in check, the fog lifted, and she felt more focused, not to mention she lost fourteen pounds in those forty days by lowering her body weight set point, described in the next chapter.

The Vast Experiment

We are unwitting crash-test dummies for the chemical industry. Over the past sixty-five years, Big Chemistry has created tens of thousands of chemicals with varying adverse health effects on the brain, body, and environment. Some were banned decades ago because they caused cancer or negative brain outcomes, but they persist in the environment and affect women worse than men. One example is the pesticide DDT, associated with a four-fold increased risk of breast cancer when one is exposed in utero.[8] Another is lead, which the first-century Greek physician Pedanius Dioscorides noted "makes the mind give way" and has been shown to induce more oxidative stress in women and loss of balance or homeostasis.[9]

Toxins make you sick. They are chemicals that become poisonous even at low doses or when metabolized inside of you. You get exposed through air, food, drinks, skin, or even high stress. Toxins can be synthesized in a lab—like bisphenol A (BPA), a hormone disruptor found on receipts and reusable plastic containers.[10] Or toxins can come from a plant or animal, like a poisonous mushroom or snake venom. Toxins can be made inside of your body, such as when your appendix gets swollen and bursts, releasing inflammatory toxins everywhere in your belly and bloodstream, or they can be released from imbalanced microbes (bacteria, fungi, or parasites) in your gut.

But most of the toxins that I'm referring to in this chapter are the type that you are exposed to in small amounts over the years, without knowing it. Your liver is the main organ in charge of triaging (or prioritizing the treatment of) toxins, but not every toxin is created equal. Alcohol moves to the front of the line, no matter what. Some toxins get walled off protectively in your fat (and are then released at higher levels when you burn fat and lose weight, perhaps leading to a weight-loss plateau). Other toxins don't get triaged at all, but specifically shut down your mitochondria, the parts of your cells that produce energy. Still other toxins instigate your immune system to go into battle and start attacking your own tissue, like the thyroid.

What's more, tiny exposures—when they accumulate, mix with other toxins, and backlog the liver—can cause serious brain/body problems. Lead is frequently present in your tap water, even though lead was banned from gas and paint. Phthalates (fake estrogens) are commonly found in your moisturizer—and women are exposed to them more than men because of our more liberal use of skin-care products.[11] Toxins from fungus, like mold from the leak behind the dishwasher in your kitchen or the yeast overgrowth in your gut from eating too much sugar, cause recurrent sinus or vaginal infections and send along toxins to the brain known as *neurotoxins*. The list goes on, but I'll spare you the overwhelm.

In the United States, thousands of unregulated chemicals that are foreign to the body are readily available. The Environmental Protection Agency (EPA) is required by law to test tens of thousands of these unregulated compounds currently on the market, as well as the two thousand new chemicals introduced each year. Guess how many they test each year? Yeah, not many. The EPA reviews about twenty chemicals at a time, leading to a large backlog as toxin levels rise in our environment.

Yet my aim is not to blame or get on a soapbox about how the chemical industry is like a modern version of the tobacco industry. My first goal is to be practical, to show you which toxins might trigger or be associated with your own brain/body breakdown so that you can look around your home to see which ones may be causing mischief. My second goal is to rid your body of the toxins that have set up residence in your tissues (such as in your fat and bones), perhaps as long ago as in your teenage years or twenties. My third goal is to help you understand what's getting you into trouble with toxins. The most common reasons I see in my practice and my own body are:

- Too high a dose or accumulation of toxins
- Too many toxins over time with negative synergies between them (the "cocktail" effect)
- Weak genes
- Not enough focused detoxification (by eating vegetables, clearing the liver pathways, using supplements, sweating, saunas)

You may have one or more of these tendencies and not know it. In this chapter, I will guide you through discovering why you have a problem, how you may build up either *exogenous* toxins from the environment or *endogenous* toxins from your body's metabolic processes, and how to help boost your detoxification functions.

Is Your Brain Body Toxic?

Do you have now or have you had in the past six months any of the following symptoms or conditions?

☐ Have you lived in an urban or industrial area (or more specifically, in a pollution zone such as near a freeway, a hazardous waste site, a contaminated water supply, building construction or demolition, or nonorganic farming)?

☐ Do you drink tap or well water, or water from plastic bottles?

☐ Do you eat food that is not organic or common foods that are genetically modified, such as corn, soy, alfalfa, squash, or zucchini?

☐ Have you had any medical exposures (general anesthesia, metal fillings, or vaccinations)?

☐ Have you taken over-the-counter medications such as diphenhydramine (an antihistamine, such as Benadryl), acetaminophen, ibuprofen, or naproxen; acid-blocking drugs; or synthetic hormones (birth control pills, fertility medication, estrogen, progestin, testosterone, prostate medication)?

☐ Have you had any exposure to mold or heavy metals?

☐ Do you use common skin-care or cleaning products?

☐ Have you experienced poor memory, difficulty with concentration, brain fog, slow processing speed, poor physical coordination, slurred speech, and/or learning difficulties?

☐ Have you experienced heavy stressors such as marital separation or divorce, retirement or loss of job, business failure, major personal illness, death or major illness in a family member (including spouse), marriage, or birth of a baby?

☐ Have you had persistent sugar cravings? Episodes of binge eating or drinking of alcohol? Cravings for certain foods?

☐ Have you been eating fewer than seven servings of vegetables in a day, produce or other foods that are not organic, or processed meats like bacon, hot dogs, or sausage?

☐ Have you suffered from skin problems including hives, acne, flushing, or excessive sweating?

☐ Have you suffered from emotional problems such as mood swings, anxiety, fear, anger, irritability, or depression?

☐ Have you had low energy during the day, including fatigue, sluggishness, apathy, or even restlessness or hyperactivity?

☐ Have you experienced digestive symptoms such as nausea, vomiting, constipation, diarrhea, gas, heartburn, and/or bloating?

☐ Have you felt pain such as headaches, joint tenderness or achiness, arthritis, stiffness or limitation of movement, or muscle aches or pains?

☐ Have you experienced respiratory symptoms such as sore throat, hoarseness, chronic coughing, stuffy nose, sinus problems, hay fever, excessive mucus production, chest congestion, asthma, bronchitis, or shortness of breath?

INTERPRETATION

If you said yes to three or more questions, you *may* have an issue with low-level toxin exposure. Six to eight, and you probably have moderate toxicity in your brain and body. Nine or more, and you may have a severe toxic burden. The protocol at the end of this chapter will help you remove toxins, reduce future exposures, and help heal damage from neurotoxins.

Losing Our Minds to Toxins

How do toxins get to the brain, and how do we get rid of them? The reasons toxins accumulate in the body were mentioned earlier, but the main ways that toxins get into the brain are more specific: through an overtaxed liver, weak detox genes, a sluggish lymphatic system, a leaky gut, and/or a leaky blood-brain barrier. That means not only do you need to detox your body, but you also need to detox your brain. Going forward, don't think of them separately. Treat them both together as one.

The main way to remove toxins from the brain is through the function of the glymphatic system, the trash collection that occurs while you sleep. What happens is that the cerebral spinal fluid in the brain increases substantially and washes away toxins and metabolic waste products that build up in between brain cells during waking hours.[12] But certain toxins, like alcohol or general anesthesia, can slow down the glymphatic system, and may inhibit removal of toxins.[13]

Additionally, the immune system connects to the brain via the lymphatic system, a vast network that transports fluid throughout our bodies. The lymphatic system helps to get rid of toxins, so if yours is sluggish, you may be vulnerable to accumulating toxins.

The good news is that your brain sits behind the blood-brain barrier (BBB), that extensive filtering system of capillaries that carry blood to the brain and spinal cord and prevent the passage of specific substances that could harm your brain. The bad news is that many toxic chemicals contain characteristics that allow them to pass through the barrier and gain access to brain tissue, leading to neurodegeneration, neurotoxicity, brain fog, dementia, and cancer. The table on pages 69–72 shows how toxins may affect biology and the ways we get exposed to them.

TOXINS OVERVIEW

TOXINS AFFECT OUR BRAIN IN A VARIETY OF WAYS:
- Brain development
- Cell signaling
- Hormone disruption
- Cognition
- Mitochondrial function

WE CAN BE EXPOSED BY:
- Food
- Drink
- Air
- Skin

TAKE STEPS TO AVOID TOXINS:
- Avoid plastic water bottles and food containers.
- Eat organic and GMO-free.
- Use organic skin-care products.
- Stop eating canned food.
- Replace tuna with salmon.

Certain toxins (listed on page 68) cross the BBB and change the very structure and function of brain tissue. Exposure is not just a problem for people who work at high-risk industrial jobs, although they have the greatest risk. Dozens of toxins fly below the radar and impact office workers, women trying to conceive, stay-at-home moms and dads, retirees in moldy homes . . . truly, *all* of us.

Note to Brain: Toxins Can Make You Fat and Slow

We're just starting to understand the full spectrum of toxic threats to the brain and body. What's clear is your body doesn't know what to do with all of these toxins. They first clog the liver, then get stored in fat, and ultimately back up into your brain. Since the brain is almost two-thirds fat (the fattiest organ in the body), it makes sense that it's likely the most vulnerable. Recall what I mentioned in the introduction—that the brain is the most calorie-hungry (in scientific terms, "metabolically active") organ in the body: it is only 2 to 3 percent of body weight, but consumes 25 percent of total body glucose and 20 percent of total body oxygen. Basically, your brain is a metabolic hog. Due to the fact that the brain uses so much of your body's resources, it is astoundingly vulnerable to any toxins that lower metabolism. These include foreign chemicals that lead to unwanted weight gain (called *obesogens*), which disrupt insulin and put you at greater risk for obesity. Ironically, when you burn fat or lose weight, the toxins stored in those cells can be released into your bloodstream, ready to once again tire out your mitochondria or block hormone receptors like insulin or leptin—making you hungrier and storing more fat than you burn as your liver works to recapture the freed toxins.

Let's spend a moment on obesogens, because the link between a toxin and your weight is an important way to understand the impact of toxins on your overall brain/body health. You may get exposed while sitting in your car or favorite chair. One study in mice showed that exposure to a flame retardant found in upholstered furniture and car textiles caused 30 percent more weight gain.[14] Japan banned this chemical in 2014, but it is still being produced and used in the United States and worldwide to the tune of twenty-eight thousand tons per year.[15] A large study in the United States shows that exposure in adults to bisphenol A (BPA), found in canned food, thermal receipt paper, and plastic bottles, is associated with increasing body weight, higher body mass index, and general and abdominal obesity.[16] How do obesogens make you fat? In rodents and humans, BPA stimulates the pancreas cells that make insulin and disturbs the insulin messaging in the liver, fat, and muscle cells, leading to pancreas dysfunction, insulin resistance, and rising blood sugar.[17] That's a recipe for storing fat. Do you really need that store receipt or plastic water bottle?

Another class of toxins is air pollution, which can constrict blood vessels and raise blood pressure, putting you at a greater risk of stroke— and once again, women seem to be at greater risk[18]—or asthma, attention deficit hyperactivity disorder (ADHD), dementia, schizophrenia, autism, heart attack, lung cancer, obesity, diabetes and high blood pressure in pregnancy, plus babies with short telomeres (reflecting a shorter life), small lungs for life, and a shorter life . . . to name a few.[19]

We need to wake up to the fact that we're losing our intelligence, stress resilience, focus, and lean body mass to toxins. Specifically, the five categories of everyday chemicals listed below—many found in clothing, food, tap water, and furniture, most external, but some made internally in the body—are harming our brains, making us more inflamed, stressed, and fat, and creating brain trash. We need to know our enemies in order to reverse brain/body damage from toxins.

1. Alcohol
2. Heavy metals (arsenic, cadmium, lead, mercury, manganese)
3. Other endocrine disruptors (pesticides, phthalates, bisphenol A, perchlorate, flame retardants, fluoride, and toluene)
4. Chemicals released in the body from chronic stress (CRH, excess cortisol)
5. Air pollutants

In my first decade of medical practice, I rarely thought of toxins as a cause of a patient's symptoms. But as my thinking evolved, I went from occasionally considering the possibility to realizing it was the underlying root cause of many patients' poor health. Now I think of those problems and other mental health issues as a sign of brain/body breakdown and possible overexposure to toxins.

So instead of going straight for the symptom diagnosis when treating a patient, I consider what else might be contributing factors from genetics and various environmental inputs, including diet, nutrients, toxins, exercise, and trauma. For example, depression becomes a nutritional-gastrointestinal-microbial-toxic-immunological-inflammatory-hormonal-detoxification-mitochondrial-environmental-structural (whew!) imbalance to resolve, not just a lack of serotonin in the brain to fix with a pill. The same can be said of many other conditions that are seemingly isolated to the brain. The goal is to restore normal set points (i.e., homeostasis) by considering all of the environmental inputs, the patient's biological individuality, and the downstream consequences. Despite the complex roots of several of the broken seven, resolving the issue is more simple: with a proven strategy of lifestyle changes that anyone can access—including how you eat, move, think, and supplement—you can solve these problems often more effectively than you would with any prescription pill.

Your Overtaxed Liver

As I've described, your liver is the body's weigh station for toxins. It tries to make most of them less dangerous through biochemical processing inside liver cells, but unfortunately that can backfire—there are some toxins that become more harmful once the liver metabolizes them. The liver sends other toxins to be stored in your fat, like when you tuck away extra junk you don't want to deal with in the guest room closet.

As you might imagine, with the volume of toxins the liver has to triage, it can get overloaded. When that happens, fat starts to accumulate in the liver in a problem called nonalcoholic fatty liver disease (NAFLD), insulin resistance rises, and usually you suffer from impaired fat metabolism. This problem is increasingly common, affecting about 30 percent of the population, many of whom may go on to develop more serious problems like liver cirrhosis and even liver failure within ten years.[20] Some medications, both prescription and over-the-counter, may make your liver more likely to suffer harm. One such medication, gastric acid blockers (known as proton pump inhibitors, including Nexium and Prilosec), has been shown to modulate the gut microbiota composition unfavorably.[21]

For most women, the fat accumulation in the liver occurs without their knowledge. I know it when I hear symptoms of brain/body issues and when I see liver damage on a blood test—that is, an ALT greater than 20 units/L.

The upshot is that for some women, myself included, relying on the liver to do its job against all the toxins we face may not be sufficient. Instead, we need to help out the liver by providing the nutrients it most needs to do its job, reducing the input of toxins, and accelerating the release of toxins—that includes cleaning up your food, eliminating alcohol (the liver toxin that always goes to the front of the line in liver metabolism), using only 100 percent–clean personal care products, taking inventory of what goes in your home and cutting out the red-flag products that are full of toxins, cleaning up your hormonal situation, and avoiding the red list of toxins in your home and work like asbestos, cadmium, flame retardants, and formaldehyde.[22]

ARE YOU LOW IN GLUTATHIONE?

When you're low in glutathione, toxins linger in your system, potentially damaging your cells. Like me, you may run low in glutathione, the master detoxifier in the body that protects cells from toxic damage. Take my quiz and find out.

☐ Do you drink tap water?

☐ Do you eat out at restaurants?

☐ Do you use a dry cleaner for your clothing?

☐ Do you eat sugary foods?

☐ Do you have a diet lacking in foods that enrich glutathione, such as onions, garlic, and leeks?

☐ Do you sleep less than seven hours every night?

☐ Do you often feel stressed and breathe shallowly?

☐ Do you perform intense exercise more than once or twice per week?

☐ Are you low in metallothioneins[23] (a family of proteins in tissues that bind metals, protect the body from oxidative stress, and regulate homeostasis of copper and zinc)?

☐ Do you get less than 35 grams per day of fiber?

☐ Have you measured your level of heavy metals and found that you were high?

☐ Do you have a variant of the gene that codes for the enzyme glutathione S-transferase (GST)?

Interpretation: If you answered yes to three or more, there's a good chance you are low in glutathione. In the first Brain Body Protocol, you will learn how to raise your glutathione levels naturally so you can protect your cells from further damage. Glutathione levels inside of your cells not only help you detoxify the brain body, but also may impact your life span.[24]

The Role of Genes in Your Detoxification

Your biochemical individuality makes you a lovely one-of-a-kind person but also determines the function or dysfunction of your detoxification pathways—and thus your risk of neurotoxicity. While it's true that our bodies are designed to detoxify continuously, it's also true that some of us (like me) have poor detoxification genes and can get overwhelmed easily by toxins. Poor detoxification shows up as being highly sensitive to physical stimuli—for example, smelling cigarette smoke or strong chemical scents sets you off—or feeling like the nervous system is delicate. Your ability to clear toxins may be impaired based on the way your genes interact with your environment. The most important detoxification genes are listed below.

- Cytochrome P450 1B1 enzymes (CYP1B1)
- Glutathione S-transferase (GSTM1, GSTP1)
- N-acetyltransferase 2 (NAT2)
- Superoxide dismutase (SOD1, SOD2)

If you want to read more about the detox genes, refer to the Notes, where I describe each gene and how to reduce risk if you have a variation.[25] In my previous book *Younger,* I describe the 90/10 rule: only about 10 percent of an adult's risk of chronic disease is genetic and 90 percent is environmental (mostly the aggregate of lifestyle factors). This rule applies especially to the brain/body connection and detoxification. Regardless of your genetic risk, the Brain Body Diet *is* designed to bring you back to vibrant health.

The Science of a Toxic Brain and Body

One or two small exposures to toxins aren't so bad and your body may process them, but multiple exposures can create a combination worse than the sum, making you more vulnerable to their effects. It's like partying like a rock star every night for a week after age forty: One night is manageable, but by the second or third night, you're a wreck. Multiple toxins accumulate and create negative synergy: alcohol, sugar, lack of sleep, caffeine, daily hangovers. By day seven, you may feel as though you're ready to be institutionalized.

When I started learning about the fascinating science of toxic exposure, I investigated everything in my home. I was surprised to learn that I needed to ventilate my home more (mold hides behind your curtains) and replace my water filter (my old carbon filter didn't remove fluoride). I detox regularly to clean out the toxins that I can't prevent exposure to (mercury and lead) and any new ones that show up (such as cadmium).

There are many delicate balances in your brain body that can be affected by subtle toxin level shifts. Your body is full of microbes, organisms too small to see with the naked eye. Think of them as part of you—bacteria, viruses, and fungi that outnumber your human cells ten to one. When the microbes in your body are in balance (when your microbiome is in homeostasis), you are far less likely to be sick or have brain problems. For example, we all have a small amount of candida, a form of yeast, that aids in our digestion and nutrient absorption. That's a good thing. However, when you take a broad-spectrum antibiotic and wipe out both invasive *and* protective bacteria and/or eat too much sugar, you may get an overgrowth of candida, which leads to serious consequences. When candida breaches the intestinal barrier and enters the bloodstream, it can release toxic by-products. That's *not* a good thing! Even more menacing, candida can change into its fungal form and bore through the wall of the intestine to reach other parts of the body, affecting not only the immune system, but also the liver and nervous system, giving you hangover symptoms like headache and fatigue—and possibly causing cancer. So candida can work for you when in balance or against you when external toxins disrupt the system.

While toxic exposures during pregnancy and childhood are especially risky, any exposure during your lifetime is a potential problem, and exposure in childhood may continue to harm your cognitive function later in life.[26] These days almost everyone has multiple exposures. Your body doesn't know what to do when it's overexposed, so as I mentioned, it stockpiles the excess chemicals in your fat and bones, until you decide to go on a diet and burn fat, or you hit your forties and bone turnover ramps up. Then symptoms can become more pronounced as excess toxins are released into your bloodstream.

Maybe you think you have a "clean" life, but chances are your medical provider is not examining you for toxic chemicals, heavy metals,

TOXIC CHILDREN

Experts at Harvard Medical School and Mount Sinai's Icahn School of Medicine say we are experiencing a "silent pandemic" of toxins that are damaging the brains of unborn children. They point to the fact that genetic factors account for only 30 to 40 percent of neurodevelopmental disorders (whereas your overall risk of developing most chronic diseases in adulthood is just 10 percent attributable to genetics, an important concept from my last book, *Younger*), and assume that nongenetic or environmental exposures make up the difference.[27]

Their concern is that "children worldwide are being exposed to unrecognized toxic chemicals that are silently eroding intelligence, disrupting behaviors, truncating future achievements, and damaging societies, perhaps most seriously in developing countries. A new framework of action is needed."[28]

pesticides, or solvents in your short physical exam once per year. Our brains and bodies slowly build up poison each day from toxins in our food, water, consumable products, and air. I find in many of my patients that they have imbalanced gut microbes that produce toxic agents like ammonia and endotoxin, which stimulate more inflammation in the gut, then systemically the body, and then cross the blood-brain barrier and cause inflammation there.[29]

Here's a list of some of the grim statistics:

- 82,000 synthetic chemicals are allowed on the market without safety testing.

- Less than 1 percent of farmland is organic.

- 287 chemicals are found in babies before they're born.

- Toxins are linked to anxiety, phobias, attention deficit disorder, depression, hormone imbalance, weight gain, multiple sclerosis, and chronic stress.[30]

- Even things you may not think of as toxic, like birth control pills and other medications, can be altering your brain, impacting your mental health, and causing depression and dementia.

THE TOXIC AIR WE BREATHE

I never thought much about indoor air quality until I learned that parts of my home contained mold and that normal home maintenance, including changing air filters once per month, does not get rid of it. We get exposed to toxins in many other ways, too: sitting in traffic, living in or visiting urban areas, and being near construction sites. When the World Health Organization listed air pollution as one of the top ten health risks for humans, linked to seven million premature deaths per year, that got my attention!

Urban polluted air contains not just benzene and heavy metals, but also aerosolized nickel nanoparticles, which can harm the brain and the cardiovascular system.[31] You breathe these toxic particles deep into your lungs, where they may cause harm. While I commuted to work in San Francisco, I was harming my brain with another nanoparticle known as magnetite, found in the human brain and associated with inflammation and Alzheimer's disease.[32]

For the first time, air pollution emerges as a leading risk factor for stroke worldwide. How many strokes are attributable to air pollutants? One-third of the global burden in 2013, according to a new study, and a higher percentage in developed countries.[33] This study adds to the body of evidence showing the link between climate change, higher air pollution, and more strokes.[34] Higher rates of stroke were associated with specific pollutants: carbon monoxide, sulfur dioxide, nitrogen dioxide, and ozone. The problem may be that air pollution damages the cells that line the circulatory system and increases the activity of the sympathetic nervous system, leading to narrow blood vessels, restricted blood flow, and more clotting.

Surprisingly, air pollution kills ten times more people than motor vehicle accidents, according to a study in London of 3.7 million premature deaths.[35] Sitting in traffic is the most deadly: pollution inside cars is up to 40 percent higher while at a red light or in traffic jams, resulting in exposure to pollution particles that are twenty-nine times more harmful than when you're driving in free-flowing traffic. Solution: hit the recirculation button before you drive!

- The last time Congress overhauled regulation of personal-care products was eighty years ago.[36] That means if a toothpaste gives you a headache or causes your fetus's IQ to drop, you probably wouldn't know about it and neither would the government.

- Toxins make us dumb. Lead has stolen twenty-three million IQ points. Common pesticides have offed another seventeen million. Methylmercury is responsible for yet another million.[37] If the average person in the United States has an IQ of 98, spreading the loss of these millions of IQ points is the equivalent to the total IQ of hundreds of thousands of people!

Let's look at lead. Lead concentrates in the brain, liver, kidneys, and bone, and it accumulates over time. Toxic levels of lead result in lower intelligence, reduced attention span, increased antisocial behavior, headaches, lower ability to learn, a greater sense of perceived stress, digestive problems, high blood pressure, dizziness, and muscle and joint pain. People with high levels of lead in their blood experience higher cortisol levels when they wake up in the morning, so they feel stressed out even when things aren't so bad. Lead disrupts the control system for sex hormones (the HPA axis), even at levels below the safe threshold recommended by the National Institute for Occupational Safety and Health and by the Centers for Disease Control and Prevention.[38] Yet we usually assume that since lead-based paint was banned a few decades ago, we're safe now. That's not the case. You can ingest lead from various consumer products and from the environment: air, food, water, dust, and soil.

Women are more susceptible to the immunotoxic effects of heavy metals and may be more vulnerable than men to their role as endocrine disruptors, particularly against normal estrogen and thyroid function.[39] Higher levels of mercury, for example, are more common in women with "unexplained" infertility,[40] and mercury correlates negatively with egg count and yield for women undergoing in vitro fertilization.[41] (Additionally, elevated lead makes women 75 percent less successful at in vitro fertilization.[42]) Women are more likely than men to have skin symptoms like eczema, especially from elevated levels of arsenic and cadmium. Periods of increased bone turnover (old bone cells being replaced with new bone cells) occur far more often in women than in men due to pregnancy and menopause, releasing stored heavy metals like arsenic, aluminum, cadmium, and lead[43] (90 percent of total body lead is stored in the bone[44]) from exposures dating back to childhood. Not only does toxic load increase as bone loss occurs in pregnancy,

SPOTLIGHT ON MERCURY

You may have heard about avoiding fish with high mercury levels or the risk of dental amalgams and exposure to mercury vapor. Mercury becomes toxic at a certain level in the body, and that level can vary depending on your gene/environment interactions. Mercury slows down your enzymes and gunks up your mitochondria so you can't make cellular energy, called adenosine triphosphate, or ATP. The normal process produces some particles called free radicals, and ideally you want a lot of ATP and just a small amount of free radicals. But the reality I see in my practice is that about half of my patients have mitochondrial dysfunction, especially as they age past forty, so their ATP and free radicals are out of balance, resulting in a feeling of fatigue, brain fog, depression, and sometimes headaches.

In the brain specifically, mercury hurts the glutamate (NMDA) receptor, so that you lose the normal balance between the stimulating effect of glutamate and the calming effect of gamma-aminobutyric acid (GABA)— see Appendix A for the cast of characters in the brain. Mercury may cause overactivity of glutamate, so you may feel anxious and get stuck in a high-stress mode.

Mercury belongs to a class of environmental toxins that are causing imbalances and increasingly robbing my patients of normal set points— that is, control and regulation mechanisms of a specific outcome, such as stable mood, clear and calm thoughts, normal memory, rational beliefs and behaviors, a normal weight, and stress resilience. Mercury is just one toxin that might be affecting your brain, set points, and—therefore—your life. Some people, like Tamara (from the beginning of the chapter) and me, have problems with weak stress-coping genes, toxin-clearing genes, and DNA-repairing genes, all of which control your ability to revitalize the brain body. That leads to accumulation of brain inflammation and, as a result, brain trash. Nobody wants to accumulate brain trash because it can make you fat and may even give you the big "A" (Alzheimer's disease).

The takeaway is that mercury exposure causes neurotoxicity at increasing levels, depending on your detoxification genes, environment, and other vulnerabilities.[45] While there's agreement that high levels are harmful to health, as I mentioned, there is no agreement about a safe lower level that doesn't cause harm. Much to my relief, moderate levels of seafood consumption, even with their accompanying higher levels of mercury, are linked to a lower risk of Alzheimer's.[46] Pardon me while I go cook my opah.

perimenopause, and menopause, some toxins may actually reduce bone density.[47]

Mold is another toxin that can find its way from your body to your brain and may make you lose balance, feel weird "ice pick" pains or headaches, or cause brain fog, trouble with focus, fatigue, muscle cramping, joint pain, numbness or tingling, or even weight gain. It can attack the rest of your central nervous system and thin out the lining of nerve cells, making you susceptible to symptoms similar to those of multiple sclerosis[48] or even Alzheimer's disease.[49] It can cause Reye's syndrome, a condition that causes swelling of the brain and liver. Mold can even drop your platelet count so that you bleed into your brain. Lead and mold are just two toxins that most of us are exposed to every day. Every day, people! Our environmental exposures are so common that most of us are clueless about them. You'll learn where to find them and how to avoid them in a few pages.

Toxic Cocktails

Toxins linger for a very long time in the brain and body—the half-life (the time required for concentration of a substance in the body to decrease by half) of mercury is two months; for cadmium it's sixteen years; for the pesticides DDT and DDE it's two to ten years; and for PCBs, it's three to *twenty-five* years! These half-lives do not account for the synergistic effects of multiple toxins, which may make half-lives shorter or longer. These toxins directly or indirectly affect your health, and may cause brain problems.[50]

Many of these toxins make the damage to your brain body worse when multiple toxins are present—even at low concentrations—a phenomenon known as the "cocktail effect." Take lead. People with high levels of lead in their blood experience many brain symptoms: fatigue, muscle twitching, and balance problems, and women appear to experience more harm (more oxidative stress, like rust inside of cells that slows them down, and greater activation of genes responding to oxidative stress) than men.[51] In addition to lead causing higher stress levels (cortisol) in the morning, other studies confirm the link between lead and disrupted cortisol levels.[52] Since cortisol plays a crucial role in the production of new memories

BRAIN TOXINS

CELL CRUSHERS
- Alcohol
- Chronic stress

ENDOCRINE DISRUPTORS
- Bisphenol A (BPA)
- Fluoride
- Heavy Metals: Arsenic, Cadmium, Lead, Mercury
- Pesticides: Chlorpyrifos, DDT/DDE, Glyphosate
- Phthalates
- Polybrominated Diphenyl Ethers (PBDEs)
- Polychlorinated Biphenyls (PCBs)
- Tetrachloroethylene (PERC)

MOTOR SKILLS
- Chlorpyrifos
- Mercury
- Phthalates
- Tetrachloroethylene (PERC)
- Toluene

COGNITION BLOCKERS
- Fluoride
- Magnanese
- Pesticides: Chlorpyrifos, DDT/DDE, Glyphosate
- Phthalates
- Polybrominated Diphenyl Ethers (PBDEs)
- Polychlorinated Biphenyls (PCBs)
- Tetrachloroethylene (PERC)
- Toluene

and brain cells (neurogenesis)—the highest concentration of receptors for cortisol is in the hippocampus (the memory center in the brain)—it's not shocking to learn that higher levels of lead and cadmium, even below "safe" thresholds, impair working memory, the type you need to function normally day to day.[53] What is important to understand is that *no known level* of heavy metal exposure is considered safe, especially when you consider the negative synergy of multiple heavy metals.

The toxic effects of stress and its accompanying elevated cortisol—whether from toxic overload or the pressure to jam-pack your life or an unprocessed trauma—can create brain/body inflammation and trash, then send you into a brain/body failure state. Stress controls your hormones and affects your mental, physical, and spiritual health. All told, it is our greatest toxin when we don't acknowledge it and bring it under control through the nutritional, supplement, and lifestyle repairs in the Brain Body Diet.

The worst part? Most toxic exposure is preventable—and self-imposed stress is one of the easiest to reduce immediately. Once you recognize the stressors in your life, detoxifying is essential for healthy living and a healthy brain, but you'll find future prevention is easier. That's where the Brain Body Diet comes in. Follow the steps outlined below to dislodge the toxins and lower the burden in your nervous system tissue and the rest of your body.

Types of Toxins, Their Effects, Where They Are Found

Here are a few highlights of the types of toxins you're exposed to, their effects, and where they show up daily. For more details, see Appendix B.

Household Item	Toxins	Toxin and Brain Effects
Air	Ozone Particulates (dust, dirt, soot, smoke, etc.), nitrogen dioxide (NO_2), sulfur dioxide (SO_2) Heavy metals: arsenic, cadmium, chromium, lead, manganese, mercury, nickel Benzene[57] Other: dioxin, asbestos, toluene (The EPA lists 187 toxic air pollutants.)	Ozone activates the sympathetic nervous system ("fight-flight-freeze") and HPA axis.[54] Particulates (<10 μm), NO_2, and SO_2 may increase risk of ischemic stroke.[55] Arsenic, cadmium, lead, manganese, and mercury escalate neurodegeneration.[56] Arsenic can disrupt the HPA axis and impair executive function, processing speed, fine motor function, and memory, and is associated with depression.[58] Benzene exposure occurs when you inhale petroleum products, such as gas, near gas stations, which may cause chromosome mutations and cancer.[59]
Clothing	Pesticides: DDT, DDE Heavy metals: cadmium, lead, mercury Endocrine disruptors: perfluorinated chemicals (PFCs)	DDT and DDE are linked to late-onset Alzheimer's.[60] Metals—see previous. Toxins in your sports bra, yoga pants, and workout gear contain endocrine disruptors that may disrupt the HPA axis and thyroid and cause cancer.[61]

Household Item	Toxins	Toxin and Brain Effects
Electronic devices	Electromagnetic fields (EMFs)	Increase free radicals, trigger the cellular stress response and breaks in DNA.[62] Affect immune function both positively and negatively.[63] May increase Alzheimer's, brain cancers such as gliomas and meningiomas, and male infertility, but evidence modest at best.[64]
Kitchen	Bisphenol A (BPA)	BPA changes brain development; may turn off the growth of synapses in response to estrogen in certain parts of the brain.[65] Altered behavior in children exposed to significant BPA has been observed.[66] BPA triples the risk of autism,[67] and is linked to serotonin problems.[68] BPA disrupts the HPA axis, leading to problems with hormones—including changes in puberty, ovulation, and fertility.
Food	Arsenic in fish, shellfish, meat, poultry, dairy products, rice, and cereals Advanced glycation end products (AGEs) in charred food Fungi, including mold Nitrogens added to flash freeze food or food packaging to preserve quality Herbicides and pesticides, such as glyphosate and chlorpyrifos	AGEs are associated with inflammation and Alzheimer's disease.[69] Nitrogen added to food may turn into toxic nitrosamine, which is linked to Alzheimer's, diabetes, and fatty liver.[70] Eating organic foods helps significantly reduce exposure to herbicides and pesticides like glyphosate and chlorpyrifos, but there are other problems that organic foods will not circumvent, like exposures to heavy metals, mold, other biotoxins, and plastics.[71]
Tap water	Arsenic Perchlorate (rocket fuel) Fluoride Manganese Lead N,N-diethyl-meta-toluamide (DEET)	The Natural Resources Defense Council found rocket fuel (perchlorate, a thyroid disruptor and potential carcinogen), lead, and arsenic in tap water in multiple urban areas.[72] Manganese increases the risk of behavior problems, particularly in boys.[73] Fluoride may cause lower IQ, cognitive impairment, and hypothyroidism.[74] DEET, a neurotoxin, is found in tap water and insect repellents.[75]

Household Item	Toxins	Toxin and Brain Effects
Bathroom	Skin care (lotions, shampoo, conditioner, nail polish, perfumes, deodorants) and cosmetics containing estrogen-mimicking toxins such as dioxins found in inorganic tampons, parabens (a preservative, or phenoxyethanol), phthalates, sodium lauryl sulfate, triclosan Medications and supplements: phthalates incorporated in the enteric coating Sunscreen: para-aminobenzoic acid (PABA), oxybenzone Mosquito repellent: N,N-diethyl-meta-toluamide (DEET), aluminum, formaldehyde, benzene/toluene, propylene glycol	Estrogen-mimicking toxins, known as xenoestrogens, can be absorbed through the skin and bind to estrogen receptors on cells, thereby changing your estrogen levels and function.[76] Many of these ingredients are on the Dirty Dozen list of Hormone-Altering Chemicals in skin care.[77] Phthalates and other toxins may affect memory, risk of asthma and autism, and ovarian function, possibly causing infertility or diminished ovarian reserve (also known as premature ovarian insufficiency).[78] Parabens may be associated with sperm abnormalities.[79] Dioxins are linked to heart disease, cancer, endometriosis, and possibly diabetes.[80] Formaldehyde is a neurotoxin linked to poor memory and reduced learning, and may cause cancer and liver damage.[81]
New car	Polybrominated diphenyl ethers (PBDEs)	PBDEs disrupt thyroid function.[82]
Under sink	Microbes—including fungi such as mold, bacteria, actinomycetes, mycobacteria Inflammagens: endotoxins, beta-glucans, hemolysins, proteinases, mannans, and possibly spirocyclic drimanes; as well as volatile organic compounds (VOCs)	Microbes and bacteria can cause type 3 Alzheimer's disease, CIRS, and biotoxin illness.
Furniture	Flame retardants: polychlorinated biphenyls (PCBs), PBDEs*, HBCDD Phthalates	PCBs and PBDEs alter the dopamine system and may increase risk of Parkinson's disease;[83] alter learning and memory.[84] HBCDD harms dopamine signaling.[85] Phthalates are tied to attention deficit disorder, autism, reduced verbal intelligence, developmental delay, and social deficits.[86]

Household item	Toxins	Toxin and Brain Effects
Household cleaners and supplies	Endocrine disruptors— phthalates Nonylphenol ethoxylates (NPEs) Fluoride in toothpaste Alcohol in mouthwash	Phthalates, NPEs, fluoride (see previous). Alcohol is a known neurotoxin (see chapter 5).
*PCBs and PBDEs are now banned but still exist in older furniture.		

The Science Behind the Protocol

The next section introduces the first steps to the Brain Body Protocol to beat toxicity, but first I want to share the science behind my recommendations.

INTERMITTENT FASTING

Intermittent fasting is when you restrict eating to a specific window of time after an overnight fast. Most animals feed this way when left to their own devices, allowing for periods of fasting that coincide with sleep. Periodically fasting creates an alternative universe with your metabolism, where you depend less on burning sugar and depend more on burning fat (known as ketone bodies). Why bother? Because intermittent fasting prevents inflammation and decelerates disease, helping you reset key metabolic and stress pathways, remove toxins, lose weight, and, ultimately, age more slowly.[87] This process gives your body more time to rebuild healthy cells. Just like a baby growing from tiny stem cells, we have the ability to heal and regenerate our cells—and intermittent fasting promotes this state. By giving the body a break from constant fueling and digestion, we create a window to focus on structural needs and to heal.

Specifically, intermittent fasting has been shown to promote health in a variety of ways: in the brains of animals, it reduces neurodegeneration.[88] In humans, it has been shown to improve brain function in epilepsy.[89] Intermittent fasting changes circadian clock genes, since eating is associated with light/dark cycles.[90] Multiple studies and reviews describe the beneficial metabolic effects of intermittent fasting.[91] Specifically, intermittent fasting in humans for three to twelve weeks reduces body weight by 3 to 7 percent, lowers body fat by 3 to 5.5 kilograms (6.6 to 12.1 pounds), and lowers total cholesterol by 10 to 21 percent.[92] Intermittent fasting can be one factor in lowering your body weight set point.

Finally, intermittent fasting reduces inflammation, improves biomarkers of health, counteracts disease, and potentially increases longevity and healthspan.[93] We've known that intermittent fasting has these benefits, as first documented more than seventy years ago,[94] yet most people aren't doing it. I hope you'll be a believer once you see the results. You'll begin intermittent fasting this week as a way of liberating toxins that are stored in your fat, and then in the next chapter, we will delve deeper into the benefits of intermittent fasting for lowering the body weight set point.

While the data on ketogenic diet (high fat, adequate or moderate protein, low carbohydrate) are unclear regarding the benefits to the brain for most healthy individuals, I urge you to try intermittent fasting as a way to enter a fat-burning (ketogenic) state and improving metabolic flexibility. For example, finish dinner by 6 p.m. and eat again at 10 a.m. the next day (a 16/8 protocol, for sixteen hours of a fast followed by an eight-hour feeding window). This turns on longevity genes, and the production of ketones improves focus.[95] Some people need to ramp up to a sixteen-hour fast more slowly—for example, beginning with a twelve-hour, then a fourteen-hour overnight fast twice per week.

GET THE RIGHT NUTRIENTS AT THE RIGHT DOSES

When it comes to removing toxins and protecting against future exposures, there are a few key scientific principles to keep in mind. Below are the highlights, and you'll learn more about how to operationalize these principles in the Brain Body Diet. The point is to remove the obstacles to brain/body wholeness and neurogenesis, like sugar, alcohol, and hyperarousal (chapter 5), and to add in more dietary components that promote neurogenesis and detoxify, like vividly colored vegetables, polyphenols, healthy fats, sulforaphane, spices, extra dark chocolate, and teas.[96]

- Foods rich in antioxidants help the liver.

  —Antioxidants are your best bet because they help counter the harmful effects of oxidative stress by inducing neuroprotection, such as the release of shielding enzymes and nitric oxide.[97] Most important are vividly colored fruits and vegetables, such as carrots, tomatoes, and berries, which are rich in carotenoids.

  —Another class of antioxidants that are helpful for detox are plant-based nutrients like the flavonoids (polyphenols) that may or may not be as highly colored, such as celery, onions, kale, grapes, Brussels sprouts, citrus fruit, cacao, and tea.[98] It's not just one vegetable or nutrient that is most important, but a combination of various types.

  —Certain vegetables help with liver detoxification, like the cruciferous vegetables: broccoli, cabbage, and cauliflower.[99] Crucifers contain sulforaphane, which inhibits Phase I and stimulates Phase II liver detoxification—that's what most of us need for improved detoxification pathways. Sulforaphane boosts production of glutathione, the queen detoxifier that protects the brain body, may be involved in the prevention of cancer, and helps tune up mitochondria.[100] The same receptor on cells that environmental toxins use for their negative effects is also used by cruciferous vegetables. That means when you eat more cruciferous vegetables, you crowd out the bad environmental toxins and strengthen your mitochondria.

  —Allium vegetables (onions, garlic, leeks) are another class of vegetables that help you make more glutathione.

  —Organic food beats out nonorganic every time, especially for the dirty dozen (strawberries, spinach, nectarines, apples, grapes, peaches, cherries, pears, tomatoes, celery, potatoes, and sweet bell peppers). Genetically modified organisms have negative effects on the microbiome and sex hormones.[101] Even one week of eating an organic and mostly plant-based diet will improve dozens of measures of health and measurably lower your toxic burden, according to a study of pesticide residues in people eating a mostly vegan diet with some fish and eggs, but without gluten, caffeine, dairy, or alcohol.[102] Imagine what forty days will do for you!

—Cacao or extra dark chocolate (85 percent cacao or higher) contains methylxanthines, another polyphenol, which are proven to enhance the brain body, reverse insulin block, lower blood pressure, and protect the nervous system.[103]

—Liberal spice use reduces inflammation and inflammatory toxins.[104]

—Alcohol consumption impairs mitochondria.[105]

—Grains tend to be moldy and laced with arsenic, cadmium, and/or lead.[106]

- Fiber doesn't detoxify just your gut but your whole brain body. Dietary fiber is proven to help the gut microbiome, gut barrier, gastrointestinal immune and endocrine systems, and detoxification organs in the liver and kidneys.[107]

- Black tea is shown to provide a barrier to protect you from external pesticide exposure and damage from an endogenous toxin called lipid peroxidase.[108]

- Green tea has been shown to induce glutathione production, help liver enzymes involved in detoxification, eliminate oxidative stress, reduce cancer risk, bolster resistance to neurodegeneration, and boost neurogenesis—so it's not surprising to learn that it also reduces anxiety and improves memory and attention.[109]

- The main ways to raise your body's internal glutathione are to cut out sugar (including alcohol), limit carbohydrates, eat more allium and cruciferous vegetables (mentioned previously), go to bed on time, exercise mildly and moderately, and calm down and breathe properly.[110] (I know, easier said than done!)

- Supplements can help if you cannot strictly follow the protocol's food guidelines.
  —Glutathione and precursors help you detoxify.
    Liposomal glutathione or the precursor, N-acetyl cysteine

(NAC), is shown to lower inflammation and mercury levels.[111] NAC helps remove lead and mercury,[112] and breaks down biofilms,[113] which are protected niches of bad microbes such as candida that release toxins and affect the brain body.[114]

(R)-alpha-lipoic acid reverses the age-related loss in glutathione, but the data in humans are not yet as strong as for NAC.[115] NAC and alpha lipoic acid improve mitochondria function.[116]

—Selenium protects you against metal toxicity. It's a natural antagonist against the harmful effects of mercury and lead.[117] Selenium works best when your body levels are low, and may contribute to metabolic syndrome if you are replete or consuming excess amounts beyond your body's need.[118]

—Berberine moderately lowers blood glucose, reduces blood markers of fatty liver, and decreases adipokines.[119] It has better efficacy combined with milk thistle.[120] Mild weight loss is seen at higher doses.

—Curcumin fights inflammation, including neuroinflammation or brain trash, and may help protect you from toxins such as lead, among others.[121] Studies show that it can help reverse nonalcoholic fatty liver disease.[122]

—Probiotics are anti-inflammatory and protect the brain body from heavy metals and mycotoxins (toxins from mold).[123] They lower body burden of BPA in rats.[124] They support mood and probably decrease depression and anxiety, although data are still emerging.[125] Probiotics may prevent and possibly reverse harm to the liver such as nonalcoholic fatty liver and subsequent brain effects.[126]

—Though gingko may improve liver and gallbladder function (the gallbladder stores bile, which helps the body break down fat from the diet) and gingko has also been shown to improve blood flow to the brain, cognition, speed of cognitive processing, and memory, the data are mixed.[127] Because of risk of cancer in animal models, the lack of consistency in study results, and its classification as a possible human carcinogen (Group 2B) by the World Health Organization's International Agency for Research on Cancer, I do not recommend it.[128]

PUMP YOUR LYMPHATICS

The lymphatic system functions as a network of tissues, nodes, and organs—like the spleen, tonsils, and thymus—that help rid the body of toxins, waste, and other undesirable debris. The main function of a normal lymphatic system is to transport lymph, a fluid containing immune-boosting and infection-fighting white blood cells, throughout the body and upward to the neck, where the lymph empties into your subclavian veins. When it's not working, you feel puffy, like you're retaining fluid, and may be more prone to infection.

Think of the lymphatic system as the waste clearance system for the whole body. It took my traumatic brain injury to realize just how important the lymphatic system is, because it ferries toxins and waste products out of the body. Not only that, but the lymphatic system is also responsible for keeping the fluid between cells (the extracellular fluid) in homeostasis, helping proteins stay in balance, providing immune surveillance, and combating infection.[129] As I lay in bed recovering, my swollen body provided evidence of accumulated toxins that I couldn't get rid of. My lymphatics needed attention to help clear my brain/body toxins.

Various problems of modern life conspire against normal lymphatic flow: gaining weight, underhydrating, and underexercising, among others. At the time of my head injury, my lymphatics had been neglected for decades. I had a habit of not drinking enough water, established during my medical training when I didn't have time to urinate, and leading up to the day of my fall, when the bathroom was too far away. I went twelve hours without a sip of water.

How is the brain involved? In 2015, a landmark discovery was published in the prestigious scientific journal *Nature*: the brain connects to the immune system via lymphatic vessels, located in the sinuses of the head.[130]

Brain injury of any kind, whether it's gradual (eating too much sugar and the resulting neuroinflammation) or traumatic like my injury, impairs the lymphatic system in the nervous system, which means you are more likely to experience sleep difficulties, and less likely to remove toxins efficiently.[131] So to keep your lymphatic system doing its job and disposing of toxins, drink more water, keep your weight at a healthy set point (more on that in the next chapter), sleep more, exercise more to keep your circulation moving, and sit less.[132] Jump on a rebounder (a small trampoline), for example. One of the best ways to improve your lymphatic circulation and aid in the removal of toxins is with resistance exercise. Even just ten to fifteen minutes of brief muscle contractions increases lymph flow by 300 to 600 percent.[133]

KUNDALINI YOGA FOR DETOXIFICATION

Kundalini is based on hatha yoga but with a different format, and in my opinion it is better suited to the removal of toxins. In kundalini, postures are just one part of a continuous movement called a kriya—breathing, chanting, and flexing/extending the spine—to permit the kundalini, or life force, to circulate in the body and brain. Kriyas last three to eleven minutes, and there are thousands of them. Best of all, you don't need to be flexible or to have practiced yoga for years in order to benefit: even the earliest beginners benefit immediately.

I began practicing kundalini about fifteen years ago after learning hatha yoga from my great-grandmother as a child and practicing alongside my mother. Honestly, though, it took multiple reconstructive breast surgeries in 2017 for me to slow down enough to make kundalini part of my rehabilitation. After my surgeries, I couldn't make it through a tough vinyasa yoga class because my pectoralis and serratus muscles could no longer hold Downward-Facing Dog, so I resorted to the more gentle kundalini practice. Along the way, I rediscovered a very subtle yet powerful way to rebalance body and brain.[134] Perhaps that's why kundalini is growing in popularity and was named a top-ten fitness trend by the *Washington Post*.[135]

On a mechanistic level, the movements of your physical and energetic bodies pump specific muscles as well as deeper internal systems, flushing capillaries and gently stimulating the lymph system so it can pick up toxins and get them out of your tissues, as well as rebalancing your endocrine system. Practitioners say other benefits are weight loss and stress and blood pressure reduction. Scientifically, kundalini improves anxiety, depression, diastolic blood pressure, resilience, perceived stress and cortisol levels, homeostasis, obsessive-compulsive disorder, and executive function, and may reverse mild cognitive impairment.[136] Kundalini yoga can also help by removing toxic thoughts and stuck emotions. Kundalini helps to move the toxins from your field of awareness metaphorically, as well as from your blood, fat, and bones physically. We all need a better technique to clear the toxins from our subtle energetic anatomy, and kundalini is a great one.

Psychiatrist Carl Jung, MD, considered kundalini to be a blueprint for higher consciousness, which can flow only from robust brain/body health. Jung described kundalini as a method of psychic hygiene, something we lack in Western thought—a redefinition and reintegration of self. This is not something that exists outside of you, but rather is latent within you and every person, and is even your birthright. In the lore of kundalini, it's an activity that reignites capacities that could be dormant by stimulating the brain and endocrine system, reestablishing balance in the left and right brain hemispheres. After practicing kundalini after my brain injury, I got to the point where I stopped digging in an endless inventory of all the problems that exist in life, and instead started focusing on the solutions—truly a redefinition, reignition, and reintegration for me. Kundalini can be a solution to many of my problems and yours.

NEUROSPIRITUALITY

One of the best ways to detoxify stress is something that grew out of kundalini for me. After a few decades of practicing yoga and still feeling dogged by stress, I realized that I could use my basic understanding of neuroscience to grow and enhance my experience of spirituality. Before I get too metaphysical on you, look at it this way: you can use your connection to something greater, no matter what it is, to improve your brain/body connection. (In more scientific parlance, you can use your beliefs along with the basics of neuroscience to improve spiritual neuroplasticity and build a better, healthier brain/body connection.) You could use a walking meditation, prayer, or other spiritual practices to detoxify stress from the brain in just a few minutes per day. These are simple and easy shifts that lead to important change. Even further, they change the structure and function of the brain, as documented in brain scan studies. The important part of creating and strengthening new pathways in the brain is repetition. As Rick Hanson, noted author and lecturer on neuroplasticity, says, whatever holds your attention has a special power to change your brain. So find a practice that suits you and stick with it.

To enhance neurospirituality, I began a daily practice that increases blood flow to the brain, grows the gray matter (you want more!), reduces the focus on self-centeredness, and creates a connection to something greater—through a process of empowered surrender that helps me let go of my ego. This practice has measurable effects on the brain, especially the limbic or emotional system, parietal lobe, and frontal cortex—brain regions that you'll get to know intimately and learn to love in the coming chapters. These new practices improve brain/body physiology while clearing out old traumas and providing a shield against the normal stress of daily life. You'll learn the specifics in the first protocol below.

The Brain Body Protocol: Removing Toxins

Now you get the basics of how toxins damage brain and body cells, disrupt hormones, and trigger the type of inflammation that leads to brain fog, weight gain, hormonal imbalance, and brain trash, among other life-depleting symptoms. It's time to lighten up your toxic load. You may think you're safe because you live far from a freeway or coal-burning power plant, but as you've read, the dangers lurk in your dry-cleaned dress, restaurant food, and probably your favorite workout clothes. As a physician taking care of women who don't know that toxins are causing many of their symptoms, I can tell you there's a good chance that they are—by harming your liver, mitochondria, brain, or all three. The bad news? Almost none of my patients are free of toxins, and it costs a small fortune to test for them. If your symptoms are particularly severe and you think you may need testing for a particular metal, see the Advanced Protocol or Appendix B for suggested labs. The good news is that you can start removing the worst toxins today by starting with just one or two steps below.

Our focus of the first part of the Brain Body Diet is to clear the toxins you've been exposed to via your lifestyle, from the time of conception until now. Most of us have toxic issues that need to be cleared with positive influences like sprouts, more fiber, and glutathione-boosting foods that help you build up a reserve for detoxification. We will optimize detoxification starting with the Basic Protocol. If you feel inclined or are especially toxic, add in one item or more from the Advanced Protocol. I urge you to follow the Toxin Protocol for forty days, adding protocols in the chapters that follow based on your self-assessments at the beginning of chapters 3 through 8.

BASIC PROTOCOL

Step 1: Lighten the load on your liver.

Your liver and mitochondrial activity have a direct impact on brain function, hormone levels, and detoxification of external environmental toxins as well as internally made toxins. Throughout the forty days of the Brain Body Diet, the following are your food rules.

Consume liver-supportive and brain-boosting foods and drinks to detox your brain body.

- **Vegetables:** Consume eleven servings (five to ten cups) of vegetables per day, half cooked, half raw. If you're currently well below eleven daily servings, add one serving per day until you get to eleven, or more slowly if you experience gas or bloating. Your gut flora will need to adjust to the increased fiber.

    Include in that count *bitter vegetables* and herbs at every meal for their liver benefit: arugula, dandelion leaves, endive, radish, sage.

    To raise glutathione (the master detoxifier in the body), eat *allium vegetables*: onions, garlic, leeks.

    Eat *cruciferous vegetables* because they trigger cleanup in your liver and immune system: broccoli, Brussels sprouts, cabbage, cauliflower, kale, radishes.

    Include both *nonstarchy and starchy vegetables*. Limit starchy vegetables to one serving twice per week if you are trying to lower your body weight set point. Replace grains like rice with tubers: sweet potatoes, potatoes, yams.

Eat the rainbow. You've heard it before, but in my practice, people get lazy about eating at least *five colors of whole foods* each day. Do it to help your detoxification genes and prevent micronutrient deficiency. Examples are provided in the Notes to help you accomplish this important task daily.[137]

Add prebiotic fiber. Feed the good bacteria in your gut ecosystem and remove toxins like BPA. Include asparagus, burdock root, Jerusalem artichoke, jicama, garlic, onion, leeks, unripe (green) bananas, flaxseeds, seaweed, konjac root (you can find this prebiotic source in shirataki noodles), and yacon root.

Spice it up. Extensive research over the last ten years has shown that some spices target inflammatory pathways, and thereby may prevent neurodegenerative diseases: turmeric, red pepper and chili, black pepper, licorice, clove, ginger, garlic, coriander, cardamom, fenugreek, cumin, rosemary, anise, cinnamon.

Make sure your vegetables are *organic*—that is, free of glyphosate, the herbicide found in a lot of genetically modified food.

Add in four to five forkfuls of *probiotic foods* per day: sauerkraut, kefir, and kimchi.

- **Fruits:** Include specific fruits that support the liver and brain: berries, cranberries, grapefruit. I eat one six-ounce serving of fruit each day, unless I am treating fungal overgrowth, in which case I skip all fruit for forty days or longer.

- **Protein:** Eat enough clean protein to maintain muscle mass (typically three to four ounces per meal for women, six for men), but limit saturated fat: include beans, fish, poultry, pea protein powder, hemp protein.

- **Fats:** Consume the equivalent of two tablespoons per day of healthy fats: coconut oil, olive oil, dark chocolate (more than 85 percent cacao), avocados, olives, wild fish.

- **Fiber:** Beyond the food-based fiber, take supplemental prebiotic fiber including arabinogalactan, human milk oligosaccharides, oat bran, rice bran, inulin, pectin, and others. Slowly increase fiber intake by no more than 2 to 5 grams per day. If you experience increased gas or bloating, back off and refer to the Advanced Protocol.

- **Drink:** Every day, you should be consuming half your weight in ounces of filtered water (carbon filter or reverse osmosis), organic herbal tea, hot filtered water with a squeeze of fresh lemon or lime juice, black tea, green tea.

Commit to intermittent fasting. Limit your eating to a specific window of time, after an overnight fast, for all of the remarkable benefits listed in the Science section on pages 72 to 73, but most of all, for the way it helps you burn fat, free up toxins, and then have an opportunity to remove them. I recommend a fourteen- to sixteen-hour window for men and a sixteen- to eighteen-hour window for women. For example, finish dinner by 6 p.m., and eat again at or after 10 a.m. the next day.

Avoid foods that destabilize your blood sugar, introduce heavy metals, and hurt your mitochondria.

- Foods frequently containing mold: coffee, nuts, peanuts, wine, grains
- Red meat, processed meats, margarine, cheese, pastries, fried foods, fast food, artificial sweeteners, diet drinks
- Alcohol
- Tonic (contains quinine, a known poison to the central nervous system, including vision)
- Sugar, refined carbohydrates, processed foods, which harm mitochondria

Step 2: Take brain botanicals.

- **Berberine.** Dose: 500 mg twice to three times per day. Combine with milk thistle at a dose of 105 mg to improve effectiveness.
- **Curcumin,** the anti-inflammatory, is safe at high doses but hard to absorb, so I recommend bioavailable curcumin 1,000 mg once to three times per day.

Step 3: Detoxify your body with sweat, heat, and circulation.

Extensive studies now indicate that one of the best ways to remove toxins is to sweat them out.[138]

> ### YOGA FOR DETOXIFICATION: BREATH OF FIRE
>
> This energizing kriya from kundalini yoga is designed to free up the diaphragm and pump your core so that your lymphatics work better.
>
> - Sit in a comfortable cross-legged position.
> - Inhale and exhale fast through your nose, with your mouth shut.
> - Aim for one to three breath cycles per second, and continue for ten to thirty seconds, about fifty pumpings.
> - Your breath duration in and out should be equivalent, but as short as possible, like a bellows. Don't be afraid to make some noise.

- **Exercise** to pump lymphatics at moderate to high intensity for thirty minutes four days per week. Get your heart rate up to at least the moderate zone (50 to 70 percent of maximal heart rate—a quick calculation is to subtract your age from 220) to be sure you sweat.

- **Sit in a sauna** four to seven days of the week for twenty to sixty minutes. Go to your local gym or consider investing in a home sauna (see Appendix B for recommendations).

- **Practice kundalini yoga** to detoxify body and mind and improve circulation. Start with fifteen to thirty minutes every day, and build up to thirty to ninety minutes at least five days per week.

ADVANCED PROTOCOL

If the Basic Protocol doesn't lower your toxic burden enough or you are still experiencing symptoms after forty days, try one or more of the advanced items for another forty days.

Step 4: Perform a basic detox of your environment at home and in your car.

Clean up your bathroom, kitchen, and car to reduce your exposure to the most common everyday chemicals and endocrine disruptors:

- Buy houseplants. They reduce indoor pollution by 30 percent in nine weeks.[139]
- Use fluoride-free toothpaste.

- Be sure your water filter removes fluoride.
- Install a reverse-osmosis water filter.
- Kill mold in showers, in tubs, under sinks, and in toilets. Make a paste of organic liquid soap mixed with baking soda. Wear gloves to apply the paste, then rinse with hot water. Spray full-strength white vinegar on any residual mold, let it sit for an hour, and clean. It kills the majority of mold without the toxic effects of bleach. Areas larger than a few feet may require professional attention.
- Replace plastic food and water containers with glass, ceramic, and stainless steel. Use your stash of containers instead of plastic wrap to store and transport food.
- Recirculate air and keep car windows closed while sitting in traffic or at red lights in your car. This will keep the air circulating internally rather than drawing in pollutants from the outdoors. These settings provide the best ventilation with up to a 76 percent reduction of in-car air pollution.

Step 5: Supplement to reduce toxin levels.

If you are on prescription medications, talk to your pharmacist about any drug interactions first.

- Still the mainstay of treating acute poisoning in the emergency room, **activated charcoal** can be used at home as well. I recommend it at the end of the day, at least two hours before or after any other supplements.[140] It works by interrupting the circulation between the gut and liver (called the entero-hepatic circulation) and the gut and blood (entero-enteric circulation), so repeated doses for two weeks are recommended. Activated charcoal can also reduce gas, but be aware it can cause black stools, and because it binds supplements and medications, it can prevent absorption, so avoid taking it within two hours of prescribed medications or other supplements recommended in this book. Dose: 500 to 600 mg once or twice per day.
- For probiotic supplements, I suggest *Saccharomyces boulardii* at a dose of 250 mg to 2,000 mg per day, plus a lactic acid–based probiotic at the dose you can tolerate, starting around 1 to 25 billion

colony-forming units per day, and building up to 50 billion per day.

- **Omega-3s** provide neuroprotection.[141] Dose: 1 to 4 grams per day.

- If you consume too much fluoride in your tap water, you may be at greater risk of low thyroid function, among other problems.[142] Taking **calcium** and **vitamins C and D** was shown to be helpful in children with excess fluoride exposure.[143] Dose: depends on body level, so I recommend testing to personalize the dose. Recommended daily dosages for calcium are 1,000 mg/day for women age fifty and younger, and 1,200 for women over fifty. Recommended vitamin D dosages are 600 IU for women of all ages, but should be dosed based on genetics and serum level. Upper limit of vitamin C is 2,000 mg per day.

- **Selenium** should be known as the "mercury-fighting" mineral. Selenium deficiency causes a sluggish thyroid and extra toxicity from mercury, so keep your selenium levels optimized. Selenium has been shown to reduce thyroid antibodies in autoimmune thyroiditis,[144] but too much selenium can cause toxicity, too. Dose: 200 mcg daily for three to twelve months. When you eat fish, choose fish using the new selenium-based standard, meaning with more selenium than mercury, such as the types mentioned in the table on page 92.[145]

- To help rid the body of heavy metals, take **liposomal glutathione,** 250 mg twice per day, or take the precursor, N-acetyl cysteine (NAC), 1,200 to 1,800 mg daily.[146] Or take (R)-alpha-lipoic acid 600 mg per day to counter the loss of glutathione as you get older.

Step 6: Test your toxin levels.

I routinely use several tests for patients who have symptoms of exposure, including but not limited to allergies, gut problems, asthma, autoimmune conditions, brain fog, heart disease, cancer, fatigue, frequent infections, hypertension, learning challenges, mood disorders, and obesity. We can measure toxic metals in the blood and urine and organic acids in the urine. In the blood, we can measure toxic by-products like homocysteine and other inflammatory markers like high-sensitivity C-reactive protein.

The tests that I commonly recommend (see Appendix B) are the following:

- Online test
  —Visual Contrast Sensitivity test to look for mold and other biotoxin exposures.[147]

- Blood, hair, and urine tests
  — Quicksilver Scientific to measure toxic metals like arsenic, cadmium, cobalt, lead, mercury, silver, and strontium.[148]

- Blood and urine tests
  — Genova Toxic Effects CORE to assess levels of bisphenol A (BPA), chlorinated pesticides, organophosphates, PCBs, phthalates and parabens, and volatile solvents.
  — Genova NutrEval to find micronutrient deficiencies and heavy metals in the blood and urine.[149]

- Stool tests
  —Viome is an in-home stool and metabolic test that provides personalized food and nutrient recommendations based on comprehensive analyses of your gut microbiota and RNA messages (transcribed by the microbial genes), also known as metatranscriptomics.[150]
  — Gastrointestinal Microbial Assay Plus (GI-MAP) by Diagnostic Solutions Lab offers PCR Stool Technology to map your microbiome. It screens for pathogenic bacteria, commensal bacteria, opportunistic pathogens, fungi, viruses, and parasites.[151]

- Urine tests
  — Great Plains Organic Acid Test (OAT) to check the biochemical machinery of the body—this is one of the tests that I use to look at overall metabolism in a single snapshot with over seventy markers, including dysbiosis, fungal overgrowth, vitamin and mineral levels, oxidative stress, neurotransmitters, and oxalates.[152]
  — Great Plains Toxic Non-Metal Chemical Profile (GPL-Tox) to screen for 172 different environmental pollutants using eighteen different metabolites, all from a single urine sample.[153]

Step 7: Draw toxins out of the body.

There are many ways to remove toxins from the body, some proven and some unproven.

- Cupping therapy is a traditional Chinese medical treatment that has been practiced for thousands of years, and is thought to remove toxins and inflammation. The World Health Organization defines cupping as a therapeutic method that involves the application of suction by creating a vacuum, usually with a cup placed on the skin of the affected part of the body.[154] More recent evidence proves that cupping reduces inflammation (by lowering natural killer cell numbers, their activity, and their cytotoxicity), lowers pain, and increases skin temperature and blood oxygenation.[155] Acupuncturists and physical therapists use cupping to decompress the fascia (the head-to-toe continuous sheath of the body that encloses everything inside your skin, including muscles, nerves, and organs), which is not possible with other techniques. Cupping appears to be safe, as long as you have it performed by a qualified clinician who knows how to avoid certain blood vessels, limit the length of time the cups are left on, and avoid sucking with excess force.[156] One of the side effects of cupping is that it can break delicate capillaries in the skin, leading to bruising and petechiae (small purple spots).[157] Personally, I've found cupping to be extremely helpful for the relief of inflammation, pain, and swelling.

- Some treatments are situation-specific:

  —Low stomach acid can induce toxins by causing imbalanced gut microbes. One way to help is to take betaine (trimethylglycine), 1 to 1.5 grams two to three times per day before meals, either anhydrous (which is better for estrogen metabolism) or betaine HCl (which is better for digestion).

  —For Tamara's high mercury, I prescribed a daily dose of 2,3-Dimercapto-1-propanesulfonic acid (DMPS) at a dose of 125 mg every night, along with a mineral supplement. We paid attention to keeping her bowels moving every day so that she would not reabsorb the mercury she was removing. After twelve weeks, her mercury level was in the normal and nontoxic range. Now she periodically tests her mercury level, about once per year. She uses liposomal glutathione, 250 mg twice per day, as needed if her mercury starts to climb. (See Appendix B for recommended labs.)

— For details about additional over-the-counter[158] and prescription medications[159] for binding and chelation, see Notes.

• Other forms of toxin therapy *not* recommended: bentonite or montmorillonite clay, diatomaceous earth.[160]

Step 8: Diagnose and treat brain/gut problems.

Depending on your gut function and symptoms, you may benefit from a more extensive gut assessment and repair of the gut/brain axis. First you want to identify the gut issues that cause or worsen the gut-derived toxins affecting the brain body, including loss of gut integrity, maldigestion, partially digested food, food additives, the wrong bacteria (or bacteria in the wrong place), the wrong microbes (such as fungal overgrowth or parasites), toxins from normal bacteria (such as lipopolysaccharides from gram negative bacteria), loss of normal liver detoxification, and inflammation. Many of the tests mentioned in Step 6 will uncover these problems. Based on your results, in functional medicine we follow the "4R" program of four stages—remove, replace, reinoculate, and repair— designed to address underlying root causes of symptoms affecting the brain body. If eating the foods and taking the supplements recommended earlier in the protocol are not helping you feel better in terms of gas, bloating, and other gastrointestinal symptoms, consult a functional medicine practitioner. Depending on the severity of your issues, it may take up to six to twelve months to heal your gut.[161]

Step 9: Increase your neurospiritual practices.

Spiritual practice helps to reset the brain body, particularly the overactivation of the stress caused by toxins.[162] My daily practice is to get up in the morning, make hot water with lemon or green tea, and sit down in a comfy chair in the living room to review my day. I start by measuring my heart rate variability as I described in my previous book *Younger*. I have a wristband that measures my heart rate variability continuously, alerting me on my smartphone when high cortisol is once again hijack-

WALKING MEDITATION

This is not a hike or workout. Instead, it's an intentional form of walking slowly and meditatively, where you walk ten to thirty small and natural steps, then retrace your steps.

1. **Choose your place.** I walk out the door of my house to a bike path. Any quiet street will do. You will be walking slowly, so it's ideal if you're not having to greet a lot of neighbors or getting passed by speed walkers and fast hikers.

2. **Begin stepping.** Walk ten or so steps, then pause and practice deep abdominal breathing. For instance, inhale for five counts, pause for ten counts, then exhale for five counts. When you feel ready, turn and retrace your steps or keep walking forward for another ten or so steps. Pause and breathe again.

3. **Consider the mechanics of each of your steps.** This is where the mindfulness comes in. We are usually so automatic about walking, but now we're going to drill deep into each part and get more intentional. The components are: the lifting of your right foot, the moving of the foot forward, the placing of the foot on the ground, the shifting in weight to that forward foot as the back heel lifts. Then the cycle continues on the other foot. Notice each component. Round it out so it's smooth and effortless, noticing the tendency to hurry and letting it dissipate.

4. **Become aware of sensations.** Allow your arms to hang at your sides, hold the dog leash with one, or clasp both or one behind you. Pay attention to the breath moving in and out of your lungs. Keep your neck neutral, parallel to the ground. Notice nearby sounds or those created by the movement of your body. Trace the landscape with your eyes. When your mind wanders, bring it back to your present sensations: sounds, visual cues, breath.

5. **Integrate.** Walking meditation grows on you, but slowly at first. As you become more familiar with walking meditation, you can bring mindfulness to walking at any pace, even to running, as I've described in previous books with chi walking and chi running. The aim is to create the conditions that support gentle and gradual detoxification of the brain body, allowing a state of dynamic wellness and wholeness.

ing my calm (see Appendix B for the current wearables that I'm using). Instead of amplifying stress with coffee or indulging thoughts about the problem or shutting it off with addictions, I measure and tame it. Today I was 50 percent stressed (probably because my house is on the market), and after a thirty-minute guided visualization, I was 18 percent stressed.

When I'm tired, a guided visualization suits me best, or a few yin yoga practices. When I have more energy, I perform centering prayer. Studies show that word-based centering prayer stimulates the prefrontal cortex, plus the language part of the brain (the frontal lobe, the area behind the forehead) and the limbic areas, and makes you less self-centered.[163] It also activates the brainstem, which is how the brain connects to the body, and thereby translates calm not just into the brain but into the viscera of the rest of the body. Finally, studies show that meditation, including centering prayer, decreases sense of self as shown by reduced blood flow to the parietal lobe, the seat of self-orientation.[164] Centering prayer is the form of active surrender that I mentioned earlier. Here's how to do it.

- Select a sacred word that symbolizes your connection to inner divinity. Examples: *grace, calm, trust, faith, peace, ease.*
- Sit comfortably, and close your eyes. Silently repeat your sacred word to invite a connection to the Divine.
- When you find yourself becoming attached to thoughts, return to the sacred word, a symbol of your consent to surrender.
- Remain still with eyes closed for a few more moments.

If sitting in a comfy chair every morning, measuring your heart rate variability and visualizing a recent beach vacation, sounds like too much work, here's an alternative: take yourself on a mindful walk. Recently I've begun a daily walking meditation with my dog. It takes ten to thirty minutes, and you don't need a dog to reap the benefits. See the sidebar on page 90 for how I do it, adapted from Jon Kabat-Zinn.[165]

Last Word

An unhealthy environment creates an unhealthy brain body. At our essence, we are self-regulating biochemical machines with complex

DETOXIFICATION

What	Why	How
Detoxifying food	Antioxidants crowd out environmental toxins and rebalance liver detoxification pathways.	Consume more foods containing antioxidants, including cruciferous, bitter, allium, and vividly colored vegetables. Add tea and probiotic food like sauerkraut, kefir, and kimchi to your daily regimen.
Sauna	Saunas remove toxins like arsenic, cadmium, lead, and mercury.[166]	Sit in a sauna for twenty to sixty minutes, four times per week. Replace electrolytes and trace minerals after you emerge.
Copper in balance with zinc	You want enough copper, but in balance with zinc. High copper is neurotoxic and causes many of the same symptoms as mercury toxicity—anxiety, and even criminal behavior.	Make sure you have approximately 100 mcg/dL copper and zinc; an optimal ratio is >1.3 (copper to zinc); >1 is normal.
Glutathione	It protects cells by cleaning up excess free radicals, the enemy agents with unpaired electrons that damage DNA, cell membranes, and proteins.	Take liposomal glutathione 250 mg twice per day for a goal glutathione (GSH) level of 5.0–5.5 µm.
Restore mitochondria	Your mitochondria's job is to make energy in the form of ATP. In the process, there's free radical production. You want a lot of ATP and just a small bit of free radicals.	Avoid sugar, mold and other biotoxins, heavy metals (in grains, amalgams, and personal-care products), and stabilize your blood sugar. Measure your methylation activity and genes; if needed, take methylators.
Keep selenium in balance	Selenium should be known as the "mercury-fighting" mineral. Selenium deficiency causes a sluggish thyroid and extra toxicity from mercury, so keep your levels optimized.	Maintain serum selenium levels of 110 to 150 ng/mL. When you eat fish, choose fish using the new selenium-based standard, meaning with more selenium than mercury, such as the types listed:[167] albacore tuna yellowfin tuna skipjack tuna bigeye tuna spearfish swordfish wahoo opah

metaphysical qualities, but toxins impair the function of the machine. A friend's grandfather was a fruit farmer in the Central Valley of California. The chemicals he used to spray his fruit trees included DDT, which very likely may have contributed to his diagnosis of dementia late in life. What was surprising were his doctor's words of solace to his wife and family, including my friend: "His brain stopped telling his body to heal." In the throes of dementia, his brain forgot to activate the healing response. The brain helps the body heal, but sometimes that signal gets interrupted. Please don't let that happen to you.

Even when you're trying to detoxify, life can get in the way and interrupt the biochemical machine. While writing this book, I had two trips back to back. One was to New York. I stayed in a hotel on the waterfront with organic mattresses and sheets, clean filtered air, and filtered water in every room. The restaurant served organic food. I felt normal upon my return to San Francisco, because the hotel was much like my home environment. A few days later, I went to Sacramento for my daughter's volleyball tournament. We stayed in a hotel on the freeway, in a room that reeked of toxic cleaning products. I opened the sliding glass door and noticed smokers on the deck next door and the freeway fifty yards away, and promptly shut it. I sat in an upholstered chair to write, but then got to thinking about how it contained flame retardants, and shut my laptop. My sinuses became congested, my eyes were itchy, and I felt hungrier than normal—in fact, intermittent fasting felt close to impossible. As I drove home, I noticed in the mirror that my eyes were rimmed in red and the whites of my eyes were bloodshot. My weight increased four pounds. I was inflamed.

My experience was hardly a controlled experiment, but sometimes anecdotal self-experimentation in your own body (the n-of-1 study) can be as important as the latest large clinical trials. Find out what happens in your own brain body when you are exposed to toxins and healing begins to slow down. Start to notice how you feel when you are one week into the Brain Body Diet. Attune to the signs that you're reversing toxicity, liver stagnation, and inflammation—your face looks less puffy, you feel less stiff in the morning, and the whites of your eyes look brighter, more white. Maybe you're less angry or anxious.

Just as Tamara was able to remove mercury and other inflammatory toxins—and to optimize her self-regulating biochemical machine—you can similarly remove toxins that may be blocking normal function, disrupting homeostasis, and creating a brain/body failure state. The Brain Body Diet helps you reverse the damage by allowing the brain to help the body heal again.

3

Body Weight Set Point

How to Correct Hormones, Burn Fat, and Lose Weight Permanently

Now that you've learned how to manage some of the toxins that are threatening your brain body, let's turn to a subject that most of us are all too familiar with: how to control weight. You and I know that sometimes our approach to eating is irrational, but did you realize that it's your brain body talking and *not* a lack of willpower or knowledge? You'll learn in this chapter how the brain regulates the weight of your body and, more important, what you can do to work with your brain to achieve the set point you desire.

Attaining the right body weight set point is life-changing—imagine not worrying about weight every day, or not binge eating and then feeling bad about yourself. Picture all of your clothes in your closet fitting you, right now, today.

What did you weigh at age eighteen? According to a recent study from Harvard University, a woman's weight gain from age eighteen to middle age (forty to sixty-five, but defined as age fifty-five in the study) determines her risk of most diseases, including high blood pressure, diabetes, heart disease, and obesity-related cancer. All of these conditions affect the brain body because of the same root cause: *inflammation*. For the 92,837 women followed for about thirty-seven years, the average weight gain was twenty-eight pounds. Women were at greater risk than men who gained a similar amount of weight over a similar period. Even moderate weight gain, defined as 5.5 to 22 pounds, reduced the chance of healthy aging by 22 percent for women.[1] We knew already that excess fat predicts cognitive decline, and visceral fat deep in the abdomen is the most important health predictor in women.[2] That's because excess body fat secretes hundreds of hormones, peptides, and cytokines—such as leptin and adiponectin—collectively known as adipokines that affect the nervous system, liver, and immune system and can be associated with cognitive deficits, dementia, and Alzheimer's disease.[3] Short version: moderate weight gain between the ages of eighteen and fifty-five foretells poor aging later for your brain body, particularly for women.

I may be one of those unfortunate women. I weighed 125 pounds at age eighteen. Although I'm not yet fifty-five years old, I've spent half of middle age higher than that number by ten to twenty-five pounds. Not only does a rising body weight put me at risk of all of those major diseases, but it shifts many subtle measures in my microbiome, immune system, cardiovascular system, and gene expression (the way my genes talk to the rest of my body and brain). It gets worse. Two years ago, I gamely signed up for a "bod pod" to measure my body composition. Any confidence I had regarding my fastidious lifestyle vanished when I faced the truth that my body fat was the highest ever. I was never in the "athletic" range (14 to 20 percent), but now at 30 percent fat, I was no longer in the "fitness" (21 to 24 percent) or "moderately lean" (25 to 29 percent) category. Not only that, but I was inflamed: my face and ankles were puffy, my belly was bloated, my low back more stiff, and my mind felt less sharp. What happened?

My story is hardly unique. It's the plight of 80 percent of the women in my functional medicine practice. The amount of fat in the body tends to be relatively stable and maintained within a narrow range, but with age, the tendency is for total body fat to rise, and in lockstep, for weight to increase. As your weight rises, so does your body weight set point (your brain-based control and regulation of a stable body weight). It dawned on me that my poor genes just carried out their orders from twenty-five thousand years ago: make her fat so she can survive. I struggled for several years as I faced my rising adiposity (a nice way of saying the fat concentration in my cells) and body weight. Then I learned about the link between the brain and weight—specifically how my brain was blocking my weight loss via its set point.

The upshot is that even a small amount of weight gain worsens inflammation, and the reason may trace back to the gut. Approximately 89 percent of people with obesity have bacterial imbalance or dysbiosis, as indicated by the diagnosis of small intestinal bacterial overgrowth (SIBO).[4] These include overgrowth of bad bugs that relate to high blood sugar, insulin resistance, and lipid abnormalities. When you're inflamed, weight gain occurs for a few reasons: fluid retention, insulin resistance, decreased thyroid function, poor sleep, diminished fat breakdown, and stress hormone imbalances. Weight loss may not completely reverse the problem, according to a study from Stanford University.[5] (Don't give up! You'll see later in the chapter that weight loss can reduce inflammation.) After several years of dutiful research, I discovered a protocol for how to stop banking fat as I get older, and I'll share it with you later in this chapter.

Subtle shifts are what we are about to address in the next part of the Brain Body Diet so that you can start feeling better right away, lose weight, shift mood toward the positive, and get the bigger payoffs of a healthier, stronger brain body in the years and decades to come. Our protocol goes deeper into specific hormones of the various set points—including body weight—gene/environment interactions, and, most important, the central role of the brain.

The brain regions that regulate food consumption and energy use also monitor how much fat you have in your body and respond to changes by offsetting your food behaviors and metabolism. All of this happens without your conscious awareness or control. Instead, you just hear a message in your head along the lines of, "You deserve another cookie," which may get you to eat something that raises your set point. That's what makes lowering one's set point such a struggle: if you lose weight, your brain will tell your body to burn calories more slowly (i.e., lower your metabolic rate) and tell your mind to eat more. Your brain body adapts to weight gain and then resists weight loss. As an example, according to a recent study of *The Biggest Loser* weight-loss reality show, participants' resting metabolic rate was still down 23 percent six years after the competition.[6] The slowdown of metabolic rate, called *metabolic adaptation,* is often much greater than you might expect for a change in body composition—and as the study shows, persists much longer than you might expect.

Conversely, if you gain weight, you'll most likely be less hungry and burn more calories because of the added weight, but insulin could be stuck in the fat-storing position, so you continue to pack on the pounds as your body aims for that higher set point (sometimes homeostasis is totally annoying). Women and ethnic minorities are disproportionately vulnerable to a rising body weight set point and obesity.[7] As you'll soon understand, a vital ecosystem exists between your genes, behavior, hormones, and environment when it comes to your body weight set point. That means it's not as simple as giving up sugar or forgetting about stress (although they are important steps): understanding the brain/body circuits underlying these interdependent factors is crucial to achieving an optimal set point for you. In this chapter, you'll learn how your brain works behind the scenes like a puppet master—and more important, how you can become the master of the brain/body connection that determines your set point.

To explain what you need to know about the brain/body axis, we will focus on learning about the *body weight set point*: how it controls body weight and is regulated by thoughts, beliefs, hormones, neurotransmitters, and microbes in your gut, many of which may conspire against you as you age. When you understand the targeted dietary and lifestyle changes (including supplements) that can help you achieve a sense of harmony between your brain and your body, you'll be able to reduce the undesirable effects of metabolic adaptation. Overall, you will find in this chapter an evidence-based plan that I will show you how to implement with the determination and perseverance that lead to an enduring and lower body weight set point.

A final thought before we begin: go easy on yourself. Even though you perceive yourself as a single entity with a singular mind, the left brain looks in the mirror, sees the flaws, starts the analysis, and begins the diatribe, usually a rigid and degrading sequence of thoughts and criticisms, like a broken record. This is the type of extreme left-brain-dominated thinking that caused me to suffer. I don't indulge my harsh and critical left brain anymore. In contrast, the right brain looks in the mirror and sees the whole being—right here, right now—smiling back, grateful, nurturing, nonjudgmental, and optimistic. The right brain knows the truth as expressed by Jane Fonda: we aren't meant to be perfect, but we are meant to be whole.

Lowering your body weight set point requires a brain/body-based strategy *and* compassion. That includes the understanding that your worth is far more than just your weight or how you look in your jeans. Feeling disgusted when you look at yourself, even just in your mind, doesn't help. The truth is that shaming or loathing yourself only perpetuates the presence of more stress, cortisol, and other fat-storing hormones and brain chemicals. You don't have control over your first thought, but you have control over your second thought and that first action. Let that be about loving yourself unconditionally, without judgment or indulging the negative tactics of your inner saboteur.

Expanding your self-love to unconditional status requires a spiritual element, usually involving the understanding of your spiritual hunger, as well as a shift from left-brain domination to a place of contented balance between the two brain hemispheres. We will address this balance in the protocol. You'll learn how to outsmart your set point accurately (a left-brain function) and how to maintain your new set point with more compassion and serenity (a right-brain function). You'll also align your conscious goal—to be lean and healthy—with your brain's unconscious goal—to keep fat on the body so you don't die of starvation.

Do You Have Brain-Driven Body Weight Issues?

Do you have now or have you had in the past six months any of the following symptoms or conditions?

☐ Do you have a body mass index of 25 or greater, or are you unhappy about your weight?

☐ Are you noticing that your weight creeps up each year even when your lifestyle stays the same?

☐ Do you know what to eat but have trouble eating it?

☐ Do you experience cravings for sugar, bread, dairy, or grains?

☐ Have you diligently followed a diet and gotten partial results (i.e., lost weight), but then hit a plateau?

☐ Do you overeat even when you know better?

☐ Do you eat when stressed or feel other emotions like anger, sadness, or overwhelm?

☐ Do you have trouble sensing when you are full?

☐ Are you strict with yourself about what you can and can't eat?

☐ Do you have a food plan that makes it difficult to eat anywhere but at home, leading to isolation from family and friends?

☐ Do you eat differently in public versus in private?

☐ Have you gained and lost at least twenty pounds more than once in your lifetime (excluding pregnancy)?

☐ After you lose weight, do you regain weight, even on restricted calories?

☐ Have you had recurrent episodes of eating large amounts of food, perhaps quickly, perhaps to the point of discomfort?

☐ Do you fear becoming fat and exercise or purge to make up for overconsumption of food?

☐ Do you feel self-loathing, guilt, or resentment when you stray from your food plan?

☐ Do you feel that restricting your food and tolerating hunger is the only way to maintain control and prevent weight gain?

☐ Do you feel like most of your energy goes into controlling your weight?

INTERPRETATION

If you said yes to five or more questions, you may have an issue with a rising body weight set point. Seven or more, and it's highly probable that you have a problem. Of course, an increasing set point isn't just cosmetic or isolated to how your clothes fit, but intersects with other physical issues such as the broken seven, blood sugar problems, metabolic syndrome, obesity, fatty liver, and (in women) postmenopausal breast cancer. While the symptoms of brain fog (chapter 4) overlap with other brain chemical imbalances, if you follow the protocol in this chapter, you will most likely feel better and be able to lower your body weight set point.

The Problem: We're Fat but Don't Know Why

It's sad how poorly we understand why we get fat. The old thinking that I learned in medical school was that overeating and sedentary behavior were to blame.[8] Later in my life, doctors still told me to eat less and exercise more. However, if that approach were true, why do 98 percent of diets fail? The traditional equation is overly simplified and fails to consider stress, sleep, hormones, behaviors, microbiota, gene/environment interactions, and, most important, the brain/body interface.

Some experts continue to blame "overnutrition" (i.e., overeating) and recommend gastric bypass surgery, but the procedure is costly, risky (complications in 17 to 37 percent of patients), and often unsuccessful[9] (failure rates are 15 to 60 percent because postsurgical patients can continue to overeat by snacking continuously, and often the root cause of maladaptive eating behaviors has not been addressed[10]). Other experts blame our microbiota-harming lifestyle. We eat a Western diet and what food author Michael Pollan calls "food-like substances": processed and adulterated food. As a result, we've lost bacterial diversity, and grown too many pathogens like *E. coli, Yersinia enterocolitica,* and *Pseudomonas aeruginosa* that promote the release of inflammatory messengers called cytokines.

Some experts villainize carbs and tell us to eat more bacon and steak. Others claim the problem is that we end up with too many of the microbes that extract excess energy from food and cause inflammation, leading to leaky gut, metabolic disorders, more inflammation, and weight gain.

Some researchers blame gut microbiota and the microbiome talking to the neuroendocrine system, especially the HPA (hypothalamus-pituitary-adrenal) axis (the main stress regulation system). All you might notice is that you feel revved up and want pizza for dinner. (When overly stressed, the HPA axis may promote the growth of bacterial pathogens and yeast, thereby altering the gut-brain axis, making us inflamed and craving sugar, bread, grains, and dairy.[11]) Stress can cause the gut wall to be more permeable, allowing bacteria to cross the barrier and activate an immune response, which in turn alters the microbiome and can disrupt the blood-brain barrier. You guessed it: the HPA axis then goes wacky.

Neurobiologist Stephan Guyenet, a researcher who investigates the reasons for rising set point and how to fix it, points out another theory: many of the factors involved are not conscious.[12] He notes that the human brain is hardwired to look for certain properties in food, and "it has a way . . . of sweeping aside your natural limits on intake."[13] Yet if the diet lacks one of those reward factors (like starch, sugar, fat, and protein), the brain is not as interested in eating as much of that food—so he says it's the hyperpalatable food (lots of sugar and fat to boost tastiness) that contributes to a higher body weight set point. As in: "Ah, pepperoni pizza and beer, yes! Kale, not so much."

Who's right? Is the correct answer all of the above? My belief is that the root of the obesity epidemic is in all of these problems, a combination of complex and subtle interactions of the brain and body. Here's what we know:

- Overeating may make you fat, but it is not the only factor. Despite dramatic changes in day-to-day food consumption, weight remains relatively stable over the short term for most humans and animals. Put another way, calorie input is not the only factor when it comes to weight.[14]

- Dieting leads to weight loss, but 98 percent of the time, the weight loss is not sustained, in part because of slowing metabolism and increased hunger and body weight set point. That means your frustration is scientifically warranted! Weight loss changes more than one hundred genes, most of which make you hungrier and more inflamed.[15] As we covered in the last chapter, weight loss actually raises the body burden of toxins that make you fat—as you burn fat and liberate toxic obesogens,[16] you need safe ways to dispose of them as you lose weight.

- Moving less does not cause obesity, although it can increase fat concentration and loss of muscle mass. Exercise is good for your brain and general health, but it isn't a cure for obesity. At best, exercise helps modestly with weight loss and may be more important to prevent weight regain or maintain a lower set point.[17]

- Reduced sleep and chronic stress are part of the perfect storm of weight gain. Social and emotional factors affect food intake, exercise, mental health, set point, and weight over time.

- Cutting out carbs, while keeping calories the same, may not help you lose weight as much as cutting back on fat.[18] Sorry, paleo and keto devotees. In a meta-analysis of thirty-two controlled feeding studies, researchers concluded that while the premise of low-carb diets is that they increase energy use and promote fat loss, when the diets substituted carbs for fat, lower-fat diets came out ahead in terms of energy expenditure and fat loss. (This matter is far from settled, but the data are in line with what I see in most of my female patients. Men seem to tolerate more fat consumption than women.) That doesn't mean you need to eat a low-fat diet like we did in the 1980s, but rather that the latest high-fat craze may not be the best for every woman's waistline.

- Additionally, the popularity of low-carb eating that began around 2003 may not be ideal for all women, owing to its effects on mood, thyroid, and HPA function, which reflect loss of brain/body homeostasis. It's a delicate balance for each person.

- Getting the right food plan for your gene/environment combination is not just about cutting calories, cutting fat, or exercising more. The quality of foods matters, as does the setting for eating the food and the company around you. We are not eating our food during picnics in forests, but while commuting in cars on the freeway or over stressful lunch meetings.

- Fascinating differences exist among people who successfully maintain their weight compared with those who gain weight easily. Understanding the gene/environment interactions, particularly the hormonal components, of these extremes may lead to a better understanding of rising set point and obesity.

Body Weight Set Point

When it comes to weight problems, the brain is running the show. Yet this fact has not been fully recognized, appreciated, or honored in most discourse about weight gain and fatness. First, the brain is the source of your behaviors related to when you eat, what you eat, how much you eat, the type of movement your body performs, and regulation of body weight, fat composition, and hormones. Second, your brain is not necessarily rational in how it tells you to eat. In fact, past stress can make you eat more.[19] Stress is not your brain's friend; you'll read a lot about its detriment to your most precious organ. Often the parts of your brain wired for survival will guide you to eat calorie-dense foods, even though you're not at risk for food scarcity. So even though your nutritionist may say eat more salad, your brain tells you to order a pizza and beer, even that you deserve it. Third, when you gain weight, the brain uses all the tools in its arsenal—hunger, hormones, behavioral changes, and other physiological compensations—to make sure your body fat and weight retain the extra pounds. Your brain evolved in a way that it doesn't want you to lose too much fat because you might starve to death—and rightly so, since the brain needs fat to survive. But it can be overprotective and consequently make your belly spill over your jeans.

The brain very carefully and intelligently sets a stable body weight for every adult. This is called the *body weight set point*.[20] Your body weight set point is based on genetics, the amount you exercise, your nonexercise physical activity, diet, microbiota and microbiome, and hormone profile, particularly the hormones involved in appetite, stress, and reproduction. To keep it simple, I think of the factors underlying body weight set point as falling into four categories: genetics, hormones, behavior, and environment.

The set point theory holds that your brain strongly regulates and defends your weight at a predetermined point based on your body's feedback loops. In practical terms, when you exercise more, you crave more food and the scale doesn't budge.[21] When you eat less, you get hungrier. It's like a Neanderthal is in charge of your weight, not a modern and intelligent woman.

Humans are similar to animals when it comes to their set points: *the hypothalamus is in charge.*[22] The hypothalamus is a brain structure about the size of a macadamia nut located near the center of the head, above the brainstem and just below the thalamus (the relay center for motor and sensory pathways), and acts in partnership with the pituitary gland, which hangs below it.

When you want to give up in frustration over your weight, keep a few facts in mind. It's not just you or a lack of willpower; it's a brain/body disconnection.

- Your hypothalamus orchestrates hormones and behavior as a result of environmental and body cues, so that means it governs set point and hunger, as well as other tasks such as sleep, body temperature, sex drive, and attachment to newborns.[23]

- When you overfeed a rat, its activity and metabolism increase and appetite decreases, so it doesn't gain any weight—at least short-term.[24] Humans do the same. Short-term, our bodies adjust. Long-term, not so much. The system is prone to disruption.

- Your body's fat stores are subject to dominant and mighty—even foolproof—feedback regulation. That's why lowering your weight and set point is so difficult. The medical term for this is *energy homeostasis,* or the biological process that controls body fat mass. Again, the hypothalamus is in charge.

- Defects in homeostasis lead to a rising set point. Here's how that happens. On a molecular level, eating a typical Western diet high in sugar and saturated fat alters the body and brain in several ways. Outside of the brain, eating high-sugar and high-fat food injures neurons, triggers inflammation, and makes insulin resistance more likely. Inside the brain, a similar process occurs, impairing leptin and insulin signals regarding appetite, metabolism, and weight. The net result is that both your body and your brain become injured and inflamed, then insulin and leptin resistant, and next you experience a botched set point system in the brain.[25]

- It's easier to gain than to lose. I know, that's not surprising. But do you know why? Your genes and your body's feedback signals (stress response, heart rate, metabolism, etc.) have developed such that humans defend weight *asymmetrically*: we fight against weight loss much more than weight gain. Weight gain doesn't threaten our ability to survive like weight loss could, so evolution makes it much easier to gain weight than to lose it, and humans tend to get fatter as they age. Evidence comes from the fact that for most people, lost weight tends to be regained with time.[26]

It's the *adipostat*—located primarily in your hypothalamus—that regulates the feedback loops of fat mass. You can think of the adipostat as a temperature gauge, or thermostat, but instead of regulating temperature, it regulates food behavior and energy use—how you burn or store fat. Short version: it adjusts your fat mass up or down with thoughts and behaviors depending on the cues it receives from hormones, neurotransmitters, and the environment. Most simply, it relays information about energy status from the body to the brain.[27]

Unfortunately, sometimes the adipostat gets confused—meaning it doesn't always get the right messages from the rest of the body. If the hypothalamus has been injured or inflamed, it blocks the proper signals.[28] Your body's signals come in the form of dietary choices and the response of your endocrine system with the hormones leptin, ghrelin, and insulin, and the neurotransmitter dopamine.[29] It's like a room with a thermostat that is working properly, but a window was left open so the regulation, or homeostasis, of the room temperature breaks down. External and internal factors mess up the intended communication network, many of which you don't know about, like toxins and behavioral impulses—and they make you eat when you shouldn't. The brain also

---

ADIPOSTAT

Definition: A proposed mechanism in the brain that regulates body fat within a narrow range based on food intake (energy input) and exercise (energy output). Location is in the hypothalamus, which coordinates the activity of the pituitary, especially hunger, thirst, sleep, emotionality, and other systems of homeostasis. The adipostat sets the metabolic status quo, like a thermostat for your weight, by compensating your eating and physical activity.

regulates other organs in the body, like the liver, muscle, and fat. All this conspires to make maintaining a healthy weight so challenging for many of us, unless we fix the breakdown in the communication network.

Body weight set point is hard to change, but it is well worth the effort. You simply have to adopt a new mind-set for the long haul, aided by sustainable lifestyle changes detailed later in the protocol (the usual: stress, thoughts, beliefs, and spirituality), by rewiring the brain circuits and avoiding metabolic compensation (the yo-yo dieting effect) from the various feedback loops in the brain. Then be 90 percent consistent. Consistency, as you'll see, is the key.

The Perfect Storm: Colleen

Colleen started fighting with her weight in her twenties. A software executive, she was fine with her set point through college, when she weighed about 125 to 130 pounds. But then she hit business school and the scale topped out over 200 pounds. "I felt dead after 'B' school, and I was never the same after," she told me. That's when she started to stress-eat pretzels, crackers, and microwave popcorn, drink diet soda, and grab food on the go. She developed acne and was treated for months with antibiotics, wiping out her protective microbiota. Colleen didn't eat in binges, but the combination of high work stress and eating to soothe herself led to problems with her hormones, contributing to a rising body weight set point, imbalanced gut flora, inflammation, and belly fat. She tried lots of diets, but it was always lose five pounds, gain ten. At our first appointment, Colleen was forty and weighed 218 pounds. Her blood pressure was high at 142/92.

Colleen's labs revealed a classic pattern of inflammation, probably related to her borderline high (prediabetes) blood sugar and contributing to her borderline low thyroid function.[30] Other measurements that were out of the optimal range included insulin, leptin, cortisol, and vitamin D. Before her genomics testing returned, we knew that she had the other three causes of a rising set point: behavioral (stress eating), hormonal (insulin block, leptin resistance, sluggish thyroid, high cortisol), and environmental (toxic stress).

We started a thyroid medication (see Notes for details), omega-3 fish oil at 4,000 mg per day, and a supplement to raise her HDL.[31] I referred her to an excellent therapist who is focused on insight, solutions, and action. Instead of restricting calories, Colleen gave up the main foods that were causing inflammation, including sugar, alcohol, grains, dairy, processed food, diet soda, red meat, and high-fructose fruit (such as apples, pears, cherries, and mangoes). The structure of the protocol enabled her both to maintain a lower set point and to eliminate the cravings that were pushing her to foods that made her symptoms worse, and to make positive mind-set changes. Colleen started going to Zumba class again, four days per week. In all, Colleen dropped her set point by twenty pounds, not just by changing her behavior and what she ate, but by addressing the brain-driven weight issues.

After twelve weeks, Colleen looked and acted like a new person: her weight was 198 pounds and blood pressure was normal. Inflammation resolved and all of her hormones were in the optimal range, except leptin—it was significantly lower than baseline but took longer to normalize (see Notes for specific lab values).[32] Colleen was thrilled with her progress and felt hopeful for the first time in many years about her body. I was thrilled too, because it's far more important to focus on the long view, the slow and steady progress and sustaining that progress, than on unrealistic short-term goals or perfection. Science supports this approach. What Colleen and I kept emphasizing in our work together was to keep up the daily practices, the baby steps—the change in behavior, hormones, and environment—and most of all to celebrate and reinforce her progress.

The idea is not to achieve a super-low weight for one day through extreme measures; that's impossible to maintain. When it comes to rewiring your brain, whether it's set point or calming down your stress hormones, you want to make methodical, diligent steps—a little bit each day—over a longer period. This helps your brain body. Colleen is reversing her obesity, which in middle age is associated with a two- to three-fold greater risk of Alzheimer's disease in old age and up to a five-fold increased risk of vascular dementia.[33] It took Colleen twelve weeks, but she was very close to her new body weight set point (198 pounds) within the first forty days.

The Science Behind the Set Point

THE TWO TYPES OF EATING

Scientists describe two ways of eating. One is called *homeostatic eating*—you eat for nutrition's sake, like Colleen when she lowered her set point and redefined her carbohydrate threshold. Almost no one in my family eats this way, so I had to learn about it from some of my friends. Not surprisingly, there aren't many of them who eat simply because food is fuel, and the ones who do are thin. The other type is *hedonic eating*—you eat for the pleasure and reward of food.[34] My family considers hedonic eating to be normal: I grew up in a home where my mother and grandmother constantly talked about new recipes to try, their weight, and their latest diet.

The problem is that in certain vulnerable people, like me, hedonic eating leads to weight gain and food addiction. Hedonic eating probably reflects adaptations we've made over centuries in the reward circuits in the brain. Morphine-like chemicals in food containing gluten (gluteomorphins), such as bread, or in dairy (casomorphins), such as cheese, may account for addictive properties. In fact, brain scans of hedonic eaters show alterations in the brain areas linked with reward, motivation, memory, learning, impulse control, stress reactivity, and interoceptive awareness.[35]

Hyperpalatable foods with high levels of sugar and fat are the most addictive, leading to craving, bingeing, and withdrawal in rats, similar to what we see with addictive drugs.[36] Women are four times more likely to be food addicts compared with men.[37] Some people have something called "high opioidergic tone," meaning that eating hyperpalatable food makes you feel pleasure as if you just took heroin or morphine.[38] Craving a food reward, like chocolate, is mediated by the nucleus accumbens, the reward center in the brain.[39] While it has not yet been proven conclusively, scientists hypothesize that chronic overfeeding with hyperpalatable foods weakens the body's natural reward response, which can increase your cortisol response (hello, stress!) and increase your drive for food.[40] More simply, food acts like an addictive drug. The only variable that lowers the odds of having severe food addiction is vegetable intake—veggies truly are the super-heroes of the story.

Even diet soda can make you fat. I grew up drinking diet soda of one type or another, thinking it was safe. Turns out that daily consumption of diet soda is associated with escalating abdominal obesity: i.e., your waist keeps growing.[41] Twenty-five percent of children and 40 percent of adults in the United States consume low-calorie sweeteners.[42] Low-calorie sweeteners disrupt the delicate balance of gut microbiota, making a person more likely to have blood sugar and metabolism problems,[43] increase weight and waist circumference, and are linked to a higher incidence of obesity, hypertension, metabolic syndrome, type 2 diabetes, and cardiovascular events.[44] Artificial sweeteners: a good idea gone wrong. No more diet soda if you want to lower your body weight set point! No more artificial sweeteners, and limit natural sweeteners like stevia, too, because some people have a hypoglycemic response.

While I don't think we all need to eat like robots, devoid of pleasure, hedonic eating is risky, particularly when your set point is rising and your BMI is 25 or greater. If you're falling prey to using food in unhealthy, hedonic ways, the risks are increased cravings, more stress, weakened pleasure response, and food addiction. Food isn't a friend, lover, or de-stressor.

WHAT CONTROLS THE ADIPOSTAT

Like me at age forty-eight, maybe your fat mass or weight is higher than desired and you want to lower it. That means taking on your body's set point and the adipostat—the gauge in your brain that regulates body fat based on energy input (food) and energy output (exercise)—which can be extremely difficult. Your fat manipulates your brain, which then manipulates your body in order to preserve itself. The fat/brain/body conversation has evolved over millions of years to perform this function. Evolution wants you to be a little fat, so there's a reserve when food is scarce. One author described this manipulation as a secret conversation between fat and the brain, and I agree. Losing weight and keeping it off requires us to convert that strong-willed adipostat from enemy to friend by using the steps in the protocol.

Now we also understand that obesity and extra weight are associated with chronic inflammation in the body. Here's the science on how being overweight can lead to inflammation: it causes abnormal cytokine production (cytokines, or chemical messengers, are secreted by certain immune system cells and affect other cells); increased acute-phase reactants (proteins whose serum levels increase or decrease in response to inflammatory cytokines and are thus markers for inflammation); and activation of inflammatory pathways.[45] The inflammation exists both in circulating immune cells, called mononuclear cells, and in adipose tissue (fat).[46] In simple terms, increasing levels of inflammation ruin feedback loops and may make you fat by raising your set point. The good news is that weight loss of even 5 percent reduces cytokines and inflammatory pathways and increases anti-inflammatory molecules in obese people compared with controls.[47] Plus, decreasing inflammation benefits the entire body, not just your weight-loss control center.

Genes, Body Fat, and Weight Gain

When I ran my first genetic profile, I was unhappy to discover my high genetic risk for a rising set point, weight regain, and obesity.[48] While weight gain is influenced by both genetic and environmental factors, genomics determines up to 20 percent of BMI.[49] Not surprisingly, these genes exert their influence mostly on brain signals that direct behavior, especially when to eat, how much to eat, and when to stop, and, occasionally, on stomach, fat, and pancreatic hormones. But remember: the other 80-plus percent is determined by the choices you make. While several genes have the strongest influence on set point, consider that this topic of the gene/environment interaction is rapidly evolving and complicated. You can't blame one gene; it's the gene interacting with your environment that governs your set point, and it's important to consider the entire orchestra of your genes (your *genome*) interacting with each other.[50] That said, here is a sample of the current panel of genes

> **Should I get my genes tested if I really want to understand how to lower my set point?**
>
> **Answer:** You don't need to test your genes to benefit from the Brain Body Diet and lower your set point. However, I understand the desire to learn about your personal genome and how to work with it more strategically. Remember that your genes control less than 20 percent of your set point, but if you want to know them and perhaps modulate their expression, refer to Appendix B for specific labs that I recommend.

involved in set point and weight gain (read more details in the Notes section):

- **Fat mass and obesity associated gene (FTO).** This gene is strongly associated with your BMI and your risk for obesity and diabetes.[51] When you have the variant, it gives you poor control of leptin, so you're hungry all the time.

- **Melanocortin 4 receptor (MC4R).** The gene MC4R works in the brain's hunger center, and when normal, it tells the body, "Stop eating." Certain variants make you more likely to overeat the wrong foods, especially when stressed.[52]

- **Leptin receptor (LEPR).** Snacking can be good or bad for you, but when women have the G/G variation in the leptin receptor, they are likely to snack more.[53]

- **Adiponectin (ADIPOQ).** The ADIPOQ gene variations can cause problems with your adiponectin hormone levels in the body, making you more likely to become obese, develop diabetes, and regain weight.[54]

- **Adrenergic beta-2 surface receptor gene (ADRB2).** I call this one the takes-me-twice-as-long-to-lose-weight gene. ADRB2 is associated with fat burning and distribution.[55]

- **Dopamine receptor D2 (DRD2).** Variations may make people more likely to overeat and behave addictively.[56]

- **Other:** Many other genes have been proposed and are under investigation.[57]

For Some People, Plant-Based Is the Answer

Maria, age seventy-three, juggled kids and career for decades and made an effort to eat well, exercise moderately, and keep a connection to her spirituality for sanity and balance. But over the years, each decade brought another ten pounds. Fifteen years ago, she joined Weight Watchers and managed to lose the twenty extra pounds that she found unacceptable. But she didn't bolt once she lost the weight; she stayed the course. Maria maintained her new set point by weighing in monthly to maintain her lifetime member status and to keep herself connected to the Weight Watchers community, and by internalizing good eating habits. "There are some foods I just don't eat [or hardly ever eat]," she says. Pizza maybe two or three times a year, pastries almost never.

Although she was pleased to lose the twenty pounds, she felt stuck at a set point of 147. Her weight would fluctuate around holidays and during vacations, but she was able to stay below her Weight Watchers goal weight. Then, several months ago, her husband's doctor ordered him to become a vegan because of health problems. Maria does not eat vegan—she eats eggs and some animal protein at home and usually orders fish when they eat out, but most of their meals at home now revolve around beans, vegetables, and healthy grains. Within a month, her husband's labs improved dramatically—and Maria's weight dipped below 140. Her weight has hovered closer to 140 than 150, and she believes her new set point will be 142. Maria thought she was doing everything right, but found when she adapted to her husband's new regimen, her body gave a resounding *Yes!* Sometimes, with your set point, you can change just one thing—shifting your diet to be mostly plant-based— and your set point drops. One alteration can change several of the conversations that impact your set point, and ultimately, things improve.

Toxins That Affect Weight

Many of the toxins you read about in chapter 2 were obesogens, environmental chemicals that conspire to stimulate fat production and storage. Obesogens have been the subject of vigorous research for the past ten to fifteen years. Scientific interest evolved from the observation that the rising epidemic of obesity and the massive output of industrial chemicals were not just coincidental, but most likely related. Over time, we've begun to learn that certain environmental toxins change metabolic regulation in the hypothalamus.[58] From there, environmental toxins can alter lipid balance, weight, cholesterol levels, signaling pathways, and protein production in many animals, including humans. As noted in chapter 2, most obesogens disturb insulin pathways.[59] Due to their chemical structures, many of these toxins cross the blood-brain barrier and placental barrier, and mimic or disrupt hormones. Prenatal exposure to some obesogens can have effects that last more than one generation.

If you weren't convinced already about the danger of toxins to your brain, maybe understanding their impact on your weight and set point will seal the deal. Below are the most common obesogens and where to find them (see more obesogens in the Notes section).[60]

- **BPA (register receipts, plastic bottles, and canned food):** BPA is one of the best understood obesogens.[61] Prenatal exposure can even make you less motivated to exercise, plus they change the metabolism of carbohydrates versus fats, at least in mice.[62] One type of BPA, a flame retardant (tetrabromobisphenol A), damages the cells that produce insulin, increases adipogenesis, and promotes inflammation.[63]

- **Mercury (fish and dental amalgams):** Mercury in the blood is positively associated with increased BMI, visceral fat, and increased waist circumference.[64]

- **Phthalates (perfumes, air fresheners, shower curtains, and scented lotions):** Phthalate levels in the body correlate with increased waist circumference, body fat, and obesity, including from prenatal exposure.[65]

- **PFOA (nonstick pans and microwave popcorn):** PFOA can raise leptin and insulin levels in exposed mice, even at low doses, which is associated with increased weight in midlife.[66] PFOA also affects thyroid function, and when you mess with the thyroid, you mess with body weight set point.[67]

- **Mold (in your food, under your sink, and behind your dishwasher):** Mold is in certain foods, such as grains, alcohol, apple juice, and coffee.[68] Mold toxins disrupt the function of insulin and leptin.

On a more positive note, your natural hormones may help protect your brain from toxins. Hormones made in the adrenal glands and ovaries, such as estrogen and progesterone, can pass through the blood-brain barrier and protect brain cells from oxidative stress and damage from many toxins, including mercury.[69] You can think of the brain and ovaries as sanctuary sites, protected areas that are hard to penetrate, whether by prescription drugs or other foreign substances and toxins. Estrogen and progesterone and their protective by-products can create a sanctuary in your brain from toxins. (Of course, a leaky blood-brain barrier may still allow toxins and other foreign substances to enter the brain.) Additionally, the brain has its own endocrine system and can produce sex hormones, known as neurosteroids, that can protect the central nervous system.

A CLOSER LOOK AT FAT AND APPETITE

Fat isn't all bad. When fat is behaving properly, it secretes the proper amount of *leptin*, the hormone that suppresses appetite; and *adiponectin*, which removes glucose, fat, and toxic lipids from blood. The problem is that if your weight is creeping up or is higher than is healthy for you, these hormones—maybe even a neurotransmitter or two—are most likely misbehaving. For example, while it's true that eating a normal amount of healthy fat won't make you fat, in postmenopausal women, eating more fat may raise ghrelin, the hormone that tells you to eat.[70] As noted above, you need to find your own sweet spot when it comes to the quantity of healthy carbs and healthy fat, keeping in mind a recent article from *The Lancet* showing that eating excess carbs is associated with earlier mortality.[71]

Hormones and Neurotransmitters of Weight, Appetite, and Set Point

Hormones drive what you're interested in, and food is no exception. The figure below shows the most common hormone imbalances that interfere with normal eating, weight, set point, and fat storage. You'll learn in the protocol how to bring these hormones under control. We will deal with the brain chemicals dopamine and opioid in chapter 5.

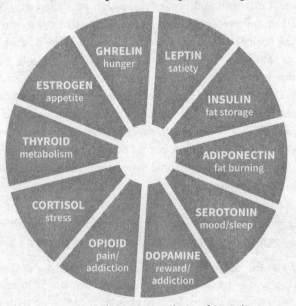

Hormones and Neurotransmitters of Set Point

GHRELIN, THE "HUNGER HORMONE"

Ghrelin is called the hunger hormone because it tells you when to pick up your fork and start eating.[72] In this way, ghrelin is the counter hormone to leptin, the hormone that tells you you're full and it's time to put down the fork. Your brain may have evolved to ignore ghrelin so you didn't starve when food was scarce, but it didn't learn to override that impulse in modern times when food became plentiful.[73] Ghrelin is produced in the stomach but is very active in the brain, especially the hypothalamus and the nucleus accumbens. (Read more about the details of ghrelin in the Notes.[74]) Bottom line: too much ghrelin is a barrier to losing weight because it increases appetite and subsequent food intake.[75] The more ghrelin in your system, the hungrier you are. As such, we want to lower your ghrelin in order to lower your set point.

LEPTIN, THE SATIETY HORMONE

Your fat cells secrete leptin, the hormone that regulates appetite, satiety, and energy expenditure, telling the hypothalamus how and when to burn energy.[76] Based on your leptin pathway, you may have a fast or slow metabolism at rest.[77] When you eat a typical Western diet high in sugar and saturated fat, your cells are at risk of becoming numb to the leptin signal, so your fat cells start to overproduce it, making you inflamed and then more fat by lowering adiponectin (see page 119).[78] The more fat cells your body makes, the less your brain is able to let you just put down the fork.

The blood-brain barrier (BBB) also plays a dynamic role in regulating leptin levels. Leptin is transported from where it's made in fat tissue to the brain via the BBB. But once you develop high insulin and insulin block, the resulting high blood sugar appears to increase the transport of leptin across the BBB.[79] Upshot: people with leptin resistance feel hungry, rarely feel full and satisfied, and tend to be overweight or obese. If your leptin is in control, you'll start to feel satisfied with modest amounts of food—the right amount for you and your set point. You want balance, with just enough leptin (not too high) and adiponectin (not too low).

INSULIN, THE BLOOD SUGAR HORMONE

You may not be diabetic yet, but you could be experiencing other telltale signs: you can't lose fat no matter what you try, and maybe you're tired because the glucose in your bloodstream can't get to your muscles to feed them and keep you strong and energized. Maybe your doctor explained your fasting blood sugar is borderline, or your triglycerides are too high, or your good cholesterol (HDL) is too low. Maybe you have been diagnosed with hypertension, atherosclerosis, fatty liver, sympathetic overactivity (too much stress), hypercoagulability, or high insulin levels.[80] All of these symptoms and conditions are related to the root cause of insulin block or resistance. Insulin block is common, found in about 41 percent of obese patients and about half of Americans.[81] The main cause is eating more carbohydrates than your body can tolerate, leading to carb intolerance and rising insulin, which in turn causes inflammation and rising body fat. (See Notes.[82])

When your insulin is blocked for too long, your brain tells your body to store the fat for future use, which means that your set point has to go up to accommodate the new stores. When your diet includes liquid sugars (cocktails, soda, juice) and excess carbohydrates in the form of bread, pasta, and potatoes, your cells become blocked to the effects of insulin. Science confirms: eating too many carbs is associated with early mortality in a prospective study of more than 135,000 adults followed for 7.4 years.[83] As we sort out the details, stay away from processed, packaged foods and refined carbohydrates, and get your carbs from one to two pounds of vegetables per day. If you're currently overweight, you are probably experiencing insulin block because your cells' ability to respond to insulin declines as fat composition rises. Insulin disposes of sugar that's in the blood, so when the action of insulin is blocked, your blood sugar rises too high or too fast or both. Rapid changes in blood sugar can stimulate cravings, weight gain, and systemic inflammation. Insulin rises, and so does fat storage, as the body increases the demand to keep blood sugar even. Your body has to do something with all of that extra blood sugar, so it turns it into fat for later use. That was a neat trick when we were hunter-gatherers surviving a famine, but now it makes us fat and unhappy.

Insulin resistance also affects your brain. When your brain is insulin resistant, it affects more than just your set point and eating behavior; it also affects your cognition, memory, reward system, and whole-body metabolism.[84] It's another grave brain/body setback. High insulin levels in women act on the neuroendocrine system and can cause it to pump out large levels of sex hormones, leading to a greater risk of polycystic ovary syndrome. So you want to keep your insulin in check to promote whole brain/body health.

ADIPONECTIN, THE FAT-BURNING SWITCH

The more fat you have, the lower your adiponectin levels. Inflammation increases as adiponectin drops.[85] Visceral fat accumulation is associated with lower circulating adiponectin levels, too. On the other hand, the more adiponectin you have, the less inflammation you have and the more fat you burn. It follows that when you lack adequate adiponectin, you have great difficulty melting fat and staying lean. That's why losing fat can be so challenging. In the protocol, you'll find the proven ways to boost adiponectin naturally and safely so that you can burn more fat.

CORTISOL, THE STRESS HORMONE

Your body secretes cortisol in response to the brain's perception of stress. Cortisol cranks up the sympathetic nervous system, so that you can be ready to fight or run. As I've described in all of my books, this is a good adaptation for the occasional danger, but cortisol levels are often far higher than the human body can properly handle. Chronically elevated cortisol levels cause fat storage in the abdominal area. Even worse, the more abdominal fat you have, the more cortisol you produce in response to stress, which then causes more abdominal fat to be deposited. Talk about a vicious cycle! Stress becomes embedded psychologically and biologically. It can affect your HPA axis function, your cortisol levels, and all aspects of food behavior: how you eat, the food you crave, and how much you eat. Women experiencing high levels of stress have a higher BMI, more emotional eating and cravings, and more visceral fat.[86] High cortisol can break down your muscle for energy, which is bad for weight loss because it lowers metabolism further. When you don't respond well to stress because of past traumas, exposure to stress increases your chances of eating more calories.[87] This is one of the key intersections between the brain and the body that is most often overlooked when it comes to weight gain and weight loss. (We'll address stress and the brain more in depth in chapters 6 and 7.)

THYROID, THE HORMONE OF METABOLISM

The thyroid affects nearly every cell in your body by telling it to turn up or down your metabolism. When thyroid function is low, you feel tired and depressed, retain fluid, and most likely will gain weight. Your thyroid gland is in your neck, but your hypothalamus controls it. You need your hypothalamus to provide adequate levels of both the storage thyroid hormone (T4) and the active thyroid hormone (T3) in order to feel your best and have a normal body weight set point. Your labs can be normal while you're still not doing a good job of converting T4 to T3 in the brain, possibly because of genes or inflammation. As a result, your brain gets confused and slows down metabolism, even though your thyroid labs are normal. (See Notes for how to check for the gene variant[88] and, if you have it, talk to your doctor about more judicious use of a T4 plus T3 medication.[89]) Furthermore, sealing a leaky gut will also help reduce autoimmune attack of the thyroid, which is the cause of most cases of low thyroid function. Experience also suggests that each person with thyroid issues may have a physiological optimal range that's more narrow than laboratory-quoted normal ranges, which implies the existence of an encoded homeostatic thyroid set point that is unique to the individual.[90]

ESTROGEN, NATURE'S APPETITE SUPPRESSANT

Estrogen has hundreds of jobs in the body, but did you know it's an appetite suppressant and it promotes energy expenditure?[91] That's part of the reason why women gain weight after menopause. Estrogen replacement can reverse the effect. You may already know that 17β-estradiol, a type of estrogen, protects tattered brain cells.[92] So it makes sense that estradiol may prevent the brain from making you eat more and burn fewer calories. I favor hormone therapy in the right person, with the right genetics. The decision ultimately varies person to person and must be individualized (see Appendix B for suggestions).

On the other hand, too much estrogen is a problem. A rising set point and obesity are associated with increased *aromatase,* an enzyme that increases estrogen production in fat tissues, leading to excess estrogen and a greater risk of certain types of breast cancer in postmenopausal women.[93] The key is to have the right amount of estrogen for you: not too much so it promotes breast cancer, and not too little so it promotes appetite and slows metabolism. Knowing what's just right is a matter of measuring symptoms and laboratory tests, as described in the Advanced Protocol.

It's Not as Simple as Giving Up Carbs

Turns out that insulin block was the primary defect leading to my increased fat composition when I tried the "bod pod." The main way I fixed it was with intermittent fasting, along with a plant-based, add-fish-and-eggs diet, as you'll learn about in the protocol. A high-fat, moderate-protein, low-carb ketogenic diet did not work for me. Later I learned that intermittent fasting protects the brain against cognitive decline created by inflammation, and it all started to make sense.[94]

I wish it were as easy as removing most carbs to reset insulin. In a one-year trial of weight loss, eating low-carb results in the same weight loss as low-fat—but causes more mood problems.[95] Other studies show impaired mood and cognitive function on low-carb eating—along with other imbalances such as decreased thyroid, low testosterone output, higher cortisol levels, gut dysbiosis, poor muscle building and athletic performance, suppressed immune function, and fatigue—sometimes leading to lower motivation to exercise.[96] On the other hand, low-carb diets and low-carb ketogenic diets may help to reset insulin levels in some people with obesity or metabolic syndrome.[97] The takeaway is to get insulin working for you so that inflammation and body weight set point are lower.

I don't want to give a rigid rule about how many carbs or how much fat or protein to eat, however, because I believe it depends on the gene/environment interaction—your DNA, your stress level, how much you exercise, and the current state of your insulin pathway. Short version: you want to match your carbs to your DNA and lifestyle. My husband is a low-fat genotype; he regulates carbs based on his daily exercise but can eat more carbs than me without raising his set point. I'm a low-carb genotype; I gain weight easily on carbs and need to watch them care-

AVOIDING THE OBSESSION WITH WEIGHT

While I want to avoid the persistent rise in set point and body weight, I also want to avoid an obsession with a few pounds, because that can lead to anxiety (chapter 6), another disaster for your brain. I'd recommend the same for you. In her essay "Fatness and the Female," Jungian analyst Ann Belford Ulanov states, "Many women today feel haunted by an obsession with weight. Though in no way psychotic or afflicted with such gross disturbances as obesity or anorexia, these women know the full force of a neurotic preoccupation with food."[98] Ulanov nailed it. We aren't talking about women who are morbidly obese. That's because it's not just about the weight; it's about a deeper spiritual hunger. "She knows she is entangled in a classical neurotic conflict: the means of dieting she employs to control her obsession with food only tie her more securely to a compulsive preoccupation with it." In other words, we displace unmet needs onto food and obsess over unattainable weight goals. As you consider your body weight set point, is it rational for your body shape? What would your wiser, older self recommend about a realistic set point for you?

fully to maintain my lower set point. For me, that means a maximum of about two ounces of carbohydrates per day (steamed sweet potatoes, yuca crackers, purple potatoes), and more if I'm stressed or exercising more. Grains raise my blood sugar too much for at least two hours—and cause carb intolerance for me, which shows up as bloating and weight gain. So you need carbs for mood, cognition, and thyroid function—just not too much. There is no one-size-fits-all rule, but one of the easiest ways to prevent carb problems with your insulin pathway is to intermittently fast, which can reset insulin, fatty liver, and obesity, shifts the microbiome in a positive direction, and turns white fat beige.[99] In this protocol, you'll lengthen the amount of time you spend intermittently fasting so that you can lower your set point by burning more fat, liberate the obesogens stored in your fat, and reset your set point hormones.[100] As you'll learn, you want to remove refined carbohydrates but continue to get healthy levels, primarily from vegetables and fruits. For maintenance, more fat and fewer carbs may be best, but you have to do your own personal research to confirm.

The Slow Creep: Kim

At age forty-two, Kim rated her health as "2/10" ("1" is sick, barely surviving, and "10" vital), way too low for a young woman in her prime of life. Her main goal was to lose twenty pounds, and in the process deal with her mood swings and fatigue. Even though her eating habits and workouts were unchanged, her main issue was the fat that showed up around her middle after beginning an antidepressant for work/life issues—including a job she hated, a boss she loathed, and a husband with whom she rarely had sex. Her primary care doctor had started her on an antidepressant, a combined selective serotonin and norepinephrine reuptake inhibitor (SNRI) called duloxetine (brand name Cymbalta, 60 mg), which did nothing except cause her to gain weight. Her doc promised that Cymbalta was a "weight-neutral" antidepressant, but the truth is that it causes nighttime sugar cravings and weight gain in susceptible individuals like Kim. When Kim asked about her increased sugar cravings and weight gain, her doctor said it's not the drug, it's you. The weight gain only made her mood worse. In desperation, Kim went to a "fat doctor" who added the appetite suppressant phentermine, 37.5 mg, to her list of medications. Kim wanted to lower her current set point, which rose on the antidepressant, back to normal. She found me during a desperate search online and traveled hours to see me for help.

Summary of what we found and the actions we took:

- **Reason for rising set point.** Sixteen to 55 percent of patients on antidepressants like duloxetine gain clinically significant weight.[101] Kim started to wean off the duloxetine with her prescribing doctor's help to manage withdrawal symptoms. I recommended other methods to support her mood and energy, like kundalini yoga every morning for fifteen minutes, working with a life coach about her job and marriage, and taking methylated folate, fish oil, N-acetyl cysteine, and spirulina.

- **Stress.** We measured Kim's hormone balance with a helpful test of her growth-and-repair in proportion to her wear-and-tear hormones, also known as the anabolic-to-catabolic ratio.[102] Her ratio was 0.8, so she had more wear and tear occurring in her body—which caused her body to sense that Kim was in a crisis and drove her body to store fat. (See Notes for Kim's laboratory values.)[103]

- **Hormones.** Kim had way too much of an enzyme called beta-glucuronidase, produced by specific bacteria in her gut, and that meant she was blocking the detoxification of toxins like carcinogenic estrogens—the enzyme kept recirculating the same bad estrogens and wouldn't let the gut remove them. Higher levels are linked to excess estrogen in the body and colon cancer. Limiting fat and meat in your diet and eating more vegetables and fiber lower beta-glucuronidase.

- **Dietary changes.** Kim cut out flour, sugar, and alcohol. Kim's fecal pH was low, meaning it was overly acidic. In Kim's case, she was eating too much conventional red meat, like burgers with her kids at a local restaurant during the week. Proper pH levels favor the beneficial microbes in the gut, deter possible pathogens, make digestion smoother, and promote short-chain fatty acid production. Besides the possible influences listed here, an acidic pH may also result from malabsorption of sugars in the intestines.

- **Genes.** Kim had several gene variations involving serotonin, which may have contributed to her rising set point on the antidepressant. Taking a bioactive form of vitamin B_6 (as pyridoxal-5-phosphatase) was very helpful at helping serotonin soothe her brain.

- **Toxins.** Kim's mercury level was very high, probably from five amalgam fillings and two crowns. Kim started the Quicksilver Protocol to reduce mercury (see Appendix B). She was working with a biological dentist to replace her mercury-containing dental work.

The Brain Body Protocol: Lowering the Body Weight Set Point

When it comes to lowering your set point, take the long view. Consistent mind-set and discipline, avoiding the yo-yo weight loss/weight gain pattern and hormonal nudges, and behavior modification are what work. When you change your environment, you change the cues to your unconscious brain and gene expression. We don't need to follow the rules of a survival game that no longer exists. We can work around our ancient brain circuits that favor a rising set point by promoting neurogenesis, reducing inflammation, and protecting the blood-brain barrier.

Just as the Toxin Protocol needs to be done for forty days to achieve results, if your set point is rising, perform the Set Point Protocol for forty days or longer. Perhaps start with one step and be consistent for a week. Once it becomes habit, add another step if you're still not seeing changes.

BASIC PROTOCOL

Step 1: Eat for blood sugar balance.

Follow the guidelines from the Toxin Protocol in chapter 2 for food with the following refinements.

- **Upgrade your set point environment.** You want your food cues at home to be good for your brain. Colleen got rid of calorie-dense trigger foods at home by donating them to a local food bank. She cleared the decks: no more visible food sitting out on kitchen counters or luring her at night. As she started intermittent fasting, she closed her home kitchen at 7 p.m. She knew that the break room at work was full of tempting foods that she used to love, like pretzels, chips, and crackers. For the sake of her brain, she stopped going to the break room while following the Brain Body Diet. Instead, for the long days at the office, she brought a bag of food with her that included cut vegetables, healthy proteins like nuts and seeds, and a big salad for lunch, or leftover vegetables and protein from the night before. If you tend to feel like eating more than you need, consider weighing food with an inexpensive kitchen scale. It's a fidelity thing: just as you wouldn't cheat on your life partner, stop cheating on yourself. These efforts set up a better food environment that will support you in intentional eating and improve the cues you send to your unconscious brain.

MACRONUTRIENTS

You know what worked for previous generations? Let's look to the 1960s, before the obesity epidemic began. Americans ate 45 percent of calories from fat, about 33 to 34 percent from carbs, and 20 to 21 percent from protein. We ate less meat, cheese, and grains (especially corn) compared with 2015. It was a healthier macronutrient combination that existed before fat became demonized by Pritikin, Keys, and Yudkin. When Americans then cut the fat over the next few decades, waistlines grew.[104] While I'm not suggesting that this macronutrient profile is the best for all, it's a reasonable starting place to then determine your best macronutrient ratios.

- **Define your carbohydrate threshold.** Eat the maximum healthy carbohydrates that you can while getting to or maintaining your new set point. That means you need to define your carbohydrate threshold through personal experimentation. Most people need about 10 to 35 percent of their total calories per day from carbohydrates, but it depends on your insulin pathway, stress levels, and microbiome function, among other factors. People with thyroid, adrenal, or mood issues—or a high level of physical activity—may need more. For most women, the typical range is 50 to 150 grams of carbohydrates (15 to 30 percent of calories on a 2,000-calorie diet), and for men 100 to 200 grams of carbohydrates (on a 2,600-calorie diet). Here's how you do it: start with about 50 grams of carbohydrates per day for women. Stick with it for two weeks, then try the middle end of the range for two weeks, then try the higher end for two weeks. (My carb threshold for weight loss is 50 to 75 grams per day as part of a 2,000-calorie diet and, for weight maintenance, about 76 to 100 grams.) For the intrepid biohacker, consider testing your blood sugar with an inexpensive home kit two hours after eating a known amount of carbs (see Notes for details).[105]

- **Minimum protein.** Eat the minimum amount of protein that preserves your muscle mass. For most people, that's 0.8 to 1.0 grams of protein per pound of lean body weight to lose fat or maintain weight, and 1.0 to 1.25 grams per pound of lean body weight to gain muscle or improve performance. For me, that's four ounces of most kinds of protein (such as fish, beans, chicken, turkey, whole tofu) at breakfast, lunch, and dinner. Or two eggs, or two ounces of nuts or seeds. Or pea protein in a shake. Or pulses, such as beans or lentils. Overall, most people do well with about 20 to 35 percent of their calories from protein.

- **The rest in fat.** Eating healthy fats improves your health. But don't eat foods that combine high fat and high carb (like French fries or chocolate cake): it raises ghrelin in postmenopausal women with insulin block. Aim for the remainder of your calories from healthy and unprocessed fats, like avocados, olives, and macadamia nuts.

- **Curb your carbs.** Studies show that counting and reducing carbs leads to improved blood sugar and weight in the short and long term.[106] If you are overweight, it's likely that you have a problem with carbohydrate metabolism, and a low-carbohydrate approach can help.

- **Eat in a way that doesn't inflame your brain (i.e., your hypothalamus).** This means getting the right balance of fat and carbs, improving the health of your gut (microbiome), and scheduling your meals. Specifically, we are keeping your hypothalamus, the boss of your hormones, cool and chill. One key is to avoid a low-calorie diet, because it makes your fat cells hoard calories and leads to overeating. At the same time, watch your body's response to saturated fats. Some people do well with healthy saturated fats, such as pastured butter and coconut oil, but some gain weight.

- **Continue to intermittently fast.** Increase from once or twice per week to five to seven days per week. Remember that intermittently fasting is much easier than dieting, because you are not restricting food—you're simply limiting your feeding window, like animals in the wild. Continue from chapter 2 with a twelve-hour eating window, such as finishing dinner before 7 p.m. and then having breakfast at 7 a.m. Try it two[107] times per week on different days (not continuous) for weight loss, and add another day if you don't see your set point drop. A longer fast of thirteen to fourteen hours,

even sixteen hours (see Advanced Protocol), is associated with a
better insulin pathway. Adjust the hours to fit into your schedule.

- **Consume a mostly plant-based food plan.** It lowers blood sugar,
  inflammation, and weight.[108] Start eating meals planned totally
  around plant-based foods. Increased soluble fiber helps to balance
  blood sugar.[109]

- **Eat more vegetables.** The only variable associated with less food
  addiction is vegetable consumption; vegetables also provide the
  fiber to reset ghrelin[110]—aim for at least one more cup per day, or a
  scoop of greens powder added to a daily shake. Ideally consume one
  to two pounds of vegetables per day.

- **Include in your diet chromium- and magnesium-rich foods.**
  Foods high in chromium include eggs, nuts, green beans, and
  broccoli. Foods high in magnesium include dark leafy greens, fish,
  extra dark chocolate, and avocados. Both can reduce your risk of
  nutrient gaps associated with blood sugar problems.

- **Add probiotic food.** You can eat more coconut (nondairy)
  yogurt, kefir, miso, tempeh, beet kvass, fermented chili paste,
  pickles, kimchi, and sauerkraut. Sauerkraut and kimchi may
  have as many as one million to one billion live microbes in each
  gram.[111] Start with a small amount, such as one or two tablespoons
  at dinner, and build up to one-half cup (four to six forkfuls)
  per day. Take care of your microbiome by eating prebiotic and
  probiotic food, consuming plenty of fiber by gradually increasing
  day by day, avoiding antibiotics if you can, and limiting red
  meat.[112]

- **Enjoy wild fish.** Eat low on the food chain, including small fish
  like salmon, mackerel, anchovies, sardines, and herring, in addition
  to the fish listed in chapter 2. If you consume poultry, make sure
  that it's pastured and free of hormones and antibiotics. Purchase
  directly from butcher counters and get poultry wrapped in paper,
  not prepackaged in plastic.

- **Watch your food thoughts.** You will still have food thoughts—
  like *I must eat a bar of chocolate now*, or *I deserve a big hunk of*

TRUE HUNGER VS. FALSE HUNGER

Most of the busy women I know are hungry. Stress makes them hungrier. Yet sometimes what feels like physical hunger is not that at all, but emotional or spiritual hunger, such as a need for affection, affirmation, understanding, competency, accomplishment, or a deeper connection. Or maybe what first seems like hunger is even something else, such as anger, loneliness, or tiredness. A tool called HALT can help you reclaim the brain/body connection:

1. Pause for a moment.
2. Ask if you're feeling **h**ungry, or is it **a**nger, **l**oneliness, or **t**iredness (HALT)?
3. Go deeper: *Is there something I need or want that I am not getting, in this moment?*

By recognizing the clues that your body gives you, you can prevent the loss of appetite regulation, hedonic eating, chronic overfeeding, and a rising set point. Not every pang of hunger needs to be treated with food. It's okay to be hungry for a period of time each day. Tuning in to and discerning the messages you get from your body about hunger can help you shift to a place of balance between the left and right hemispheres, and develop a more peaceful and satisfying relationship with food, brain, body, and set point.

pie—but you don't have to act on them. Create a gap between stimulus and response, as recommended by renowned neurologist, psychiatrist, and Holocaust survivor Viktor Frankl: "Between stimulus and response lies a space. In that space lie our freedom and power to choose a response. In our response lies our growth and our happiness."[113] Listen to his wisdom, and honor the wisdom of your body. We'll talk more about making contact with your inner self and honoring the sacred throughout this book.

- **Control stress levels.** High stress can raise blood sugar and set point.

Step 2: Reset your hormones.

- **Sleep more** to reset leptin, ghrelin, insulin, and cortisol. If you have one night of bad sleep, you will temporarily worsen your insulin and prediabetes, so it's even more important to eat pristinely that next day.[114] Aim for seven to eight and a half hours per night.

- **Add extra fiber to lower appetite, insulin, and glucose.**

  —Utilize a functional fiber containing water-soluble polysaccharides. This ingredient has been shown to reduce body weight, body fat, frequency of eating, and consumption of grains.[115] It is a proprietary polysaccharide complex that has been shown in another randomized trial to lower body fat, insulin, and glucose within three months of daily use.[116] Dose: 4.5-gram softgel orally before each meal, or 5 grams of PGX granules mixed with filtered water.

  —**Pectins** are a type of dietary fiber made of gel-forming polysaccharides derived from the cell walls of plants, especially apples and citrus. They lower bad cholesterol (LDL and very low-density lipoprotein cholesterol, VLDL-C) without affecting HDL,[117] and can reduce other toxic loads as well. Pectins appear to reduce appetite, insulin, and post-meal glucose.[118] Dose: 800 mg three times a day with meals. You can buy it at most supermarkets or online.

- **Drink a glass of filtered water with apple cider vinegar** to lower blood glucose and perhaps reset insulin.[119] Add about one tablespoon to eight to twelve ounces of water daily, ideally before you eat.

- **Increase your magnesium intake** to raise adiponectin and lower inflammation, either from food (pumpkin seeds, leafy greens like spinach and kale) or by taking a supplement. Higher endogenous magnesium levels are associated with lower levels of inflammation.[120] Even an increase of only 100 mg of magnesium per day lowers inflammatory markers.

- **Limit or remove caffeine.** Excess caffeine will raise your cortisol. Swap coffee for green or black tea, or even herbal tea if you're highly sensitive.

- **Stop snacking** to repair leptin and insulin. Eat three meals a day and when you want to snack, have a glass of water and ask: *Am I* *hungry, or angry, lonely, or tired?* Eat every four to six hours on the days when you're not fasting to help optimize insulin and leptin.

- **Practice daily meditation or visualization** for five to thirty minutes to normalize your cortisol and reduce inflammation. Consider that learning to surrender can help you heal your body and your brain. It may seem like it's more passive, but it's more about allowing the Divine to help you meet your goals.

- **Drink more mineral water** to decrease ghrelin and cravings.[121]

- **Consider medication for your thyroid.** Get your levels checked. You may need medication or a change in medication in order for your thyroid to work better in your brain and help lower your set point.

- **Intermittent fasting** lowers insulin in addition to your set point.

- **Exercise wisely** for a minimum of thirty minutes four times per week. Exercise improves your health in many ways, and has been shown to lower leptin, raise adiponectin, lower insulin, and burn fat in overweight and obese people.[122] Moderate to vigorous exercise that includes burst training or high-intensity interval training (HIIT) is ideal. Burst training can be applied to cardio exercise (e.g., intermittently sprinting on a track alternating with a jog or walking) or weight lifting (lifting a weight, such as with a biceps curl, as many times as you can with good form for one minute, followed by one minute of rest). With my girlfriend Jo, I walk or run three minutes fast (approximately 6 or 7 on an exertion scale from 1 to 10), then alternate with three minutes at a normal pace (about a 3 on the exertion scale).[123]

Step 3: Deepen your detox from obesogens.

Here's what's proven to work, in addition to the strategies described in chapter 2. Pick one or more of the following strategies.

- **Make a daily shake** with hypoallergenic protein (such as pea or hemp protein), extra fiber, vegetables (or greens powder), and 1 teaspoon of spirulina. A 500 mg dose twice per day of spirulina (to the equivalent that's in your daily shake) led to reduction of weight and appetite in obese individuals ages twenty to fifty years.[124] Spirulina is anti-inflammatory and detoxifying.[125]

BREATHE THROUGH YOUR LEFT NOSTRIL

I've written in previous books about the benefits of left nostril breathing to activate the right brain and help with sleep, but did you know left
nostril breathing also helps restrain compulsive eating?[126] Here's how
to do it.

- Sit in a chair or on a mat in easy cross-legged pose.
- Close your eyes and focus them on the space between the eyebrows.
- Use your right thumb to close your right nostril. Inhale deeply
  through your left nostril and hold at the top of your inhale for a
  few beats.
- Exhale through your left nostril and hold at the bottom of the exhale
  for a few beats.
- Repeat for three to eleven minutes.

- **Increase your daily dose of N-acetyl cysteine** to 600 mg three
  times per day, or take liposomal glutathione to boost glutathione
  levels in your cells.

- **Add prebiotic food to your meal plan,** such as including a
  green banana in your smoothie. Prebiotics are indigestible
  carbohydrates—indigestible to humans, but they feed the
  good microbes in your gut, so they can grow, multiply, and
  protect you.

- **Include probiotic food,** as mentioned in Step 1. While some
  systematic reviews and meta-analyses suggest there aren't sufficient
  data to state that probiotics reduce weight,[127] the probiotics that
  performed best for weight loss were Bifidobacterium lactis 420,
  Lactobacillus gasseri SBT 2055, Lactobacillus rhamnosus ATCC
  53103, and the combination of L. rhamnosus ATCC 53102 and
  Bifidobacterium lactis Bb12 to reduce adiposity, body weight, and
  weight gain. Overall, probiotics were associated with modest weight
  loss of up to three pounds, and performed better when combined
  with fiber.[128] They may work by lowering appetite, resolving leaky
  gut, and improving inflammation.

ADVANCED PROTOCOL

Perform the Basic Protocol, but add one or more additional items from the Advanced Protocol.

Step 4: Increase the frequency or duration of intermittent fasting.

Ideally, perform intermittent fasting daily—more frequently than in the Basic Protocol, above—for a longer period of sixteen to eighteen hours. You may need that long to see the best results because mild ketosis, the sign of metabolic flexibility, begins on average after sixteen hours of fasting. For me, that means I sometimes finish eating dinner by 5 p.m., then eat breakfast at 9 a.m. the next day. I do this five to seven days[129] per week, depending on my schedule and travel. I used to eat a small breakfast, medium lunch, and big dinner around 8 p.m., with a few snacks in between. That is the worst possible timing and strategy for insulin. Much of the food I was eating was getting stored as fat. Drinking one to two glasses of wine with dinner made it worse. Our bodies are more insulin sensitive in the early morning and far less insulin sensitive before bed, so confining the eating window to between 8 a.m. and 4 p.m., or even 10 a.m. and 6 p.m., would be ideal—although it may not be practical for you. Intermittent fasting helps reset adiponectin and leptin, improve circadian rhythm, and adjust the gut microbiome.[130]

Step 5: Reconsider your social circles.

Ask yourself: Are your friends contributing to your rising set point or lowering it? Do they keep you accountable or ply you with alcohol and candy? What matters is whether your friends are neurotic, body weight obsessed, and left-brain dominant or whether they make you laugh, lower your stress level, and help you take care of yourself. So this step should make you consider your friends and how they temper your ability to lower your set point, and spend your time accordingly.

Step 6: Take a carbohydrate blocker.

Thirty minutes before a higher-carb meal, eat a half-cup of white or brown beans, which contain *Phaseolus vulgaris,* an extract from white beans that slows down the absorption of carbohydrates by inhibiting alpha-amylase, an enzyme responsible for digesting carbs. Alternatively, take a supplement that contains *Phaseolus vulgaris*. This natural carb blocker has been used for decades for weight loss, obesity, diabetes, high cholesterol—and has the ability to reduce the postprandial spike in blood glucose levels that can store fat as well as lower insulin and ghrelin.[131] Take divided doses of up to 3 grams daily (e.g., 500 to 1,000 mg before each higher-carb meal).

Step 7: Add a supplement.

If you are on prescription medications, talk to your pharmacist about any drug interactions first.

- **Conjugated linoleic acid** (CLA) is a fatty acid that you can take to suppress appetite[132] and lower leptin,[133] and some (but not all) studies show that it may lower body fat when you're overweight or obese.[134] Two studies got my attention: CLA lowered fat in the legs[135] and reduced hip circumference.[136] Dose: 3,000 mg, once or twice per day.

- **Alpha lipoic acid** (ALA) acts as an insulin sensitizer (i.e., removes insulin block). In as little as two weeks, a dose of 600 mg helped lower after-meal glucose levels and insulin in people with prediabetes.[137] Another study showed that 1,800 mg daily for twenty weeks reduced body weight in overweight patients.[138] Finally, another study showed that in people who are overweight or obese, ALA was associated with weight loss, a smaller abdominal circumference, and lower blood pressure.[139] Dose: 600 to 1,800 mg daily.

- **Berberine** is an herb that has been shown to help reset blood sugar and lower total and LDL cholesterol.[140] When taken for twelve weeks, it reduces weight by five pounds in obese patients.[141] Berberine also helps activate thermogenesis (heat production) in your fat tissues, which is a very good thing when you want to lower your set point.[142] If you didn't start it in the last chapter, add it now. Dose: 500 mg, three times per day.

Step 8: Perform additional testing.

Review results with a functional medicine clinician (see Appendix B for specific laboratories).

- **Perform fasting blood work (in the morning, after an overnight fast):** inflammation (hsCRP, homocysteine), fasting insulin, glucose, leptin, cortisol, hemoglobin A1C, complete metabolic panel, complete blood count (CBC), thyroid panel (TSH, free T4, free T3, reverse T3, thyroid antibodies), 25-hydroxy vitamin D.

- **Test your microbiota and microbiome** for imbalances and signs of inflammation.

- **Examine your stress response.** Measure your urine for four-point cortisol and for estrogen and steroid hormone metabolism with DUTCH, and/or measure your anabolic/catabolic ratio and estrogen and steroid hormone metabolism with Genova's Complete Hormones test. Make sure to measure androgens including DHEAS and testosterone.

- **Estrogen metabolism testing** can be performed on the DUTCH test or with another lab such as Genova.

- **Genetic tests** can be performed to measure your tendencies for problems with insulin, leptin, adiponectin, ghrelin, cortisol, and estrogen. See my previous book *Younger* for more information on when, how, and why to test your genes. Specifically consider genetic testing for some of the body weight set point genes mentioned in this chapter, including the following:

  — *FTO*, the most influential gene involved in your body mass index

  — *MC4R*, the snacking gene

  — *LEPR*, the leptin receptor gene

  — *ADIPOQ*, the adiponectin gene

  — *ADRB2*, the adrenergic beta-2 surface receptor gene

  — *DIO2* and *MCT10*, genes involved in thyroid function

Last Word

For the 80 percent of my patients who struggle with body weight set point, their brain body is blocking them from losing weight, usually as part of an anciently wired survival mechanism. Then they don't eat the right foods, in the right time windows, and in the right context to match their genetics and lower their set point. Body weight set point can be complicated to understand, but not to fix. It turns out that your internal body fat sensor, the adipostat, is a more flexible regulator that can learn from past experiences and changing environments.[143] You can change your thoughts about food, repair your appetite, and restore your right mind. Your body is adaptable.

As you work through the Basic Protocol, maybe even adding one or two of the Advanced Protocol items, remember that any of the protocol steps that are new to you will not only improve your set point, but also literally force your brain to reorganize and remap through the process of neurogenesis and synaptogenesis.

In the long run, the goal is to regain a healing relationship with the four factors of your body weight set point—genes, behavior, hormones, and environment—despite the modern obesogenic lifestyle working against us. Over the years of my battle and then my surrender to set point, I've found that the most important factor is consistency, as in *lather, rinse, repeat.* The goal is not to have a perfect supermodel body, but to have the *right* body and set point for you—the one that supports your best brain function and healing. This protocol works, and the results will have you feeling like your best self—loving your body, your energy, and your mood.

4

Brain Fog

How to Burn It Off, Think More Clearly, and Make Smart Decisions

Dawn couldn't think straight. It was as if her brain had stopped in its tracks: she could not shake the vague malaise that blocked her focus, cognition, tenacity, memory, ability to multitask, and joy she had experienced in her forties. As a fifty-one-year-old architect, she found it hard to process facts and thoughts as fast as she used to, particularly when under stress and competing for a project. Some mornings she never could quite fully wake up. Dawn described it as brain fog. She had tried more coffee, a new fitness trainer, and the *New York Times* crossword puzzle; they weren't helping. Her symptoms waxed and waned, but were disruptive and scary. She felt only half-present to her life, and middle age was too young to feel this way. Recently divorced and living with her ten-year-old son, Dawn felt like she was always "on." She came to me to try bioidentical hormones next. "If it helps, why not?" she reasoned.

At first Dawn thought that growing older was the problem. As we talked, it became clear that the current biology of her brain body was creating a constellation of symptoms that fell under the category of "brain fog," including the quality of her thoughts, mood, and performance. As I took her history, I learned that Dawn grabbed a pastry and coffee on the way to work and usually a sandwich or burrito with chips and salsa at lunch. She ate at restaurants or got take-out food almost daily for dinner, washed down with a glass or two of wine. Most of these foods are laced with genetically modified organisms (GMOs). Dawn had heartburn, for which she took an over-the-counter antacid.

When it comes to brain fog, the first thing on my list to check is membrane integrity in the gut and brain: did Dawn have leaky gut? Was leaky gut then disrupting her blood-brain barrier, leading to brain fog? I was right. Over time and exposure to poor dietary choices, her gut microbes got out of balance, with too many bad bugs and not enough good bugs. This common problem, called dysbiosis, poked holes in her gut wall, which is only the thickness of tissue paper. Then her gut dysbiosis probably led to brain dysbiosis and poor brain/body function.

Dawn had classic symptoms of dysbiosis: gas, bloating, loose stool, gluten and dairy sensitivity, acid reflux, and extra pounds that stuck to her no matter what she tried. Laboratory testing confirmed what I suspected based on her history: an imbalance of bacteria in the gut, with an overgrowth of harmful bacteria and yeast, a lack of good bacteria, and a lack of microbial diversity.

Once we determined that leaky gut was the root cause of Dawn's brain fog, the right foods, nutrients, detoxification, gut and mitochondrial repair, sleep, and supplements helped her brain body feel normal again—clear, less anxious, in balance, and happier. With a few interventions from the Brain Body Diet, Dawn is now sharp and calm—maybe even better than in her forties. She even dropped a few dress sizes as her gut microbes got back into balance. These aren't shocking or outlandish interventions, and Dawn isn't unusual in her constellation of symptoms, but what's unique is that we got her brain body working *for* her again, not against her.

While many doctors don't recognize the term *brain fog* as a medical condition, it's a common problem of mildly degraded mental ability that includes diverse symptoms such as lack of focus, clarity, recall, and acuity, as well as mental fatigue. Some doctors describe it as subacute cognitive decline, meaning it's not sudden and it's not enough to warrant a diagnosis. I consider brain fog as a problem of a slow brain, and often the more subtle symptoms fly below the radar for my patients until I ask them directly.

Brain fog can be a precursor to more serious brain issues or an early sign of neurodegeneration, and it's underdiagnosed by clinicians and patients alike. Don't fall into the trap of thinking you're "just getting older." Brain fog is an important, if annoying, symptom. It is a clear warning that more harm may come if unaddressed—leading to the wayward brain symptoms of weight gain, obsession, addiction, anxiety, depression, memory loss, even Alzheimer's. For most of my patients with brain fog, symptoms occur for five to ten years before a more worrisome diagnosis.

Even though brain fog is common, it should not be dismissed as normal. Brain fog can arise from a number of root causes. The gut and mitochondria are the first places that I look for the low-level inflammation that contributes to bodily symptoms like stiffness, puffiness, and *neuroinflammation,*[1] an inflamed brain. Dawn's leaky gut contributed to her body inflammation, then caused brain inflammation, making her brain foggy. Other food intolerances such as to dairy, grain, sugar, or nightshades may be causing a problem for you. Toxins, the wrong foods, and lifestyle choices that make you inflamed—things like sitting too much but sleeping too little—can rob you of the clearheadedness that you deserve. The symptoms are an interplay of environment, biology, hormones, cognition, and discernment. This was exactly what Dawn was dealing with: the fallout of a maxed-out modern life.

The root causes of brain fog are by now familiar to you. These are the same roots that lead to the breakdown of the brain body and include toxin exposures, lack of protective nutrients and hormones, leaky gut, dysbiosis, decreased blood flow to the brain, leaky blood-brain barrier, and inflammation. Remember: inflammation is the cornerstone of all chronic disease. When these problems persist, you feel foggy-headed, which may affect your relationships, reactivity, temper, and decision-making capacity. You know—that cranky/bitchy version of you. In this chapter, you will learn how to clear the fog by continuing the removal of toxins, adding in more supportive nutrients and neuroprotective hormones, squelching neuroinflammation, and restoring homeostasis. You will re-create the brain/body resilience that you deserve.

Do You Have Brain Fog?

Do you have now or have you had in the past six months any of the following symptoms or conditions?

☐ Have you experienced loss of mental sharpness or ability to concentrate, poor mental clarity, or mental fatigue—like you're not fully present—particularly as the day rolls on?

☐ Do you have low energy or fatigue, as if you're walking in molasses? Do you struggle to exercise or experience fatigue after exercise?

☐ Do you resort to consuming more caffeine to boost your energy, but it doesn't seem to provide the perk that it once did?

☐ Have you had a pregnancy and delivery within the past twenty years, perhaps with muddled thoughts or difficulty with finding words since then?

☐ Have you experienced a previous brain injury, stroke, or cancer treatment, especially chemotherapy?

☐ Do you have difficulty with prioritization, managing tasks or multitasking, or completing to-do lists, including trouble with numbers or balancing a checkbook?

☐ Are you experiencing slow thinking or mental processing speed, or haziness in the thought process, like your thoughts are scattered or muddled? Do you have problems with verbal fluency (outside of pregnancy), like the words are there in your brain but you just can't get to them?

☐ Do you have gut problems like constipation, diarrhea, bloating, and/ or gas? Are they combined with low thyroid symptoms or function? (Dysbiosis combined with hypothyroidism can be very difficult to reverse permanently.)

☐ Have you undergone general anesthesia or the use of medications that affect cholinergic function, like the antihistamine diphenhydramine (Benadryl)?

☐ Have you had any of the following results on laboratory tests?
  —Hormone imbalances, especially with cortisol (adrenal dysregulation), estrogen, progesterone, or testosterone
  —Insulin resistance as indicated by any of the following:

a fasting blood sugar > 85 mg/dL

hemoglobin A1C > 5.0

postprandial (2-hour post-meal) blood sugar > 120 mg/dL

an abnormal oral glucose tolerance test

— Low vitamin D3 (measured as 25-hydroxycholecalciferol)
< 50 ng/mL

— Inflammation, hsCRP > 0.9 mg/dL (optimal is < 0.5) or homocysteine > 8 (optimal is 6–8)

— Chronic infection, such as Lyme disease, herpes virus, or Epstein-
Barr virus

☐ Do you suffer from irritability, moodiness, or even mild depression?
Low motivation or feeling hopelessness, anxiety, fear, or confusion?

☐ Are you experiencing forgetfulness and trouble retaining
information?

☐ Do you experience worsening of brain fog under stress, which some
call "stress dementia"?

☐ Do you have trouble falling or staying asleep? Or just don't get
enough (at least seven hours)?

INTERPRETATION

If you said yes to three or more questions, you may have an issue with
brain fog. Five or more, and it's highly probable that you have a problem.
Of course, brain fog isn't just a concern of mental clarity, but it overlaps
other brain chemical imbalances and physical issues such as low energy,
moodiness, blood sugar imbalance, broken metabolism, obesity, fatty
liver, autoimmune conditions such as lupus or celiac, thyroid problems,
or an overtaxed stress system. It's not simply a little fogginess that's at
stake. If you follow the entire basic Brain Body Protocol in this chapter,
you will feel better.

Brain Fog Basics

When I banged my head, the outer physical wound—a kiwi-sized
lump on the back of my head—healed quickly, but the brain fog

lingered for about eight weeks. Brain fog is harder to diagnose and treat because there's no medical consensus around it like there is for concussion, stroke, or infection. The symptoms were often bewildering. I'd have a good morning of relative mental clarity, so I'd go to a barre class (an hour-long combination of Pilates, yoga, and functional movement). Normally, I love the music and instructor's cues, but when I was brain injured, it felt like the instructor was screaming into the microphone and the music was oppressive. Both felt unbearable. Nauseated, I'd wonder if I might retch. Then I'd topple over while standing on one leg.

I wasn't normal, but my neurologist didn't know what to suggest, telling me to give it time. Giving my brain fog and other symptoms "more time" hardly felt like the proactive thing to do, so I called another neurologist, my friend Jay Lombard, DO. He explained that my symptoms of brain fog, nausea, noise sensitivity, and balance issues were all signs of neuroinflammation. I was forging new pathways around the damaged neurons, and it would take time along with a lot of effort—fatigue mounts as the brain exerts great effort to heal itself (yes, the brain healing itself makes the body tired). Dr. Lombard suggested an imaging test called a DTS (a specialized stress test), but I couldn't easily find someone local who could do it, and getting on another plane felt too daunting. My life felt quite constricted by the brain fog, so I tried the supplements he suggested (listed for you in the protocol at the end of this chapter).

The brain is a self-organizing system, and its primary objective is to reduce uncertainty with our thoughts, beliefs, feelings, and actions. As a result, the brain thrives on maintaining balance. So it depends on a steady stream of nutrients, from vitamins like B_6 to make serotonin, to essential fatty acids and sufficient slow-digesting carbohydrates, as well as supportive hormones like estrogen, progesterone, and testosterone. But the brain is different from organs like the liver or skeletal muscle. They can synthesize or store energy reserves from what you eat (the body can store up to two thousand calories, as glycogen or crystalline glucose, depending on your level of fitness). But the brain isn't so lucky; it can't synthesize or store energy, which makes regular food intake its primary energy source. So if you don't eat well and regularly, your brain body suffers both in the short and long term.

When you don't get the supportive nutrients you need, the result can be brain fog—the mild deterioration of mental activity. Most likely, this is not enough to earn a diagnosis from your regular doctor, but it *is* enough to dampen your quality of life. The brain is composed of delicate neurons, as I described in the introduction. So when there's a deficiency of nutrients getting to the brain (or any other physical injury to the brain is present), regardless of cause or extent, the cells go into overdrive in order to promote healing. The supportive cells—the *astrocytes* and *microglia*—get turned on, multiply, and plump up. That's the hallmark inflammation of an injured brain. That means even modest harms in the diet or small injuries from toxins, trauma, or changes in blood flow can worsen neuron function and make you feel foggy.

When I'm clearheaded, I feel at peace, calm, positive, and mentally sharp. The inflammation at the root of brain fog can make you feel blue, even depressed, fatigued, irritable, and despairing. And if you don't address it, it may devolve into addiction, anxiety, depression, or memory loss. That's reason enough not to ignore even a little mental cloudiness.

Because brain fog is an early stage symptom, severity can wax and wane. You may not feel foggy all the time. You may feel foggier under stress, after a poor night of sleep, or when you eat a cupcake or drink a cocktail. Your symptoms may be worse at 4 p.m., after a taxing day of mental processing, or you may experience brain fog all day long. I've seen the full range of symptoms in my patients. The important takeaway is to track your symptoms going forward.

Mental Exhaustion That May Turn Physical, and Vice Versa

After my traumatic brain injury, my mental fatigue would hit a point where it turned into physical fatigue. After a one-hour barre class, as mentioned, I was battered and bone tired. I'd have to go home to my dark bedroom to lie still and sleep for three hours. My brain would hit a place of zero reserves and shut down.

Think of this kind of exhaustion like a cell phone that starts to act wonky when the battery reserve gets low. Your usual applications don't respond like normal and might quit for no reason. At some point, the phone powers down.

Most folks with brain fog experience the fogginess at specific times— not all the time. For example, Dawn had more focus in the morning and tended to deplete her reserves in the afternoon, a common pattern. When she pushed herself more mentally or physically, her brain fog would increase. As we worked together, we identified the circumstances that were associated with tapping out her reserves and proactively planned more rest during the day and a more appropriate pace for her brain. Other factors that depleted Dawn's brain reserves were drinking alcohol, smoking pot, eating poorly, and sleeping less. We figured out ways to keep her fully charged.

Dawn came to me thinking she needed hormone replacement therapy. Although that does address some patients' problems, in Dawn's case, dietary, lifestyle, and supplement adjustments put her back on track. When you address the root cause of brain fog, often you feel so much better that you don't need hormonal support. You have more reserves and greater brain/body resilience. Hormone therapy may be an option in the future, but not necessary now.

Brain/Body Resilience
Depends on Your Organ Reserves

At the foundation of brain/body resilience is the concept of organ reserves. An organ's reserve is an individual organ's inherent capacity to withstand demands, including trauma, stress, and loss of nutrients. This reserve is your organ's ability to function beyond baseline needs. Loss of your organ reserves makes it tougher for your individual organs to restore equilibrium. That's true of most of your organs—liver, adrenals, heart, kidneys, intestines—and the brain's reserve is the most important and perhaps the most sensitive of all.

All organs lose function (and therefore reserves) as you age. Around age eighteen, healthy folks have ten times the function they need, so their organ reserves are at ten times their capacity and they can cope easily with physical challenges like a car accident or a high degree of athletic training. (For example, the heart can pump ten times more blood than needed to keep the body alive, because the cells are young, fresh, and rich in mitochondria, the cell's power supply.) Once you hit your thirties, you lose about 1 to 2 percent of function every year. Decline is faster if you are ill, are highly stressed, eat excess carbohydrates (sugar) and bad fats, have dysbiosis, or take certain medications. Recovery from illness is rarely 100 percent, so there's an accumulating cost of these health debits to your organ reserves and brain/body resilience.

By age forty, the cells of your organs are older, and you can tell by looking at them under a microscope: they are larger, they divide more slowly, they are less able to multiply, the membranes are stiffer, and they accumulate fat. You can even see a yucky yellow-brown pigment in the cell called lipofuscin, a product of wear and tear that accumulates in the heart, liver, kidneys, adrenals, retina, nerve cells, and ganglions (a collection of nerve cell bodies). In terms of function, the cell's stiffer membranes make it harder to deliver oxygen and nutrients to the inside of the cell, and it's not as easy to remove carbon dioxide and other waste products.

At the organ level, you've lost half or more of the function you had as a teenager by about age fifty. The organ is fatty, lumpy—no longer pretty. When you've lost organ reserves, any extra workload makes the whole body feel tired, like you're pushing a rock up a hill. For most of your organs, reserve is lost gradually, but when you have a problem like dysbiosis, reserve can be lost rapidly, leading to low brain/body resilience, like Dawn experienced.

Don't we all wish we had better reserves, a higher capacity to restore equilibrium when under stress? I never seem to have enough balance. I had my first baby at age thirty-two and second at age thirty-seven. Know what the ideal age is for having a kid? Twenty-four. If your reserves are lower when you enter a major life cycle change like pregnancy or perimenopause, you are more likely to experience symptoms like depletion and brain fog.

As a gynecologist and an expert in the female body, my opinion is that women have less organ reserve generally, and less brain reserve in particular, than men, for several reasons:

- Women have babies. Pregnancy amplifies the demands on the endocrine system, including the brain. When your amplified need isn't met with a concordant amplified supply of supportive nutrients, you may develop mild brain decline and, consequently, brain fog.

- Women suffer from depression and anxiety at twice the rates of men, and both conditions are associated with a shrinking hippocampus in the brain.

- Women experience higher rates of other physical and mental diseases than men at all ages and across all parts of the world.[2] If you look at the thirty most common diagnoses in primary care, 90 percent are more common in women.[3] We suffer from more lost days at work due to illness, longer hospital stays, higher health care costs—even when reproductive illness is excluded.[4] These issues lower women's economic resources.

- In our current culture, women experience higher stress levels. In the annual stress survey conducted by the American Psychological Association, the gender-based stress gap keeps growing wider. Women have reported higher stress levels than men for a decade, but in 2017, women's stress increased further and men's stress levels dropped.[5] According to a recent Gallup poll, women are more likely to experience frequent stress compared with men.[6] Work and children are the biggest stressors—working mothers fare the worst.

- Pregnancy extensively shrinks the gray matter, which may make a new mom focus more on attachment and less on other distractions, like work. First-time fathers have no significant change in brain volume (lucky!) compared with first-time mothers.[7]

- Of course, women don't need to survive a pregnancy to develop low brain/body reserve and brain fog. Women in my practice who choose not to become pregnant, or are infertile and unable to (often an enormous stressor for women), also develop low brain reserve. I suspect it is due to the overall increased stress on women compared with men, as revealed by our higher rates of anxiety, depression, and Alzheimer's disease.

- Finally, women are still the caretakers in our culture, and they're more susceptible to the stresses of juggling multiple roles.

The bottom line is that if you lack the organ reserves to keep up with amplified need, you may suffer. The bad news? You can measure the decline of organ reserves, but it's usually happening before symptoms ever show. The good news is that you have control over the health of your brain. The main takeaway is to honor, protect, and enhance your brain body by filling your tank with supportive nutrients and reversing neuroinflammation, so that you can bounce back from stressors like injury, illness, pregnancy, perimenopause, menopause, dysbiosis, and environmental toxins.

The Female Brain

While women may have less organ reserve, we have other health advantages over men. When you image the brain, you can tell with 85 percent certainty whether it's a male or female brain. According to the majority of imaging studies, the sexual differences include:[8]

- Women tend to have a bigger hippocampus (the seat of learning, emotion, and memory) compared with men (and relative to overall cerebral volume).

- Women differ in function of the hippocampus and stress response.

- Men have a bigger amygdala (center of fear) and hypothalamus (hormone command center).

- Men tend to have a bigger cerebellum, the part of the brain in the back of the skull that coordinates muscular activity and balance.

- When aging brains are imaged, men have more shrinkage of the whole brain, but women show more shrinkage of the hippocampus.

While this isn't a comprehensive list of differences between men's and women's brains, it's important that when you shrink the hippocampus as a result of aging or consuming too much sugar, the brain body can really suffer, and women may be particularly vulnerable.

"BABY BRAIN": HOW THE BRAIN SHRINKS IN PREGNANCY

Dawn traced the start of her brain fog to the end of her last pregnancy. Pregnancy is very taxing on the female body in ways that many don't fully comprehend. If you've had a baby in the past twenty years, you could still be suffering from brain/body depletion, which shows up as brain fog, poor energy, distractibility, emotional lability, feeling overwhelmed, feeling wear and tear, loss of libido, difficulty losing weight, and memory lapses—colloquially referred to as "baby brain."

A woman's brain shrinkage can begin before she conceives, due to severe childhood adversity, depression, post-traumatic stress disorder, bipolar disorder, head injury, high blood pressure, or sleep apnea before pregnancy, or in women with a variant of the serotonin transporter gene.[9] Having prediabetes, diabetes, or obesity can also shrink the brain, particularly the hippocampus.[10] You even lose gray matter volume if your mother was stressed in the first twenty weeks of pregnancy with you, which may impact your future mood as a young adult.[11] Additionally, infertility can take a toll by causing high stress, depletion of HPA axis activity, and depression.[12] Alterations in normal stress response are linked to shrunken brain, including in one study (mostly male subjects) high cortisol in the evening, and in another study (all female subjects) both high and low cortisol patterns, all in the hippocampus.[13]

Then, once you're pregnant, the biology swings in favor of the fetus, which acts like a parasite that takes all that it needs from the mother, regardless of how much she may need for her own function—including iron, vitamins B_9 and B_{12}, iodine, zinc, selenium, and omega-3 fats like DHA, which your brain needs more desperately as you age. As an example, about 35 to 58 percent of healthy pregnant women are low in iron,[14] and this leads to problems not only in the woman (anemia, fatigue, and low reserve for birth-related blood loss), but also in the baby's brain development.[15]

Immediately in pregnancy, there are radical hormone surges—and I mean huge. Trying to balance your fetus's needs with your own and compete for limited resources can be extremely demanding, and homeostasis may suffer. Some women have severe morning sickness and vomit so much they need intravenous therapy, are put on bed rest for months at a time, or lose significant blood before, during, or after they give birth. As mentioned previously, *pregnancy shrinks your gray matter significantly,* by 5 percent or more.[16] Recovery is possible, but it can take years. In animals, post-pregnancy changes in gene expression and cell growth persist past pregnancy, weaning, and well into old age.[17] No wonder I still feel dumb, easily distracted, and forgetful, even though my younger daughter is fourteen years old!

How does a mother's brain shrink? Researchers believe it's the dramatic hormonal roller coaster of pregnancy that leads to the gray matter changes, since sex hormones can change brain cell numbers and shape.[18] Are these gray matter changes associated with cognitive changes (i.e., feeling spacey and less smart)? Yes, changes can be subtle and not always consistent across all studies, but word recall and memory deficits are documented.[19] In other words, if you feel absentminded and forgetful, blame the pregnancy hormones. When you're postpartum, the worsening connections between nerve cells and the number of times you're awakened at night both impair your memory.[20] So if you had a baby and can't remember stuff, and don't know the name for ordinary objects you use all the time, this is why.

Another patient, Kelly, described what it feels like in her body: "My brain fog feels like I'm running at half speed, and it takes ages to understand information. I feel like my brain cells have gone AWOL. I used to be very quick, witty, and hardly forgot anything. Then I had my daughter, who didn't sleep much for the first three years. The lack of sleep and stress at the time seem to have triggered something, and I haven't felt completely well since. My doctor is not interested in getting to the bottom of it, so I'm trying my very best to eat well, sleep a lot, and not get too stressed. I take magnesium powder and have started making fermented foods, which seem to be great for me. I wonder if there's still an underlying condition that's lurking in the background, but trying to keep the stress at bay and getting enough sleep seem to have the biggest impact for now."

Certain pregnancy-specific conditions can shrink the brain further. Preeclampsia—a problem of high blood pressure and protein in the urine, and a leading cause of maternal and baby mortality—shrinks the gray matter of the brain even more, and the severity of changes is proportional to time since pregnancy, which suggests continued accumulation of damage after pregnancy.[21] Toward the end of pregnancy, 60 percent of total energy that passes from mother to baby via the placenta is to grow the baby's brain. Then birth can be challenging, followed by breastfeeding. As wonderful as it is to become a mother, these issues have lasting effects on the brain and body.

Which pregnant women are at greatest risk? Older women, women with less support, women with chronic medical problems, such as pain or obesity. That's not all—the women I see with maternal depletion appear to be at greater risk of inflammatory conditions like cancer, prediabetes and diabetes, and autoimmune disease. While the term "maternal depletion syndrome" is used to describe the wear and tear from successive pregnancies, I see depletion after just one. The biochemical fingerprint of women with maternal depletion shows particularly low B vitamins, low iron, imbalanced copper-to-zinc ratios and hormones, and lack of self-care because they're sacrificing to serve their children's needs. It's not all bad news: bonding with a baby matures your limbic system and provides incredible joy—there's a reward for the sacrificed gray matter, and with the Brain Body Diet, you can regain it. Since loss of gray matter can persist for years after birth,[22] it's important to employ mind-body practices aimed at growing gray matter, such as yoga and meditation, to prevent or reverse maternal depletion and recover gray matter (lest you've forgotten, gray matter is the part of the brain responsible for processing and cognition).

The Science of Brain Fog

Brain fog reflects a gap between supply and demand. Supply is the ability to meet a challenge, such as the needed brain blood flow to manage your career, volunteer for your favorite cause, or simply complete tasks like grocery shopping. When toxins, injury, a leaky gut wall, a leaky blood-brain barrier, inflammation, or a combination of all of these bombard your brain, demand for extra energy rises, occasionally exceeding supply,[23] as can the secretion of various cytokines (molecules that provide cell-to-cell communication and can cause inflammation).

Microglia constitute the resident immune system of the brain. They act as brain sensors to alert the rest of the brain to harm if you're veering from homeostasis. They become activated in response to deviations, migrate to the site of insult, and kick off the use of immune weapons like cytokines.[24] Cytokines make healing possible, but you can get too much of a good thing. When overactivated, microglia and cytokines add insult to injury, hurting your brain.

In functional medicine, we call the underlying problem and its downstream effects the Immune Cytokine Model; it's the reason for many of the brain symptoms you may experience, like brain fog. Microglial activation can also set you up for worse future injury. So the next time you're exposed, the symptoms are amplified. It's like being allergic to a bee sting: you get a bad reaction the first time you get stung, but susceptible individuals can have a life-threatening reaction the next time. The same is true for the microglia in your brain. These immune cells in the brain have a long memory of past insults and injustices, and the consequences of activating the microglia tend to get worse with time, unless you make a concerted effort to change the situation. At first you end up with brain fog, but over time, the fog can turn into depression, anxiety, memory loss, multiple sclerosis, Alzheimer's, or Parkinson's.[25] Yet the fix, to turn off the excessive microglial activation and calm down the brain body, is relatively easy if you know what to do.

DIGESTING BRAIN FOG

Once again, the microbiome (consisting of the DNA belonging to the microorganisms in your gut) is important. Microbiota in your body do not directly change the biochemistry of your brain, but they modulate the immune system to either promote or worsen the health of brain cells.[26]

A good example is a toxin called lipopolysaccharide (LPS). When the microbiome is out of balance, this toxin from bad bacteria escapes into the bloodstream, causing brain fog and body-wide inflammation. If unaddressed, elevated levels of LPS can lead to inflammatory conditions like insulin resistance, weight gain, diabetes, obesity, and depression.[27] LPS toxicity is an important example of how the body's response to a situation can lead to intoxication, in this case autointoxication, also called LPS endotoxemia.[28]

The problem with LPS was first recognized about one hundred years ago by a microbiologist who found that your own gut bacteria release the endotoxin. That is, LPS is an endogenous toxin. The way it works is that LPS is naturally found on certain bacteria in the gut, and it stimulates a very strong immune response. This is good! When LPS gets in the wrong place, it causes profound inflammation in the body by triggering the immune system to activate on whatever it's sticking to, leading to constipation and diarrhea, and then it exerts its negative effects on the brain, primarily through the microglia and by increasing the brain/body response to stress.[29] This is bad. LPS in the blood can cause leaky gut, then leaky brain (by disrupting the blood-brain barrier), then neuroinflammation,[30] leading to brain fog and, later, potentially depression, anxiety, and increased pain.[31] Fortunately, there are ways to reduce LPS, including cutting back on saturated fat and eating more monounsaturated fat (which doesn't raise LPS),[32] and eating more prebiotic and probiotic food.[33]

Sonia is a forty-eight-year-old who told me that the best thing for her brain fog was switching from a high-fat, very-low-carbohydrate, ketogenic-type diet to a whole-food, higher-carb, lower-fat diet with her carbs coming from fruit, vegetables, and tubers, like sweet potatoes, yams, or potatoes. She attributes her brain fog to a sluggish liver on keto and blood sugar problems. Maybe too much LPS in the wrong place was a problem for her, causing inflammation and weight gain. The excess fat was doing her brain a disservice, and there are reports in rodents of long-term adherence to a ketogenic diet being associated with worsening insulin resistance, hepatic inflammation, and fatty liver.[34] She begins her day with a banana and celery juice, then has roasted vegetables like celery, carrots, and onions with some pastured turkey and avocado for lunch. She's much better off than when she used to drink butter coffee and eat pastured hamburgers. I'm not suggesting that keto is bad, or that a higher-carb diet is right for everyone—I'm diet agnostic and don't believe one size fits all—but Sonia is an example of someone who found the right fit for herself through trial and error, and trial and success. She probably needs more carbohydrates for optimal thyroid and adrenal function. Your body is unique, and in the Brain Body Diet, you'll find what works for you.

SUGAR AND OTHER DANGEROUS TOXINS

One of the worst causes of brain fog is consuming too much refined sugar—the white stuff extracted from sugar cane and sugar beets—which may propel you to sugar highs followed by sugar crashes and brain fog. Look, you had to know this was coming.

In the past three decades, American adults increased their consumption of added sugar by 30 percent.[35] I saw evidence of this firsthand when I met a man from Atlanta who loved to drink Coke, not Diet Coke but regular Coke. I had a few dinners with him, and watched as he drank Coke after Coke during the meal. Astounded, I asked him about it. "I'm from Atlanta, the home of Coca-Cola," he said proudly. "I drink at least five Cokes per day." *Whaaaa?*

Coca-Cola spends billions on advertising, and the investment worked on this man. The advertising assault of soda companies got him (and many of us) drinking refined sugar by the quart without blinking an eye or considering the downstream health costs. At 39 grams of refined sugar per can, he was consuming well more than one cup of sugar per day. He may have never even crashed from his sugar highs because he just kept forcing his blood sugar into the max zone. That's not good for the brain; here's why:

- A higher intake of refined sugar has been associated with lower cognitive function, memory, and intelligence.[36] It harms the brain and mitochondria and increases the risk of insulin resistance, fatty liver, metabolic syndrome, type 2 diabetes, and obesity.

- Added sugar decreases the brain's ability to repair injury. Sugar even limits the ability of the body to process omega-3 fatty acids, so you might not even get the anti-inflammatory benefits of omega-3s if eaten with added sugars.[37]

- Consumption of refined sugar can exert long-term molecular changes in the brain, especially in the hippocampus, so your memory, stress level, and emotional regulation take a hit.

- Obese adolescents respond differently to sugar than lean adolescents. After drinking glucose, blood flow decreases to the prefrontal cortex (involved in executive function) and increases to the hypothalamus region involved in appetite. That means poorer decision-making and greater hunger. On the other hand, lean adolescents drinking glucose show *increased* blood flow to the prefrontal cortex and *no* change in blood flow to the hypothalamus. On top of that, obese adolescents have abnormal suppression of ghrelin (the hunger hormone), increased insulin after drinking glucose, and reduced connections between the executive, homeostatic, and pleasure brain regions. This suggests that obesity is associated with less executive control in response to sugar and that the appetite and pleasure centers of obese adolescents are overly responsive.[38] By now, we all know sugar is addictive, which makes it easier for me to completely avoid it rather than to consume a little (as you'll see in chapter 5, my genotype leaves me susceptible to addiction).

- Eating refined sugar is a risk factor for depression,[39] perhaps the reason for Coke Guy's depression.

- Eating more refined sugar early in adulthood may inhibit long-term expression of certain genes, such as the gene FOXO3, which regulates longevity in many species, including flies, yeast, worms, and humans. The extra sugar early in life, even if corrected later, drives long-term reprogramming of gene expression.[40] Drinking refined sugar is associated with shortening life by five years.[41]

- Rats fed refined sugar experience harm to the hippocampus. In particular, rats fed high-sugar diets had increased levels of certain cytokines in their hippocampus.[42] The hippocampus may be particularly vulnerable to harm from refined sugar because of its location and lack of blood supply.[43] Remember that the hippocampus is in charge of emotional regulation and memory consolidation, so when it becomes toxic from sugar, brain fog, confusion, and poor emotional control can result.

You might wonder if all of this talk of rodent research is relevant, since you are not a mouse or rat. Turns out the genes responsible for building and operating the mouse brain and the human brain are 90 percent the same, so the mouse brain is a powerful tool for understanding problems in the human brain.

Other toxins can rob you of a clear brain. Many toxins mess with homeostasis and send mixed messages to your body. Here are a few examples:

- **Glyphosate.** A broad-spectrum antibiotic and herbicide used to kill weeds, glyphosate is marketed by Monsanto as a product called Roundup. Globally, 1.2 billion pounds are used each year, and because it is water soluble, 99.99 percent of glyphosate ends up in water, air, rainfall, and human urine.[44] Glyphosate inhibits the shikimate pathway, a process necessary to make the amino acids tryptophan, phenylalanine, and tyrosine—essential components of making hormones and cell membranes. Glyphosate can disrupt the gut barrier, potentially increasing the risk of inflammatory disease, from Hashimoto's thyroiditis to depression, and possibly neurodegenerative brain problems.[45] In 2015, IARC stated that glyphosate is "probably carcinogenic to humans."[46]

- **Solvents.** Many volatile solvents (benzene, toluene, styrene, and xylene) are neurotoxins that reduce brain function—they disrupt axons (nerve cell extensions) and harm myelin (the sheaths on nerve cells that allow rapid communication), so they slow down nerve transmission. Several solvents are effective as anesthetics and are used both medically and as recreational drugs. The most common symptoms of neurotoxicity from solvents are impaired vision, balance issues, paresthesia (a burning or prickling sensation usually in the arms or legs, like a tingling or numbness), and a decrease in cognitive function (chronic toxic encephalopathy). Symptoms are most common in solvent workers (painters, etc.), but it doesn't take high-risk occupational exposure to be compromised. You can have a problem with glutathione production, like I do, or a genetic variation in your detoxification genes (see page 61).

- **Early life adversity.** Excessive stress, accidents, or abuse may be toxic to your brain plasticity later in life, depending on the activity of your brain-derived neurotrophic factor (BDNF).[47] Childhood adversity can dampen how much BDNF you make,[48] and changes in cortisol and BDNF indicate emotional distress, which can increase your risk of cardiovascular disease and diabetes. Early life adversity also harms gene expression in the hippocampus, particularly of the glucocorticoid receptor that helps with stress management. (Sugar consumption causes a similar effect.) In rats, early life adversity can change brain pathways in the hippocampus similar to the effects of sugar.[49]

- **Lead.** Perhaps ingested from your chocolate or tap water, lead may make your brain slow and cause you to be unmotivated, or "slow going." Evidence also shows that lead blocks the uptake and effect of dopamine, the brain reward chemical that influences your ability to focus, concentrate, and think quickly.[50]

- **Diesel exhaust.** A major component of air pollution, diesel particles are toxic to your brain body: they can hurt your lungs when you inhale them, then enter your blood circulation and cross the blood-brain barrier, where they harm the dopamine-producing nerve cells and overactivate microglia.[51] Air pollution can cause the symptoms of brain fog: lack of concentration, difficulty focusing, and slow thinking. The parts of the brain most sensitive to diesel exhaust are the hippocampus and the olfactory bulb, which provides your sense of smell.[52] As you will see in the Protocol section, hijiki, a brown sea vegetable found on the coast of Japan, China, and Korea, may help.[53]

Dawn had several of these problems: she worked with lead as an architect (an occupational hazard), and her levels were high. She often ate meals at restaurants with clients and got exposed to glyphosate (from eating foods that contain ingredients genetically modified with herbicides or pesticides, which is very common at restaurants), which disrupts the integrity of the intestinal wall. She had early life adversity—childhood sexual abuse—and probably had lifelong problems with her BDNF pathway. She commuted all over the Bay Area, meeting with clients and traveling to projects, constantly exposing herself to diesel exhaust. She had nonceliac gluten sensitivity, and this drove up her levels of inflammation.[54] Finally, we tested her ability to detoxify. Half of the population has a problem with the detoxification gene called GST: glutathione S-transferase (discussed in chapter 2). She had the null genotype, so her body has a tough time clearing toxins well. It's like she was drunk on neurotoxins, and it was the primary cause of her brain fog.

Other patients have had similar experiences, particularly finding the relief from brain fog by eliminating grains, dairy, and sugar, and eating a nutrient-dense, whole-food diet. The reason that these dietary changes may reduce brain fog is that they can lower the level of inflammation in the gut, body, and brain. Inflammation is the root of all chronic disease, and gluten and sugar are potent stimulators of the immune response—another example of a good thing turned against you when the immune system is out of balance.

Additional factors that commonly cause brain fog are medications, sitting too much, sleeping too little, and electromagnetic fields (EMFs).

1. **Medications.** Sleeping pills, antacids, antidepressants, stimulants, antipsychotics, antihistamines, chemotherapy, and blood pressure medication are associated with brain fog and may trigger brain inflammation. Antacids increase bacterial overgrowth, impair your ability to absorb nutrients, and may alter your ability to fight infection.[55] If you take one or more of these medications, discuss with your prescribing clinician how to counteract the effects on your brain or switch to something more natural yet effective.

2. **Sitting too much.** First of all, sitting kills. It can trigger or worsen thirty diseases, including heart disease, diabetes, and obesity.[56] Second, this is yet another situation where women fare worse than men—increased sitting time raises insulin, leptin, leptin-to-adiponectin ratio, and markers of inflammation such as CRP and IL-6 in women but not men, even after adjusting for exercise.[57]

   Finally, bad posture while sitting, defined as forward flexion and rotation, loads the spine 400 percent more than good posture.[58] Can you imagine that much pressure on any other part of your body? We sit with our head shoved over the shoulders. We stand over the balls of our feet instead of the middle of the foot, as recommended by biochemist and structural integrationist Ida Rolf, PhD. Poor posture and too much sitting are important causes of hidden inflammation to the brain body, particularly when we work against rather than with gravity. Certainly, something's got to give. Poor posture can slow down how fast you walk and create another form of unnecessary inflammatory load that can worsen brain fog. With techniques for better posture and movement, you can increase your gait speed, lower brain fog, and maybe even ease depression.[59]

ROOT CAUSES OF BRAIN FOG

When you can't think clearly, it's important to identify the root causes affecting you, so you can move on to an effective solution. Most of
my patients have multiple reasons for brain fog: they got poisoned by
organophosphates (a pesticide used in farming), they don't get enough
magnesium or B_{12}, and they lack the gene COQ12, and as a result their mitochondria are weak. The following culprits diminish your ability to make
the hormones and brain chemicals of a healthy brain body and block
your return to homeostasis:

- **Toxins**
  - Poor detoxification, usually a result of low glutathione or weak
    mitochondria
  - External toxins, including BPA, lead, mold, and diesel exhaust[60]
  - Internal exposures, such as leaky gut, LPS, or adipokines[61]
  - Too much stress (perceived and oxidative)[62]
  - Poor glucose handling (high fasting or postprandial blood sugar),
    high insulin

- **Increased blood-brain barrier permeability,** which can be from gut
  dysfunction, toxin exposure (hello, alcohol!), or lack of sleep[63]

- **Reduced blood flow to the brain,** short-term or long-term ischemia
  or stroke

- **Insufficient supportive nutrients**
  - Wrong calories (too much sugar, excess inflammatory fats), other
    inflammatory foods, food intolerances, celiac disease[64]
  - Dehydration
  - Decreased neurotrophic factors, like BDNF[65]
  - Imbalanced hormones

- **Neuroinflammation**
  - Food intolerances such as gluten and/or dairy sensitivity
  - Leaky gut
  - Dysbiosis
  - Oxidative stress, overactive immune system, and inflammation
  - Autoimmune conditions such as celiac disease

- **Medications,** such as statins, antihistamines, benzodiazepines, chemotherapy, and others listed in the text[66]

- **Other chronic conditions,** such as fibromyalgia,[67] chronic fatigue syndrome,[68] autism spectrum disorder,[69] and mast cell problems (such as mastocytosis or issues with mast cell activation)[70]

3. **Resting too little.** If I had to recommend just one thing for you to heal your brain body generally and brain fog specifically, it would be to rest more. Most of us need more time for rest and recovery to counter the impact of stressful lives, yet it's the overlooked factor that I want you to start measuring. Rest builds resilience and clears out the fog. The right dose of rest varies person to person, but most women I know tend to cut corners, whether it's the active unwinding that we need every day, or the earlier bedtime that we know is a good idea. Nearly half of Americans wake up exhausted at least once per week.[71] When you cut sleep short, inflammation rises and *pokes holes in the blood-brain barrier.*[72] That translates into less attention, stamina, strength, and performance because you're less effective at repairing and rebuilding your brain body. Elite athletes know it: LeBron James, Michael Phelps, and Roger Federer get about twelve hours of sleep per day while training.[73] Twelve hours, people! I bet they don't have brain fog. If those busy guys can find the time for twelve hours every night, or eight to ten hours at night combined with a nap, we mere mortals can too. If you're not sure about how you're sleeping, track your deep, light, and REM sleep as well as awakenings, like with a Fitbit or Oura (see Appendix B). How does it help clear brain fog? Sleep seals the holes in the blood-brain barrier, allowing the glymphatic system to remove toxins, clear out the cobwebs, and tidy up your brain, so you feel smarter and refreshed when you wake up.[74]

4. **EMFs.** Physicians are increasingly treating health problems from unidentified causes, and that makes me wonder about toxins and EMF exposures. We've all noticed the exponential increase in the use of electronic devices over the past decade, which has led to un-

precedented exposure to electromagnetic fields (EMFs). If you haven't noticed, keep hiding under that rock—your brain might benefit! EMFs can increase free radicals in the body (discussed in chapter 2), trigger the cell danger response, damage DNA, affect gene transcription, and modulate immune function, and may increase the risk of certain brain cancers. Studies, empirical observations, and patient reports clearly indicate interactions between EMF exposure and health problems, although physicians and scientists in Europe appear more concerned than my colleagues in the United States.

People are now getting diagnosed with electromagnetic hypersensitivity, a condition involving headaches, fatigue, brain fog, and difficulty with concentration, sleep, and depression, and sometimes flu-like symptoms.[75] The prevalence ranges from 1.5 percent in Sweden to 13 percent in Taiwan.[76] Even though the evidence is modest, lack of proof is not proof against the dangers. I side with the Europeans on this topic until we know more and suggest limiting the use of high EMFs in your home and work—cell phones, house-wide Wi-Fi—and getting off your electronic devices at night so that the brain/body connection has a chance to recover.

PROTECTING YOUR BRAIN DURING AND AFTER CHEMO

Even if you have to endure cancer treatment such as chemotherapy, you may still reduce inflammation and augment neurogenesis by taking omega-3 fatty acids while under treatment.[77] Brenda is a good example. A sixty-four-year-old accountant, she was diagnosed with cancer in her left breast. She needed two multiple-hour surgeries under a general anesthesia with a known neurotoxin for a mastectomy and axillary lymph node dissection, followed by use of an expander, and then reconstruction. She was given tamoxifen to prevent breast cancer recurrence, and that caused fatigue and brain fog and interfered with her hormones, including estrogen, thyroid, and cortisol. By following the detoxification principles of the Brain Body Diet, cleaning up her food and gut, adding brain-supportive nutrients like omega-3s and phosphatidylserine, and correcting her insulin resistance, her brain fog cleared and there are no further signs of cancer.

The Role of Hormones in Brain Fog

Four key hormones, when they are in balance, prevent brain fog. However, when these hormones are out of balance, the brain may not properly sense and adjust your hormone levels (as described in the last chapter with the thyroid), and the body may suffer. The fog may roll in with any or all of them; the weight climbs, memory sputters, and energy drops.

- **Low thyroid.** When your thyroid function is low, your brain function is low, often causing brain fog, slow processing speed and reflexes, cognitive impairment, weight gain, fatigue, depression, irritability, constipation, and intolerance to cold, among other symptoms. Increasingly I find in my patients that they don't convert enough active thyroid hormone (T3) from inactive thyroid hormone (T4). One reason is poor conversion of T4 to T3 in the liver, but another common reason is that you have a gene that's not working well, as I mentioned in chapter 3. I have two common genetic variations that limit my ability to convert T4 to T3 in the brain.[78] So even though I have normal-appearing thyroid blood test results (thyroid stimulating hormone, free T3, and free T4), I feel far from normal and experience many thyroid symptoms, from brain fog, to fatigue, to weight gain. Most clinicians have no idea about this genetic variation, how it impacts brain T3 levels, and how to test for it. I'll show you how next in the protocol.

- **Low estrogen or estrogen resistance.** Starting around age forty, the female brain slows down in metabolic rate, known as cerebral metabolism, and symptoms of brain fog may develop. Estrogen is one of the most important nutrients that protects your brain from decline.[79] Estrogen is also involved in libido and sexuality for women.

- **Cortisol problems.** When cortisol is too high or too low, or both within the day, you may experience brain fog. The root cause is high perceived stress. The control system, the hypothalamic-pituitary-adrenal (HPA) axis, gets out of whack when allostatic (stress) load exceeds reserves, causing brain fog, anxiety, depression, addiction, and memory problems. Additionally, high stress can harm mitochondria, leading to low energy, reduced stamina, and less mental flexibility.[80] You may not feel stressed, but a move, a demanding schedule, or sick parents have a way of sneaking up on your mitochondria and slowing down your brain body.

- **Insulin block.** When you eat too many refined carbohydrates for your system, your insulin may spike, which makes blood sugar go from high to low, causing brain fog. As a result, you store fat no matter what you try. The key is to keep blood sugar relatively stable around 70 to 85 mg/dL when fasting, and an average of

---

EXERCISE GROWS YOUR GRAY MATTER

You know who has the least brain fog? People who exercise regularly.[81] Exercise increases gray matter, particularly in the hippocampus and prefrontal cortex. Middle-aged and older adults who engage in sports and other physical activities tend to retain high executive functioning and cognitive function over time.[82] The improvement in executive functioning with exercise may be higher in women compared with men.[83] Intensity of exercise matters more than quantity, although moderate levels (including tai chi and brisk walking) may be the best for women.[84] What's more, having more gray matter *keeps* you exercising. Conversely, people with poor executive function tend to exercise less and less over time.[85]

In a study from the University of Pittsburgh, healthy people who walked six to nine miles per week over thirteen years grew the gray matter in their brains.[86] Aerobic fitness boosts cerebral blood flow to gray matter, which correlates with gray matter volume.[87] Even in people with mild cognitive impairment, aerobic fitness correlates with gray matter volume and may help prevent progression to Alzheimer's disease.[88] (Exercise just twice per week in midlife cuts your risk of developing Alzheimer's or other types of dementia later in life by more than half.[89]) Physical activity creates a virtuous cycle: more brain volume predicts better adherence to future exercise.[90] That's good, because age-related brain changes like a shrinking hippocampus appear to be attenuated or prevented in exercisers—further support that aging in the brain is optional.[91]

about 85 to 92 all the time. For my patients and myself, that means defining the best carb threshold so that you're not getting too little (linked to mood problems and hair loss) nor too much (linked to insulin resistance). The best way I've found to reset insulin is with intermittent fasting, described in chapters 2 and 3.

The Brain Body Protocol: Clearing Brain Fog

Brain fog happens to everyone on occasion. However, persistent brain fog is what we're addressing in this part of the Brain Body Diet. The key areas that we will address to keep you clearheaded are neurogenesis, reduction of neuroinflammation, and protection of the blood-brain barrier. Specifically, we will build upon the foundation from the last chapter.

BASIC PROTOCOL

Step 1: Eat for clarity.

Toxins can make you foggy, and it can take one or two weeks before you start to clear the fog once you remove toxins, depending on your toxic burden. The best way to start is with your food. You don't need to be overweight to develop brain fog and experience other health detriments, just undernourished. The focus in clearing brain fog is to decrease inflammation and increase neurogenesis by eating anti-inflammatory foods and the right type and doses of healthy carbohydrates, proteins, and fats (see chapter 3); then boost the production of BDNF through lifestyle choices.

As I say elsewhere in this book, I can't give you rigid proportions of carbs or fats or proteins because so much depends on the interplay between your genes and the environment. You are your best guide, so choose foods that you determine your body is most likely to process well. When in doubt, check your blood sugar two hours after eating food that you think may cause brain fog.[92]

- **Eat sea vegetables** like hijiki, which may block the damage to the brain from air pollution.

- **Consume good fats** such as coconut oil, MCT oil, olive oil, olives, avocados, nuts.

- **Cook with turmeric** because it is anti-inflammatory.

- **Consume healthy fiber** to feed your good bugs and prevent dysbiosis.

- **Eat probiotic food** like sauerkraut, miso, and kimchi.

- **Avoid sugar.** Search for it in all of your foods. Beware that it hides in ketchup and salad dressings. Eliminate artificial sweeteners. Still drinking diet soda? Stop that right now. It's not a treat; it's a setup for imbalanced microbiota and brain fog.

- **Avoid alcohol.**

- **Cut out dairy and grains.** Eliminate them for forty days total, then add them back and see how you react. Other common food intolerances include soy and corn, so if you're still feeling foggy after eliminating dairy and grains, try eliminating them as well.

- **Turn off all electronic screens at least one hour before you go to bed.** Limit cell phone use. Consider removing Wi-Fi throughout your house and use a hardwired internet connection.

Step 2: Grow your gray matter.

- **Strength train your brain.** For women, fifty to eighty minutes of strength exercise three times per week increased hippocampal volume.[93]

- **Walk this way.** Physical exercise improves brain function and structure at the molecular, cellular, body-wide systems, and behavioral levels.[94] Even a modest amount of walking helps to clear brain fog and make a bigger brain.

- **Run for your hippocampus.** Running in particular produces brain cells that are quantitatively and qualitatively better in the hippocampus, the center of learning and memory, and an important target for healing when you have brain fog.[95]

- **Meditate.** Practicing meditation for ten minutes or more per day grows gray matter throughout the brain, and especially in your

THINK YOUR BRAIN BIGGER

Yes, meditation provides a sense of peace and relaxation, but benefits extend further into the realm of neuroprotection and can *grow the size of the brain*. Here's how it works: meditation rebuilds your hippocampus by boosting gray matter density, which is believed to provide cognitive and psychological benefits that persist throughout the day and counter the brain fog.[96] Additional studies have confirmed:

- a larger hippocampus and smaller amygdala in meditators, even in those new to meditation.[97]
- long-term meditators with a daily practice of ten to ninety minutes had bigger volumes of certain brain structures, particularly the hippocampus.[98]
- the insula, the brain center of body awareness, is bigger in meditators.[99]
- meditation increases the gray matter throughout the whole brain, and especially the right hemisphere.[100]
- meditation can slow, stall, or even reverse the usual brain shrinkage and cognitive decline associated with age over thirty.[101]
- for each year over the age of fifty, the brain of a meditator is nearly two months younger compared to the brain of a control. Two systematic reviews call the effect "medium" in size and impact.[102]

I'll take it. What type of meditation? Doesn't seem to matter as long as attention is focused: Zen, vipassana, loving-kindness, mindfulness, Samatha, Sahaja—meditators in these studies were engaged in control of breath, visualization, attention to external and internal stimuli, withdrawal of sensory perceptions, and letting go of thoughts.

hippocampus and right brain so that you can focus better, feel well-adjusted and resilient, and keep your brain young.[103]

- **Yoga.** There's significant overlap between yoga and meditation, but it's worth adding that yoga increases the size of the hippocampus and other structures in the brain beyond the limbic system (frontal, temporal, occipital, and cerebellar regions), and the number of years of practice correlates with larger volume. Yogis do not show the usual age-related gray matter shrinkage seen in controls.[104]

STRUCTURAL INTEGRATION

Sometimes bad posture or habits create adhesions, particularly in the muscles and fascia, but they can be released so that the tissue can repair. Many of the experts in the field of structural integration, like biochemist Ida Rolf and physicist Moshe Feldenkrais, emphasize front-to-back balance, as well as inside-to-outside balance, and then side-to-side balance. The concept behind integration is how the various segments of the body—feet, ankles, knees, hips, ribcage, shoulders, neck, head—line up and function within the field of gravity. Structural integration teaches us how to move in a more relaxed manner.

The goal is to stand straighter, with more ease and minimal tension, sit taller, increase flexibility, reduce inflammation and pain, move more fluidly, breathe more easily, and prevent brain fog. To stand with correct posture:

- Plant your feet hip-width apart. Ground evenly into all four sides and the bottom of each foot. Feel your body supported through your feet near the center of the foot, not the ball of the foot.

- Lift your head gently, lengthening the crown to the sky while keeping your chin parallel to the floor and expanding cervical vertebrae. Lengthen your torso, front and back, and widen your shoulders. (Sometimes I need to tuck my chin and jaw back a little toward my chest to get to a neutral position, especially if I'm working on my treadmill desk and have jutted my head forward in order to see my laptop. I tend to look down at my smartphone or even my laptop, so another cue for me is to keep my chin parallel to the ground.)

- Breathe naturally and deeply.

- Permit your shoulders to widen your back. Don't squeeze your shoulder blades together or allow them to hunch up toward your ears. Ease them down your spine.

- Allow the natural curves of your spine to support you and your neurological network. That includes a gentle cervical, thoracic, and lumbar curve. My tendency is to tuck my lumbar vertebrae too much, so an alternate method to help me is to lie over a foam roller, with the roller horizontal across my low back.

According to my colleague Paul Van Alstine, an advanced certified Rolfer in Anchorage, Alaska, standing posture and the internal "lift" that you see with amazing posture are effortless and unconscious. Standing correctly results in a nearly perfect balance in the resting tone of the slow-twitch muscle fibers and joint positions.

- **Avoid sleep debt** because we lose gray matter with sleep deprivation.[105] Activate the glymphatic system's removal of toxins from your brain by aiming for seven to eight and a half hours per night, and catch up with a nap if you don't meet your nightly quota. Be sure to breathe through your nose, which warms, filters, and moistens inspired air.

  Sleep-disordered breathing exists on a spectrum between healthy nose breathing on one end and sleep apnea on the other. You may have issues even if you don't snore. Try mouth tape if you're a mouth breather—the mouth is for eating, not breathing. Mouth breathing impairs sleep quality, elevates blood pressure, and can deprive the brain body of needed oxygen. If you wake up with the tape falling off, see your dentist or talk to your clinician about further testing.

Step 3: Keep your gas tank full.

Don't let your energy reserves dip too low. I used to run myself ragged trying to be all things to all people. Then I decided not to let my inner gas tank fall below three-quarters full. I started to eat foods that I processed well, not the ones I craved (cheese, French fries, challah) that caused microbiota imbalances and leaky gut. I stepped up to the fact that I had a grain and dairy intolerance and just eliminated them from my diet. I detoxified codependent relationships and behaviors out of my life. I began tracking my stress level (as measured by my heart rate variability) several times per day to make sure I'm calm and not spending my energy too fast. I perform the walking meditation described on page 90 in a forest when I can or my neighborhood street when I can't. I stopped living vacation to vacation and started to take an inner vacation every day with guided visualization (see Appendix B for my favorites). No one can do this for you. You have to take responsibility and do it for yourself.

Step 4: Stand and sit up straight and move more.

Brain fog can lead to lack of movement, and stasis can cause more neuroinflammation and brain fog. Moving more, and moving more functionally, can help. The ideal posture allows for dynamic movement, and it is not effortful. It's not rigid or ramrod straight, like a soldier at attention with the spine in a straight line and abdomen sucked in, but natural, fluid, and efficient. Your spine is lengthened, flexible, and decompressed, like a child's spine. You don't stay in any one position for too long. Your body is inherently plastic and capable of change beyond what you may expect is possible. Standing, sitting, and moving correctly heal the body.

ADVANCED PROTOCOL

Step 5: Supplement your way to a clear head.

If you are on prescription medications, talk to your pharmacist about any drug interactions first.

- **L-Glutamine.** L-Glutamine is necessary for maintaining intestinal barrier function, immune response, and amino acid homeostasis, particularly during times of stress.[106] When given orally or intravenously, L-Glutamine is like a seal for the gut wall: it increases the height of intestinal villi (finger-like projections into the lumen of the small intestine, which allow greater nutrient absorption through more surface area), stimulates gut cells to grow, and maintains gut integrity, which in aggregate may reverse leaky gut, leaky brain, and brain fog.[107] Dose: 1,000 mg three times per day before meals.

- **Phosphatidylserine.** Your body makes phosphatidylserine; it's necessary for healthy nerve cell membranes and myelin, the insulating tissue around nerves. Phosphatidylserine appears to reverse the biochemical alterations and structural problems associated with aging and brain fog. Clinical studies show phosphatidylserine improves attention, arousal, memory, and verbal fluency in aging people with cognitive deterioration.[108] It seems to work best in people with relatively good cognitive performance, according to one study.[109] As you get older, you may not make enough phosphatidylserine. The good news is that when you take phosphatidylserine as a supplement, your body absorbs it well and it crosses the BBB. Dose: 300 to 800 mg per day, for at least twelve weeks.

- **Citicoline.** Sometimes written as Cytidine 5′-diphosphocholine or CDP choline, citicoline may help with brain fog or mild cognitive deficits, such as those resulting from a stroke.[110] It's considered an old supplement that may have new tricks for clearing neuroinflammation.[111] Recently, it has been found to increase expression of the longevity gene, SIRT1, in the central nervous system, and helps multiple cognitive domains.[112] Dose: 1,000 to 2,000 mg daily.

- **Omega-3s.** The omega-3 fatty acids eicosapentaenoic acid (EPA) and docosahexaenoic acid (DHA) protect the brain body from inflammation.

  — Getting adequate DHA can change cell membranes in good ways. In animals, DHA supplements restore brain DHA levels, enhance learning and memory tasks in older animals, and reduce amyloid beta, the bad protein associated with Alzheimer's disease. Further, DHA may buffer your brain from the harm of stress, protect synaptic transmission in the hippocampus, and create neurogenesis, also in the hippocampus.[113]

  — Both DHA and EPA reduce inflammation. Not surprisingly, the combination of DHA and EPA helps patients with mild cognitive impairment, but not in Alzheimer's disease as a single treatment. That suggests there might be a timing issue: sooner may be better.[114] Taken together, DHA and EPA may limit age-related brain decline by boosting your body's own repair mechanisms.

  Dose: about 1,200 to 1,500 mg EPA and 500 to 1,000 mg DHA daily while avoiding added sugars and starches (remember, sugar reduces the effectiveness of omega-3s). These doses reduce inflammation and improve depression scores, and seem to be better than higher doses.[115]

- **Vitamin B$_{12}$.** After age forty, absorption of vitamin B$_{12}$ wanes, and it's worse if you're mostly plant-based like me.[116] Subclinical B$_{12}$ deficiency occurs in up to 26 percent of the population.[117] Dose: Methylcobalamin 500 to 1,000 mcg daily.

- **Prebiotics/Probiotics.** As we covered previously, taking prebiotics and probiotics can restore your microbiome and, along the way, reduce insulin levels, insulin resistance, microglial activation, and inflammation—all of which can help clear brain fog.[118] (Read more about prebiotics, a type of plant fiber that feeds good bacteria, in the Notes.)[119] My recommendation is to focus on prebiotics to feed your good microbes and probiotic food like miso, tempeh, sauerkraut, and kimchi to maintain your microbial diversity. Additionally, probiotics may worsen brain fog, especially if you have dysbiosis[120] (see Notes for further information and research[121]).

Step 6: Heal maternal depletion.

The idea behind this step is for mothers to replete the nutrients they are most likely to be missing, including the following:

- **Iron, copper, and zinc.** You don't want to be too low or too high with these nutrients. Copper is often too high, while zinc is often too low. See a functional medicine doctor to order the appropriate tests.

- **Vitamins D and B$_{12}$** and some of the trace elements, such as selenium, manganese, and magnesium, can also be important.

- **Macronutrients such as protein, fats, and carbohydrates.** One of these that is almost universally deficient in mothers is the omega-3 fatty acid DHA.

It's hard to balance the hormones if you haven't addressed the other aspects of food, stress, toxins, and exercise. But if you've performed the rest of the protocol and are still experiencing brain fog, ask your clinician to look at organ function—typically brain, gut, and liver, and sometimes the immune system. Collaboratively run a few tests, such as blood, saliva, or urine, to investigate how your hormones are driving symptoms such as brain fog, difficulty concentrating, poor libido, lethargy, and hypervigilance.

Step 7: Measure and lengthen your deep sleep.

More sleep is the gateway to better focus, a clear mind, and memory. While you may not aspire to twelve hours per night like LeBron James, start first with tracking your sleep stages and then biohack your way to more deep sleep.[122] Adults need one and a half to two hours of deep sleep every night, which is about 20 percent of your total sleep. Deep sleep is when you produce human growth hormone, the growth and repair hormone that counters the effect of wear and tear. More importantly, deep sleep is the time when your brain is refreshed, and cleared for learning the next day.

My goal for you in the Advanced Protocol is to double your deep sleep, also known as slow wave, non–rapid eye movement (REM) sleep. Here's how to do it.

- Obtain a tracker such as a Fitbit Versa or Ionic, or Oura ring. Measure your deep sleep for one week. Determine your average. If it's less than 90 to 120 minutes, continue this Advanced Protocol.

- Stick to the same bedtime every night, even on weekends. Consistency helps you improve deep sleep.

- Cool the room. My husband prefers 67 degrees Fahrenheit, and I prefer 64, so we compromise.

- Power down bright lights and screens a minimum of one hour before bed. This is a good time to take a hot bath with magnesium (see Appendix B).

- Avoid eating or workouts within three hours of bedtime. This is where intermittent fasting can help you gain deep sleep.

- If you have trouble winding down and falling asleep, perform five to ten (or more) rounds of left nostril breathing, covered on page 132.

- Measure your deep sleep for the next seven days and see if it's improved, however much. If still less than 90 to 120 minutes, or you just don't feel refreshed, try one of the following supplements for seven days, then compare your average deep sleep for the week. Switch to the next supplement if unimproved.

—**Ashwagandha.** Ashwagandha has been used for several thousand years to induce sleep, relieve stress, and treat neurodegenerative disorders.[123] Dose: 250 mg.

—**Magnesium.** Magnesium improves sleep in people with insomnia.[124] Dose: 500 mg at bedtime.

—**Melatonin.** Melatonin controls your sleep and wake cycles. Screen time and light at night disrupt melatonin production. I recommend supplemental melatonin to improve sleep, correct jet lag, help shift workers, repair mitochondria, and improve brain/body function when compromised.[125] Dose: 0.3 to 3 mg at night.

Other herbs that are proven to improve sleep: valerian, hops, and lemon balm. When I first began tracking my deep sleep, I averaged 48 minutes per night. After following this protocol, I am now at 90 to 120 minutes, sometimes longer, and my fog is lifted. There is no such thing as too much deep sleep. Just ask LeBron.

Step 8: Meditate, supported by technology.

Technology-supported meditation improves body awareness, cognitive function, attention, mood, psychological well-being, and somatic symptoms (headaches, pain, discomfort, etc.).[126] It can be helpful to "gamify" meditation with a device like the Muse, a compact electroencephalography (EEG) system that fits like a headband and works like a brain/body biofeedback device by providing brainwave information to an app on your smartphone (see Appendix B for more information). Dose: twenty minutes per day for three days (minimum); ten minutes per day for six weeks (ideal).

Step 9: Test for toxins, hormones, and infections.

Toxic body burden is at the root of brain and body dysfunction. See Appendix B for recommended labs that assess the most common toxins at the root of brain fog, neurodegeneration, and chronic inflammation. Then use the corresponding protocol to detoxify. Sometimes even low-grade infections like Epstein-Barr virus or Lyme disease could be at the root of brain fog,[127] so consult a functional medicine clinician to see if that may be a problem for you. Talk to your clinician about measuring your fasting blood levels of thyroid (including thyroid stimulating hormone or TSH, free T3, and free T4), estradiol, progesterone, cortisol, insulin, and glucose. Most women who need thyroid medication for a TSH>2.0 benefit most from combination therapy with T3 and T4 so that you get sufficient T3 to your brain.[128] If you have a problem with the gene for DIO2, you may benefit from more judicious use of T3 and T4 combination therapy.

Last Word

By clearing brain fog, you reverse the early signs of declining cognitive function and may prevent more serious brain issues. Nip it in the bud now: small and even transient cognitive impairments resolve when you are intentional about removing toxins, reducing neuroinflammation, and adding in protective factors. You allow your brain to function at its best so that you don't regret a clouded decision made at work, an eruption with your teenager because you were too mentally fatigued to concentrate, or just feeling half-present to your own life. For Dawn, eating only organic food removed glyphosate from her system. We added probiotic food like miso, sauerkraut, kimchi, and tempeh; we removed grains and dairy. She began taking glutamine before each meal, and once per day made a functional medicine shake that contained prebiotics to feed her good bacteria. She started intermittent fasting twice per week for fourteen to sixteen hours, and began her eating window at 10 a.m. Within one week of following the Brain Fog Protocol, Dawn's mental fog dissipated. She swapped coffee for green tea, and her work improved. She feels less of the rush of modern life, like she's more present to how each day unfolds. On her last appointment, Dawn described how she is now comfortable streamlining her life. She looks and feels her best, able to show up to her life. Dawn not only got her health back, but she also made her scattered sense of self whole again.

Don't lose any more of your precious life to brain fog.

5

Hooked

Rewiring the Obsessive Brain Pathways to Soothe Inner Turmoil, Be More Present, and Generate Lasting Peace

"Women today are asked to be wholly in one place and then to go home and be wholly in another, with no model for wholeness. Unless there's an ego strong enough to integrate the two, it leaves a hole in the center, and into that hole falls addictive behavior." When I heard this quote years ago from Christiane Northrup, MD, I stopped in my tracks. I sensed that Dr. Northrup was talking specifically to me, about something baffling, shadowy, and shameful—I felt suddenly exposed.

Since hearing the quote, I've thought a lot about what women are up against when it comes to work and financial pressure—always in battle with the competing priorities of family, raising children, attending to spouses, supporting aging parents, and, last on the list—if at all—finding time for self-care. We're expected to be perfect at work and perfect at home, and few of us are wise enough to see the conundrum or refuse to buy into it. We go about our way with limited guidance, biding our time until retirement, armed with few good or realistic models for how to integrate it all into a sacred, cohesive whole.

Not only do we lack a model of wholeness, but most of us develop cravings and addictions as described by Dr. Northrup: shopping, social media, wine, vacations, caffeine, affirmation from excessive work, exercise, cannabis, or opioids can all be symptoms of the "hole" inside of us. The overwhelm of daily life and cycles of exhaustion—both physical and emotional—make it nearly impossible to find the homeostasis we need. But the ups and downs of a busy life and the struggle to find balance don't need to be a life sentence—the cravings, addictions, and manic states aren't simply "a fact of life." We have the science and the tools to reclaim the lost balance in our lives, and in this chapter I will walk you through the specific protocol to help eliminate these behaviors that rob you of equilibrium. You *will* get your life back.

Living in an insane and demanding world creates "the pleasure trap," also known scientifically as *reward deficiency syndrome,* the "hole" that Dr. Northrup describes.[1] We crave the chemical reward of pleasure, that dopamine hit. Call reward what you will: freedom, escape, comfort, peace, release, bliss, relief from pain. For most of us, the pleasure trap begins when we seek relief in the wrong form when we are young and no wise adult is around to offer an alternative. Then we get older, and the stressors and toxins of modern life turn us into the unaware and unsuspecting saboteurs of our own health. We get stuck in a self-destructive rut, but go along with it because denial seems easier than change.

We all need better options to restore homeostasis, which knits together brain and body into a nourishing whole. If you crave homeostasis but feel stuck in a pattern of eating the wrong foods or shopping too much, it's not because you are lazy or undisciplined or inherited bad genes, but rather because we are anciently wired for the primitive drives that today create self-sabotage. The key to escape the pleasure trap is to reclaim your power by outsmarting your inner saboteur and base drives.

Most women are not aware of being stuck in the pleasure trap. They believe addiction affects other unfortunate people, but not them. They think addiction is a lack of willpower, or, like I was taught in medical school, "purely" a mental health problem. They have no idea that people just like you and me pass through a specific physiological condition prior to addiction called *hyperarousal,* which is a state of heightened physical and emotional tension marked by anxiety, stress, exaggerated startle response, insomnia, fatigue, and accentuated personality traits (hint: not the good ones!). Not only are many people convinced that addiction is all in the head, they aren't aware of the latest discovery that addiction is a head *and* gut problem. Once again, gut/brain imbalance—specifically, gut dysbiosis—is linked with addictive behavior in addition to other brain/body disconnections. When you finally understand exactly the brain/body states that lead to addiction, you can switch gears and heal the drivers of addictive behavior before it's too late.

Furthermore, I find that my patients don't realize that their brain dopamine activity may be abnormal—either too low or too high, but certainly in a state of altered balance—putting them at risk for addictive behavior as their brain bodies seek homeostasis from external sources. Think of dopamine as the *that-feels-good, do-it-again-please* neurotransmitter. It's the star of the pleasure-reward system in your brain and the brain chemical involved in motivation, sex, satisfaction, and habit formation. Dopamine is central to your reactions to behaviors that naturally produce dopamine (such as exercise and meditation) and substances that stimulate dopamine production but may cause harm (alcohol, caffeine, cigarettes, opioids, etc.). When you are in hyperarousal, there's an internal pattern of your brain body driving you to seek outside substances to satisfy the feel-good brain receptors that aren't, well, feeling good.

On a more somber note, when you have a genetic tendency toward altered dopamine activity in the brain, it can lead to impulse control problems, low motivation, addiction, and—when dopamine-based neurons degenerate—Parkinson's disease. On the other hand, inheriting a gene isn't required to have a problem with addictive behavior, and moreover, you're not stuck with the genes you have.

In this chapter, we will focus on how problems with the brain body lead to the pleasure trap, hyperarousal, gut dysbiosis, and issues with dopamine. For the scientifically inclined, I'll briefly review how altered dopamine balance interacts with the brain's pleasure centers to create impulsive, obsessive, compulsive, and addictive behaviors. Our goal is to mitigate the biochemical discomfort that leads to problematic behaviors. This is a missing part of the addiction and recovery model. A holistic model includes all of it—nutritional, physical, emotional, and spiritual health. We will address the root cause of the pleasure trap by getting your brain body back in balance, so that you can finally end the cycle of suffering, repair the damage and replenish the brain body, feel whole again, and ultimately live the life meant for you, full of purpose and meaning.

Are You Stuck in the Pleasure Trap?

Do you have now or have you had in the past six months any of the following symptoms or conditions?

☐ Have you overconsumed foods or drinks that harm you?

☐ Have you experienced negative effects on your physical (including sleep or injury), financial, mental, or spiritual health from any of the following stimuli: caffeine, food, social media, alcohol, cannabis, shopping, medication, or exercise?

☐ Have you continued to use a substance or activity even when you noticed it was worsening your physical, mental, or spiritual health?

☐ Have you had difficulty experiencing pleasure?

☐ Have you had any trouble with paying attention or concentrating, poor motivation, or distractibility?

☐ Have you experienced trouble with getting out of bed and moving your body in the morning?

☐ Have you had mood swings? Have you felt aloof, more introverted than usual, or a tendency to isolate yourself? Have you experienced persistent negative thinking, procrastination, self-doubt, anger, and/ or resentment?

☐ Do you have a family history of addiction, such as alcoholism, obesity due to overeating, or drug use disorder in your parents, siblings, grandparents, aunts, or uncles?

☐ Have you experienced any memory loss or blackouts when you can't remember what you ate for lunch yesterday or what happened after you drank a bottle of wine?

☐ Have you used any mind-altering drugs daily, such as caffeine, sugar, cannabis (particularly now that it's legal in so many states), or alcohol?

☐ Have you failed to meet your responsibilities at home, work, or

school—such as calling in sick or poor performance—because of
the use of any of the stimuli?

☐ Have you spent a lot of time involved in activities to obtain your
stimuli of choice, such as thinking about food and planning
how you're going to get it? Or how you can get your next
prescription—or more wine, a new purse, or jewelry?

☐ Have you used a mind-altering drug—such as alcohol, Xanax, or
cannabis—when it was hazardous, such as driving your car?

☐ Have you experienced any social or relationship issues, including
fights or other forms of conflict, due to the effects of a stimulus, and
continued to use it anyway? Have family or friends expressed concern?

☐ Have you been using your substance or stimulus (food, spending,
exercise, social media, alcohol, pills, other types of bingeing, etc.)
in greater amounts than intended? Have you wanted to cut down or
unsuccessfully tried to cut down on your use?

☐ Have you experienced powerful cravings or urges to use your
substance or stimulus? Have you been needing greater amounts of
your substance or activity in order to obtain the desired effect?

☐ Do you have difficulty stopping a behavior once you start, like
drinking wine or checking social media before you go to bed?

INTERPRETATION

If you said yes to five or more questions, you may have an issue with
the pleasure trap (i.e., reward deficiency syndrome). Seven or more,
and it's highly probable that you have a problem. While the symptoms
of reward deficiency and altered dopamine activity overlap with other
brain chemical imbalances, if you follow the entire Basic Protocol in
this chapter, you will feel better.

Woman on a Tear

Marni idles high, meaning she experiences an uncomfortable high-
speed churning of her nervous system while at rest. She lives alone in
Mill Valley, California, a wealthy enclave within the Bay Area. She is

forty-one, right-handed, linear, detail-oriented, logical, ambitious, hard-driving, and successful, and she has always excelled at numbers and math, meaning that she is probably dominant in the left hemisphere of her brain. She works in finance as an investment banker, a stressful job. She carries a high level of tension in her psyche and body and gets a weekly massage to try to settle down.

When she comes home after a long work day, Marni loves to unwind with a glass of wine. Drinking wine, though, gives her night sweats and ruins her sleep, so when she turned forty, she decided to drink only on the weekends, believing it would be a simple change. Lately though, she drinks on other days too—work has been so demanding that she needs the relief. What began as a mild interest in a drink now feels more like an overwhelming desire.

"I'm drinking a bottle every night. Isn't wine good for you?" she asks. Maybe for some people, since wine in moderation lowers the risk of cardiovascular disease, but not necessarily for Marni if it robs her of quality sleep and gives her a hangover (clear signs of harm to the brain/liver connection). Behind the scenes, alcohol not only kills brain and liver cells but detrimentally affects the microbiome. Alcohol can be destructive to a strong, confident, and self-possessed woman when it causes sleep debt and damage to the brain. (Remember: the blood-brain barrier thins out as you age, so toxins like alcohol hit you harder.) In chapter 2, alcohol was identified as a neurotoxin, but alcohol is also a carcinogen that increases a woman's risk of breast cancer, even at a modest dose of three servings per week.[2]

Marni exercises to blow off steam: barre class six days a week, running on the weekends, and spin class as often as possible. She is nursing a stress fracture from running, but she doesn't want to slow down. "It's addictive," she tells me, "and I feel so good afterward, almost human." Oh, except for the pain in her foot.

Every day, Marni has a bar of chocolate. It started as a single square to perk herself up in the afternoon, but she gradually developed the habit of eating the entire bar. "Don't ask me to give it up. I can't live without my chocolate. It's the only carb that I allow myself. I exercise so I can eat the way I want."

Sensing a pattern, I asked if she binge watches television. You bet. She doesn't want to admit it, but she has watched all seasons of about twenty long-running shows in the past year, typically three episodes in a night, when she knows she could be sleeping. I ask her about spiritual practices, and she looks at me bug-eyed, as in, "Are-you-friggin'-kidding-me?"

"You mean meditation or yoga? Absolutely not. I can't sit still. I feel like an alien surrounded by hippies. I don't get it. Literally, going to a yoga class makes me want to kill somebody."

Marni's high idle speed is a sign of hyperarousal. Her go-go-go work life pulls her out of balance, creating a lifestyle that's too compressed and crosses a line somewhere in her brain body: demands exceed supply. Wine, chocolate, and exercise are her only coping mechanisms. When the brain body is in hyperarousal, it craves a downer as a demand for homeostasis. Most people reach for alcohol, marijuana, benzodiazepines like Xanax, and opiates—and initially, they work . . . until they don't. When the stressed brain body can no longer healthily process these downers, they backfire, lead back to hyperarousal, and cause harm to the brain body in the form of higher cortisol load, leaky gut, leaky brain, reactive hypoglycemia (blood sugar crashes), fat storage, inflammation, brain fog, blackouts, and cancer.

Marni insists that her liver has always been fine when tested annually by other doctors, but I disagree: she looks inflamed, puffy, teeth clenched, and highly stressed. Sure enough, her blood test shows that her liver enzymes are elevated, a sign of toxicity that we reviewed back in chapter 2. Her morning cortisol, the chief stress hormone, is too high, because alcohol raises cortisol. The very thing you hope to get from alcohol—relief and lowered cortisol—is a lie.

Marni may or may not qualify as an alcoholic or another type of addict, but she has a *spread addiction,* addictive behaviors spread across multiple stimuli—alcohol, exercise, and chocolate.[3] There are no driving-under-the-influence arrests or blackouts, but she is hooked on legal substances, and which one varies throughout the course of the week. She looks outside of herself for chemical gratification to ease discomfort. She restricts herself on some days and overexercises and binges on others. It's not a matter of how much she drinks or how often, but rather what happens on the inside. Her whole self is shrinking, and she keeps trying to figure out how to fit alcohol, excess exercise, and chocolate into her life. Is her spread addiction holding her back from greatness? Yes. Quietly, Marni explains—quite prophetically—"Something or someone is in control, but it isn't me."

You may or may not have a life like Marni's, but I want to ask gently: Are you in hyperarousal? Have you crossed the line into a heightened stress state and seek relief? What do you reach for to calm down? Addict or not, Marni is concerned and, for the moment, interested in help. Hopefully the same is true for you.

Getting Hooked

When most people think of addiction, they picture a person on the street with track marks from heroin or a brown bag of alcohol, or maybe even the occasional "high-functioning" professional with alcohol use disorder. The truth is that many women, myself included, have addictive tendencies. Even if you don't identify as a problem drinker or drug user, pay attention to early signs of hyperarousal and its temporary fix, spread addiction. You could be like me and not make enough dopamine due to genetic reasons, you could have low dopamine receptors causing social isolation, or you could have dopamine resistance (similar to insulin resistance, dopamine resistance is when your reward pathways become numb to dopamine, so your cells can't make proper use of it, driving the dopamine system out of whack).

Addiction is defined clinically as *compulsive engagement in a habit despite adverse consequences.* In Marni's case, the consequences show up as eroding sleep from alcohol, injuries from overexercising, and liver damage. In my functional medicine practice, I commonly see these symptoms and often wonder what's wrong with us as women that we need to numb out across so many facets of our being. Women tell me in hushed tones, behind the closed door of my office, that mothering feels easier with a glass of wine ("Mommy juice") or that they can't imagine life without marijuana every night. This is hyperarousal and a cry for balance. You have to be in hyperarousal for a compulsive habit to form in response to acquiring a dopamine reward from a substance or stimulus,[4] and unless other coping tools are used as described in the protocol, it can happen to you.

Hyperarousal is a form of left-brain domination, and dopamine rules the left side of the brain in left-brain-dominant people—remember that the left hemisphere tends to govern critical, deductive, and analytical thinking, while the right hemisphere tends to support more intuitive and creative thinking, reading and expressing emotions. Ultimately, the goal of wholeness is that the two sides of the brain are in balance, with each half collaborating and dopamine in homeostasis.

When dopamine levels are altered you can feel tired, moody, apathetic, unfocused, distracted, and uncoordinated, like learning and memorization are no longer as easy as they used to be. Serotonin, which rules the right side of the brain, is central to the regulation of mood, sleep, and appetite, although the mechanism for both of these neurotransmitters is far more complex than previously understood. Still, we can shift the way these neurotransmitters interact in the brain—we can improve the communication system and balance between left and right hemispheres and reduce inflammation as a way of dealing with the common problems of addiction, anxiety, and depression (chapters 6 and 7).

Your left and right brain hemispheres are connected by the *corpus callosum,* and the brain constantly changes, updates, and moves information between the hemispheres—the beauty and result of plasticity. (Before my concussion, I was more left-brained: linear, focused on the *how,* not the *why,* analytical, detail- and fact-oriented, considered the parts rather than the whole, and very driven. After the concussion, when I presumably traumatized and deactivated my left brain hemisphere, I was more creative, emotional, sensitive, loving, and focused on the whole, integrated picture.) Drugs tend to light up the left hemisphere,[5] and people with substance use disorder show increased activation of the left hemisphere in response to immediate rewards, suggesting a reward bias in the left hemisphere.[6]

The Pleasure Trap of "More"

I read an interview with actress Emily Blunt after she played a New York City suburban alcoholic: "I don't have an addictive personality whatsoever, so it was like wearing somebody else's skin," she said.[7] I did a double take. I was surprised that she considered the addictive personality to feel so foreign. Once I started researching the pleasure trap, I began finding that addiction is a lot more common than we realize, and it inflicts harm on our brain body when it carries on unaddressed. We need to redefine it as brain/body disconnection and not as a moral failing.

Now, you may believe that you're in the 63 percent of people who don't qualify as having a drug addiction or aren't at risk for one, but I'd like to stop you right there. Addiction is more broad and complex than the narrow definition you might be thinking of—an alcoholic or someone with substance use disorder. In more subtle cases, the related issues of impulsiveness, compulsion, and obsession can stem from the same brain pathways that recognized addictions do. I suggest we look at addiction as the problem of wanting *more*. You don't have to be a full-blown addict to suffer from the condition of wanting more. It's a problem of dopamine dependence—the neurotransmitter that states, "That was awesome! I want more!"

I know very few women who aren't obsessed with, compulsive about, or addicted to certain behaviors or substances, some not only socially acceptable but culturally bound. Perhaps you are obsessed with how much you exercise each day, or getting your coffee or sugar fix, or you suffer from orthorexia, an *unhealthy* preoccupation with eating *healthy* food. While we're on the topic of "positive" addiction, another example is ultramarathon running of fifty to one hundred miles at one time in a day. These, too, have the same addictive effects—producing dopamine and hurting the brain body by starving it of rest and recovery from stress.

Maybe you can relate more to a different label: martyr, fixer, perfectionist. Conceivably a bathroom scale has become your Higher Power—the arbiter of your worth—instead of its rightful role as a simple tool to measure physical change. (For years, I used my bathroom scale to measure my willpower, habits, and moral standing—and that became an obsessive problem.)

I interpret the term *addiction* as referring to the unhealthy drive or craving behind the behavior, a hollow core into which we pour all the wrong things. For me, the craving for "more" applies to specific foods and work. For others, it's alcohol, shopping, opioids (such as methadone, OxyContin, fentanyl), carbohydrates, shoes, Pilates, personal development, technology, Botox, busyness—even love and sex. I believe addiction stems from a spectrum of maladaptive desire for more of something to make up for a lack of something else very deep and hidden. I think of it now interchangeably as inner emptiness, the pleasure trap, the reward deficiency. Sometimes it feels like hustling or outrunning fear.

In the vast majority of my patients, maybe 90 percent, this missing core feeling is repressed, and instead you simply feel the "rev," the high idle, the stressful churning of modern life.

In many ways, the promises of modern medicine lull us into a false sense of security about our own health, potentially robbing us of our power over dietary and lifestyle choices that are the foundation of true health and wholeness. I want you to start to break through that wall of denial because your current and future health is at stake. In my opinion, this inner emptiness is at the core of any decision you make that's not good for you: the glass of wine when you know you'll suffer in the morning, the extra piece of chocolate cake, the vacation you cannot afford, the eye roll when your partner wants to talk about something important. It may be the most important determinant of your health—deeper, more fundamental, and scarier than your gut bugs or hormone levels or genes. It may even be the silent hand controlling your microbiome, hormones, and genes—and how they talk to your brain body.

Regardless of what you call or consider to be the root cause of your pleasure trap, there's always a cost to falling into it. The fruits of this type of drive may include academic or athletic or financial success, but not peace. Symptoms can be vague: exhaustion, striving, keeping secrets, image management, persistent thoughts of *not enough* (or its cousins, extreme self-reliance and arrogance), negative mind-set, or number obsession (bank account, stocks, weight).

The problem starts out as a symptom ("I just ate seven cookies") that ultimately becomes its own illness ("I binge on sweets every day, then feel guilty, so I make myself vomit"). When in hyperarousal, we want to escape our lives at the end of the day (usually out of pain, guilt, or fear), but the underlying root cause of a heightened stress state isn't obvious. Most women don't know when they're in hyperarousal, and most doctors don't notice, either. Then our chosen behavior reinforces itself. We get stuck, and without help, we don't heal. Our brain bodies decline further. We sense something is off, but often don't have the awareness that we are actually harming ourselves, much less our brain/body connection.

Ultimately, the label matters less than the concept that women are perhaps more vulnerable to impulsiveness, obsession, compulsion, and addiction. It's more about the brain body behaving badly as a result of the gene/environment interactions, family background, and personality. What's happening behind the scenes of your skull is a reinforcement of maladaptive neural pathways.

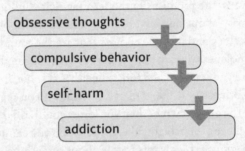

Ruthie, one of my patients with reward deficiency syndrome, had binge eating disorder and struggled with feelings of rebellion: *I know what to do for myself, but I'm just not going to do it. There's no hope that I'll ever lick this problem, so I might as well indulge.* Fortunately, she's now recovered at age fifty-two after performing the Brain Body Diet. And *I* learned how to work around my own genetic tendency toward dopamine problems, reward deficiency, and a desire for *more*. You can too, even if your dopamine is out of balance or functioning poorly, and find freedom from problem behaviors that cause you harm.

If you're unaware of addictive patterns in your brain, you may be unwittingly grooving a downward neurological track of unhealthy habits, leading to a lazy, desensitized brain that begets future pain. On the other hand, when you rewire addictive tracks, your brain bounces back in full-on neuroplastic glory, better than ever. You begin this process of awareness by noticing when you're in a hyperarousal state. See the sidebar on page 187 and check off the symptoms that you experience most days of the week.

Hyperarousal is an imbalanced state involving the "cats," or catecholamines—epinephrine, norepinephrine, and dopamine—their transporters, and their receptor systems.[8] This lack of homeostasis with dopamine and related brain modulators is just one example of a situation that can promote a brain/body failure state like addiction. Certainly biological, social, and environmental factors are at play, but as scientists (myself included) try to understand why this is happening, women are experiencing a more rapid progression of their addiction from casual and moderate use to problematic use, suffer greater withdrawal response with abstinence, and are more vulnerable to a poor treatment outcome, compared with men.[9]

Perform an honest assessment of whether you tend to get hyperaroused. It's a faulty physiological setting that leads to the pleasure trap and may lead to addictive behaviors. If I put on my neuroscience hat for a moment, addiction can be viewed as abnormal dopamine firing in the

---

HYPERAROUSAL

Hyperarousal is a stress state of increased biological and psychological tension.[10]

Signs include:

☐ Agitation

☐ Anger and angry outbursts

☐ Anxiety and/or panic

☐ Being easily frightened or startled

☐ Difficulty concentrating

☐ Experiencing fight-flight-freeze reactions

☐ Feeling overly sensitive, or conversely, a "numbed-out" emotional state

☐ Feelings of guilt or shame

☐ Flashbacks

☐ Gastrointestinal symptoms like diarrhea, constipation, or irritable bowel syndrome

☐ Irritability

☐ Insomnia

☐ Lower pain tolerance (so you feel more emotional or physical pain)

☐ Self-destructive behavior (such as driving too fast or drinking too much)

brain's reward center, the nucleus accumbens, which lights up when you seek reward. Dopamine triggers reward, but then your opioid receptors create pleasure, or the hook.[11] When you deny the craving—for sugar, alcohol, your smartphone, and the like—the dopamine levels in the nucleus accumbens drop precipitously, similar to when a user withdraws from a drug. When you relapse, dopamine, serotonin, and norepineph-rine activity soars.[12] So we need to work around this faulty physiological setting that promotes craving by restoring homeostasis, thereby avoiding the extreme of hyperarousal.

Recovery and healing *are* possible. It's not a matter of just going to a health coach or buying an app to have the healing done *to* us; it's a choice in each moment that we make to live a certain way, congruent with our highest values. It's an inside job where you focus on resetting dopamine with specific strategies of lifestyle medicine, including food, supplements, and daily practices. The takeaway is that you can change your dopamine levels simply with what you eat and don't eat, drink and don't drink, supplement, and how you consciously think and move.

In the protocol, we'll address what to do when dopamine com-munication goes awry. You will learn about the ways to override the dopamine- and serotonin-mediated commands in order to recover from problem behaviors and create long-term adaptive changes in the brain. You will learn how to activate the right hemisphere—the seat of intuition, creativity, and happiness—and restore dopamine balance.

Science of Pleasure, Reward, and Getting Hooked

As a journalist at the *New York Times* put it, if serotonin was the "It" neurotransmitter of the 1990s, dopamine is the "It" neurotransmitter of today.[13] Dopamine helped our ancient ancestors survive by providing an energy kick when a new and pleasurable experience presented itself. It makes us feel fully alive and excited. Over time, the dopamine cir-cuits have evolved to ping in response to many other things: the latest iPhone, the wild ride of the stock market, sugar, cocaine—they all pro-vide a dopamine rush that can become addictive in certain people. One theory is that if you don't make enough of the feel-good brain chemicals like dopamine on your own, you develop an unconscious pattern of seeking substances to match to those receptors, like a key in a lock that opens the door of pleasure. People with addictive tendencies—from dopamine imbalance, gut dysbiosis, inflammation, genetics, or all of the above—can't "just stop." It's not that simple to re-create homeostasis; there's a brain/body gap that must be addressed. Willpower isn't the issue; the problem is an out-of-whack brain body.

Dopamine has hundreds of jobs in your body, including boosting focus, learning, memory, sleep, motor control, and mood (in collaboration with serotonin). Nonetheless, the full understanding of the functions of dopamine is a work in progress. What we know about dopamine:[14]

- Dopamine is central to motivating completion of short-term and long-term goals.

- When you complete something you've set out to do or when your needs are about to be met, dopamine is released in the nucleus accumbens.

- The complete reward circuit hormones include not just dopamine, but also serotonin, glutamate, γ-aminobutyric acid (GABA), endorphins, and others. Beyond the nucleus accumbens, other important areas of the brain in the reward system are the amygdala, hippocampus, medial prefrontal cortical regions, and ventral tegmental area.

- Overall, certain drugs that raise dopamine levels enhance the entire function of the reward circuit in the brain, and thus produce the "high" that drug users seek; ultimately, rewarding stimuli can remodel the reward circuit to cause addiction in vulnerable people, like me.[15]

- Certain people are genetically programmed to be low in dopamine activity and are at risk for reward deficiency syndrome and/or dopamine resistance.

- Healthy people with low levels of dopamine receptors in the striatum of the brain tend to feel aloof and detached. On the other hand, higher levels of dopamine receptors can make you more extroverted and feel socially supported.[16]

MÉNAGE À TROIS: THE GUT, BRAIN, AND MICROBIOTA

We used to think of addiction as only a mental health problem, but there is increasing recognition of the physiological components. There is growing scientific evidence that the microbiota in your gut play a role in mental health, including addiction:

- Gut bacteria act on the gut-brain axis to control the brain function and appetite at the root of food addiction, eating disorders, alcoholism, and other substance use disorders.[17]

- About 40 percent of people with alcohol use disorder have increased intestinal permeability, dysbiosis, or altered metabolomics (changes in microbial metabolism) in their feces.[18]

- Dysbiosis correlates with the cravings, depression, and anxiety associated with alcohol use disorder, though it's not yet clear if the disordered gut ecology is a cause or effect of drinking.[19]

- Animal studies show a link between gut microbiota and cocaine use disorder.[20]

Taken further, the gut ecosystem is involved in not just the genesis of addiction, but downstream issues like altered physiology, thought, and social functioning. So addiction is not just in the head—it's in the head and gut, which means healing the brain/body connection is essential to healing addiction. We need to target the population, diversity, and function of your microbiota as part of treating the whole person with addiction. Specifically, certain bugs correlate with eating behavior. For example, *Prevotella* prefer carbohydrates, while *Bacteroides* prefer protein and animal fat.[21] Similarly, the diversity of bugs in your gut regulates host food intake, too.[22]

Your risk of addiction is related to stress—that is, to a stress-response system (hypothalamic-pituitary-adrenal or HPA axis) that's gone haywire. Stress can lead to disordered eating behaviors and substance use disorders in vulnerable people, depending on genetics and perhaps microbiota.[23] Gut microbiota are involved in normal and abnormal HPA function, and the effect works both ways:[24] namely, bacteria produce neurotransmitters. An example is that *Bifidobacterium* produces GABA, which can modulate anxiety, and *Enterococcus* secretes serotonin, which can modulate mood.[25] LPS increases the activity of the HPA.[26]

In summary, microbiota can change your mind. Gut bacteria may tell you what to eat and what not to eat or drink, how much, and how often. They can also make you more likely to get addicted to certain foods and drinks and unable to cope well with stress through various pathways, including the HPA. The key is to modulate your microbiome through the Brain Body Protocol so you have more choice in these matters.

WHY THE BRAIN PREFERS ALCOHOL TO KALE

Triggers, such as eating sugar, light up the nucleus accumbens, as previously mentioned. The brain records the experience as a "good thing," whether or not it is, and tells the body to do it again: more is better. Usually, a "good thing" is an action that improves survival or reproduction, but the brain can be easily fooled by stimulants that shortcut our biology (like drugs or gambling) and flood the nucleus accumbens with dopamine, even though the activity doesn't serve survival or reproduction and may actually be harmful to the brain and body. When you feel intense pleasure, the hippocampus records the memory, and the amygdala starts scanning the environment for another chance to feel that good again.

Over time and with repeated flooding, the dopamine receptors call a time-out, making everything less rewarding and pleasurable.[27] Eventually, your production of dopamine is reduced, but the craving persists for the drug or behavior. Other sources of dopamine that require effort and even delayed gratification, like broccoli and connection, become less valuable compared to the shortcut stimulant. You may require higher doses and quicker access to the "drug." Ultimately, you may want the drug even when it no longer provides any pleasure or satisfaction, a hallmark of serious full-blown addiction.

At a minimum, 10 percent of us behave addictively and misuse food, substances, and processes, and that includes women who look like you and me. There is scientific agreement that alcohol, opiates, nicotine, cocaine, methamphetamine—and even conditions like food addiction, anorexia, and bulimia—are linked to a decreased number of dopamine receptors in the brain.[28] Not only that, but certain genes (e.g., TaqA1) are associated with more carbohydrate and fast-food cravings (but curiously, not higher rates of obesity).[29] So you may be intrinsically wired to be low in dopamine receptors and crave things that are bad for you as your brain body seeks balance. That's why a strategy like the Brain Body Diet is so important to work around the faulty wiring that many of us have.

PHASES OF GETTING HOOKED

On the road to addiction, there are three distinct phases:[30]

1. Getting high (binge and intoxication)
2. Avoiding the low (withdrawal and "negative affect"—the emotional tone a person expresses)
3. Craving (preoccupation and yearning)

Getting high through bingeing and intoxication raises dopamine activity. In people stuck in the pleasure trap (revisit the quiz at the beginning of this chapter to remind yourself), there is neuroadaptation at every phase that leads to a greater chance of developing substance use disorder, which can be mild, moderate, or severe, but includes some degree of health problems, such as difficulty sleeping. Addiction is the most chronic and severe form of substance use disorder—you keep getting high despite wanting to quit—but you can encounter problems long before you reach that stage.

Withdrawal and feeling negative about it is the uncomfortable experience of low dopamine activity and altered homeostasis. Studies show that the cycle of repeated use and withdrawal leads to smaller synapses and greater prevalence of depression.[31]

Cravings result from the desire to raise dopamine again in the face of down-regulated dopamine signaling. In other words, dopamine activity is quieter because the reward circuit has been dulled in its sensitivity to pleasure, from a substance (food, drug) or an activity (video gaming, shopping, relationships). This problem is based in the prefrontal cortex, and involves a few other areas, including the insula and amygdala. As a result, a person with reward deficiency syndrome craves a dopamine hit. As the cycle continues, executive function declines, including the ability to self-regulate in response to the reward, as does decision-making, cognitive flexibility, and ability to monitor your own error. The net result is that you are unable to resist the strong urge to use the stimulant again.

At the physical level of the brain, addiction is a disregulation of reward and pleasure. You first change certain brain chemical levels, like dopamine and opioid peptides, in the brain. Then you develop too many stress neurotransmitters, such as corticotropin-releasing factor, in the amygdala. Some people in recovery consider their addiction as an allergy—like an allergy to alcohol—but not in the traditional sense of the word. Instead, allergy is a sign of your body turning against itself. Your body turns against you by craving the very thing that hurts it.

When the normal homeostasis involved in making decisions breaks down, at least two physiological conditions occur simultaneously in the brain, leading to reward deficiency syndrome and ultimately substance use disorder:[32]

1. A "hot" or hyperactive amygdala, which creates impulsivity and exaggerates the reward impact of available triggers
2. A "cold" or underactive prefrontal cortex—your reflective system, the part of your brain that can predict the consequences of your actions. You lose resourcefulness.

What's fascinating to me, and something I've experienced as I've recovered from my own spread addiction, is that when you have these two brain problems, you're totally unaware that you have a problem. My inclination when I ate, drank, or worked too much was to deny it, minimize it, or at the very least, have a difficult time explaining my behavior. Perhaps you have this same lack of awareness, too: this is why you shouldn't ignore dopamine problems. You could be disregarding or minimizing misuse you don't even know you have—and damaging your health and physical, mental, and spiritual well-being.

The Dope on Addiction Vulnerability

The most complete picture of addiction and why we're vulnerable is complex. Addictions produce both positive features including euphoria, relief from anxiety, relief from withdrawal, and reward, and negative features including aversion, dysphoria, anxiety, and withdrawal symptoms. Stress, anxiety, and depression are tightly associated with addiction. Sometimes they precede misuse; sometimes they result from misuse—the effect is bidirectional. Usually the 90/10 rule applies to the genetic component of chronic disease, meaning that only 10 percent of your risk is genetic and 90 percent is environmental, but not in addiction. The latest theory is that at least half of your risk of addictive behavior is genetic, and half is environmental. To see this 50/50 rule in action, consider workaholism. Your choice to work to excess may be personal, but how your brain responds to working excessively and the validation from peers and bosses may be strongly influenced by genetics (see the sidebar on pages 195 to 196).

I have a problem with the COMT gene, and it made me a hyperfocused workaholic until I hit my head. Most of my friends were workaholics (except the therapists and coaches). Living in the Bay Area, working fourteen-hour days was a default lifestyle choice. I started my own company and was willing to give up almost everything to see patients and help women feel less insane as I upped my own hours and insanity. Missing back-to-school night? My husband can go; I'm busy changing the world. New business opportunities? Yes, please! Daughter needs to go to volleyball in the city? I can do that too. My girlfriends and I would meet for a run and lament about our husbands who complained about us typing emails in bed, how work was all we ever talked about, or that we weren't having much sex. Oh, the irony!

Now my right and left hemispheres are more balanced, and I am no longer obsessed and compulsive about work. I work less, listen more, and tune in to the sacred throughout the day. Despite my genetics, my dopamine activity is near normalized because of my diet, supplements, and chosen activities (more on this in the protocol). I finally feel more congruent about the way I work and the message I am sharing. I understand that working more than full-time each week doesn't increase productivity[33] or make me feel whole.

The bottom line is that we are in a new era of addiction medicine that considers the whole person, including early genetic diagnosis of your vulnerability toward addictive tendencies and the pleasure trap, and screening for problem behaviors. (What if you want to undergo genetic testing? See Appendix B for a list of recommended resources.) If you're

GENETICS

Vulnerability to addiction has its origins in a complex interplay of gene and environment. You can predict who's at risk for some addictions by looking at genetic variations, though genetics are not the whole story. A few examples: childhood maltreatment interacts with the monoamine oxidase A (MAOA) gene to predict alcoholism and antisocial behavior. The Met158 variant in the "corporate warrior" gene (catechol-O-methyltransferase, or COMT) can increase the risk of and resilience to alcoholism.[34] On the other hand, childhood trauma is associated with food addiction and binge eating and, for women, doubles the risk of food addiction, but the genetic connection is not firmly established.[35]

We can predict with about 97 percent accuracy who will become a person with an opioid addiction based on genetic testing by looking at the genetic variations involving four brain chemical pathways: dopamine, serotonin, endorphin, and GABA.[36] Overall, genes are moderately to highly predictive of your risk of addiction, and so far, there is no single addiction gene. Consequently, it can be helpful to consider a panel of candidate genes if you feel you're at risk. Some of the current genetic variations under investigation are listed below. (Note that several of these genes are described and discussed in relation to their effect on disease and behavior related to healthspan—the length of time that a person is healthy, not just alive—in my previous book *Younger*.)

"Corporate warrior" gene. COMT regulates dopamine levels and is involved in reward processing.[37] Females may respond differently than males to the change in dopamine activity, at least in animal studies.[38] There are three possible genes: Val/Val, Val/Met, and Met/Met. If you inherit one of the Val alleles (variant form of the gene), you may have more trouble with inhibition—that is, saying no when you mean no to a stimulus.[39] On the other hand, Met/Met carriers may seek more novelty.[40]

Dopamine genes. Several genes change dopamine activity and may make you vulnerable to reward deficit syndrome. These include the dopamine transporter and the dopamine D1, D2, and D4 receptors. See Notes for further details.[41]

Alcohol processing genes. Genetic risk factors associated with alcohol problems include common variants in genes that code for how your body processes and breaks down alcohol. If you have a mutation in your ADH1B and ALDH2 genes, the ones that would protect you against alcohol dependence, then you'll be at a greater risk for becoming a problem drinker (and smoker).[42]

Serotonin transporter gene. SLC6A4 (also known as 5-HTTLPR) is involved in serotonin activity, another player in the reward system. Genetic variations may result in lower rates of serotonin reuptake, lower stress resilience, less response to antidepressants like selective serotonin reuptake inhibitors (SSRIs), greater adverse reactions to SSRIs, increased environmental sensitivity leading to sleep difficulty, and a fussy temperament, plus a higher rate of alcohol use disorder, cocaine use disorder, (possibly) nicotine use disorder, post-traumatic stress disorder, and obsessive-compulsive disorder.[43] I think of it as the gene that makes it more likely that a person may have an overactive or "hot" amygdala.

Stress-response gene. FK506 binding protein 5 (FKBP5) is a gene well known to be associated with cortisol regulation, the stress-response system (fight-flight-freeze), the HPA axis, and risk of PTSD. (In the brain, significant overlap occurs between addiction and PTSD.)

Monoamine oxidase A. MAOA metabolizes several neurotransmitters, including norepinephrine, epinephrine, serotonin, and dopamine.[44] Variants of MAOA genes are associated with aggression, anxiety, and addiction.[45] Specifically, MAOA genes are associated with nicotine use disorder in women.[46] Certain polymorphisms of MAOA are associated with heroin use disorder and greater harm from cocaine.[47]

at risk for reward deficiency, careful management of your lifestyle is essential to avoid the more risky addictive behaviors—including violating food and work/life boundaries—and to nurture a connection to something bigger than yourself.

OTHER FACTORS

The other side of genetic risk? Environmental factors: neurological vulnerability (more so with women compared to men), family disturbances, parenting issues, and troubled intimate relationships.[48] Subsequently and perhaps as a result of altered dopamine activity, addictive behavior may make relationships worse because there's a lack of disclosure, authenticity, and honesty, and that just fuels a negative spiral. Sometimes use disorder is the downstream result of running from negative emotions and seeking temporary relief; other times it stems from a hyped-up nervous system. Then the three basic survival mechanisms get overactivated: anger (fight), fear (flight), and camouflage (freeze). These are the basic modes of your sympathetic nervous system that raise blood sugar and blood pressure so you can cope with the perceived threat, but in my opinion, addiction takes hold when they are activated too often and/or for too long. I know because I've been there.

At fifteen, I discovered restricted eating (nine out of ten addictive behaviors start in adolescence[49]). I lost weight, but I also lost muscle mass as I starved my brain and cells throughout my body. For the next twenty years, I restricted my food until my willpower ran out; then I binged and purged, sometimes with exercise and sometimes by making myself vomit. I obsessively weighed myself. Daily. Multiple times. The results either filled me with euphoria—which was rare—or despair, the more common response. Being a chronic dieter and bulimic didn't work; it just made me more obsessed with food and weight in a wretched, chaotic, and soul-sucking way.

My story isn't unique. Eighty percent of women are dissatisfied with their bodies and feel they don't measure up to some impossible standard. We diet, restrict food, or develop bulimia in order to keep ourselves "small," to outrun the collective pain of being alive, and to silence the noise of our inevitable sorrow and despair in a male-dominated, misogynist world. Taken one step further, Jungian psychoanalyst Ann Belford Ulanov describes that in her own clinical practice with women, obsession with fatness is about a search for the transcendent—"God, the unknown, or the holy"—as a reality that functions in our lives all the time, and manifests as compulsions as well as ordinary daily struggles. More practically, those internal thoughts may sound like this:

- *My belly is too fat.*

- *I feel out of control with my eating, which makes me super sad, so I'll keep bingeing to avoid feeling overwhelmed by the emotion. Now I feel even worse.*

- *My breasts are too small and droopy.*

- *This is the last time [I use this substance or process]. I'll stop tomorrow.*

- *I ate too much last night and hate myself. I'll make up for it by restricting my food today.*

- *It doesn't matter that I swore off alcohol today; I'm desperate for just one glass of wine. I'll be better tomorrow.*

- *It's too hard to do this (healthy food, healthy quantity, exercise, meditation). I don't see the benefit in working so hard. I quit.*

- *There's no hope for me; I might as well indulge.*

- *I know what to do, but I'm not going to do it. The sacrifice is too much.*

- *I deserve this piece of cheesecake. And another.*

Ultimately, these thoughts lead to poor decisions and obsession, and they block the opportunity for freedom and grace. On page 200, you will see my unscientific illustration of my addictions.

One way I recognized my food addiction is that I experienced a weird sort of craving when I ate just one bite of certain foods (items containing flour, sugar—even paleo cheesecake), and the result was that I ate more than I intended. My old relationship to food was similar to that of an alcoholic with her wine or vodka. When I wasn't bingeing, I thought about food all the time. After I binged, I was full of remorse and helplessness. This cycle repeated itself thousands of times: binge, remorse, preoccupation, despair. Sadly, the despair arose from shame and guilt, so I'd start the cycle all over again, each time convinced that I simply needed to try harder or learn a new strategy to navigate food in a different way. That would help me manage it better *next* time and, of course, with different results.

But it didn't happen.

WOMEN AND ADDICTION

We live in a culture of acceptable lies when it comes to alcohol, body image, debt, and men. We exaggerate our assets and minimize our liabilities. I used to do it, too: I would go out on a Friday and feel like a rock star after a few drinks, and not be honest about the bad behaviors and experiences that followed: the munchies and overeating, driving while a little buzzed, the crummy sleep, the difficulty functioning the next day while hungover, the weight gain, the blood sugar problems, the unsustainable cortisol levels. We overvalue the fun and undervalue the cost. We don't say to ourselves: "Darling, you're hurting yourself. You don't need to keep researching the topic and collecting more data. You're aware of the cost, and it's too high." We don't value the cost of addictive behavior and realize our risk as women.

- Women are more likely to be food addicts compared with men. In a study of US female nurses, food addiction was associated with other problems, including atopic dermatitis, food allergies, hay fever, and asthma.[50]
- Women are prescribed opioids more often than men[51] and are the fastest-growing group of people with opioid use disorder in the United States.
- Women are more likely to be dependent on methamphetamines compared with men.[52]
- Women more rapidly escalate from casual drug use to addictive behavior, show more marked withdrawal with abstinence, and are less successful with treatment compared with men.[53]
- Women tend to run low in progesterone starting in perimenopause (starting around age forty-three, give or take five to ten years), and research has shown that oral progesterone reduces cravings. It helped women but not men to experience less negative emotion and a more relaxed mood when provoked by stress.[54]
- Social, behavioral, and biological factors that may result in addiction are worse for women.

Sound familiar? To my surprise, I later learned that my food addiction was just a symptom of a bigger issue: my low dopamine and an inability to bring my altered dopamine state into balance. Food was simply one symbol of my troubles. I binged not just on food, but on excessive self-reliance, Jimmy Choos, and stress.

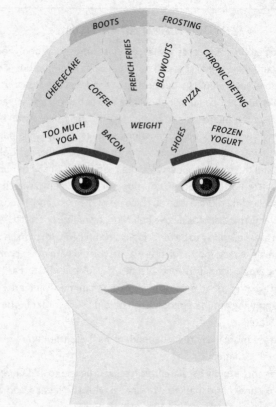

My Previous Addictions

What Addiction Looks Like

I recently read Glennon Doyle Melton's bestseller *Love Warrior*, in which she describes the painful ways that her addictive behavior developed as she grew up—in high school when she was obsessed with being thin, making herself smaller and conforming to the ideals that boys had of who she should be—and how she recovered. One line slayed me: "Be the person you needed when you were younger." Obsession, compulsion, and addictive behavior keep you from being that person. Here are other ways that addiction holds you back from full expression of your uniqueness, from your greatness:

- creates negative emotional states and compromises your executive functioning, thereby inhibiting you from looking for the good in your spouse or kids, stopping you from feeling resourceful at work, or prompting you to get short-tempered when your mother tells you the same story three times in a day.[55]

- causes deficits of hippocampus-dependent learning and memory, meaning you can't recall how bad it was last time when you drank too much, spent too much, or impulsively binged.[56]

- gives you a higher risk of being allergic to yourself (suffering from autoimmune conditions). Not surprisingly, US women with food addiction are more likely to have skin conditions, such as eczema.[57]

- makes you crave your substance during withdrawal, which is associated with increased stress and raised cortisol, making you also crave sugar or other unhealthy substances even more.[58]

- puts you at risk to get consumed with the internet and technology such as smartphones. Internet addiction is linked to reduced immune function and is associated with depression, anxiety, social isolation, and sleep problems, which all prevent your brain from reaching its highest potential.[59]

- creates conditioned learning that's hard to turn off, meaning internal and external stress can cause relapse.

- may lead to distortions in perception, like negative thinking, procrastination, self-doubt, anger, and resentments. It also plays a role in many mental health conditions, including depression and attention deficit disorder.

As I've tried to understand my own reward deficiency syndrome and addictions, I didn't find satisfying answers in conventional medicine. So I turned to Ayurveda to shed light on the roots of my addictive tendencies.

In Ayurveda, the ancient model of wholeness and integration from India, separation is the cause of disease, meaning that disease occurs when you feel separate from who you are as a whole, integrated person. Separation causes homeostasis to break down. Our true nature is that we are spiritual beings in a physical frame. One Ayurvedic physician told me that in his early practice twenty-five years ago, 60 percent of his patients had physical issues, 30 percent had emotional issues, and 10 percent had spiritual issues—but now, 80 percent of his patients have a spirit that is out of balance. That separation, or spiritual illness, is easier to see in addiction. Ayurveda provides a great reminder that when it comes to addiction and wanting more external gratification, recovery must be rooted in lifestyle. That's how you can reclaim homeostasis— through the small disciplines of daily life, carving a new set of healthier grooves in your reward circuit system. The old dysfunctional feelings and attachments don't go away—they are part of the human condition. But for me, I need to practice daily tools to keep my peace and emotional sobriety.

You Have a Choice: Pain or Gain?

At the root of addictive behavior is often heightened emotional sensitivity (i.e., hyperarousal). Sometimes the nervous system is too amped up.[60] Addicts of any sort have difficulty with trust. One of my patients described her poorly developed sense of trust like she's a little girl in the middle of a busy street, with nowhere to turn, wondering: *Where are the responsible adults charged with my care? Why aren't they protecting me?* It's mind-blowing to learn as an adult how to provide a sense of trust for yourself. You can become a benevolent, soothing presence—for yourself first, and then for others. First, you have to understand all aspects of the roots of addiction.

The psychological aspect is an obsession with control. You develop a misperception that you can control your substance or activity. The fact is that deep down, you know you shouldn't be indulging, but you do it anyway, desperately seeking solace.

The spiritual aspect can be considered a connection disorder. There's a sense of disappointment with life; you keep looking outside of yourself for what you're missing. Like me when I was fifteen, you seek people, places, vacations, things, behaviors, or experiences that can bring true fulfillment and joy. It's the disease of looking elsewhere that leads to disconnection from yourself and others and from something bigger—a

Higher Power, God, or your own version of a greater good, a divine code, or love. You fall into the trap of looking for external solutions to make yourself whole, chasing fleeting pleasures, accumulating wealth or possessions, or seeking release in a "drug" or process. The result can be a chemical addiction (food, cigarettes, cannabis, amphetamines, cocaine, heroin, opioids) or a process addiction (gambling, continual debt, underearning income, codependence, rage, anxiety)—both types activate the pleasure centers and deluge the brain in dopamine. (Yes, you can become habituated to negative emotions such as anxiety and rage; your dopamine goes up, then reward kicks in, and you get a rush of almost paradoxical pleasure.)

Psychiatrist Carl Jung believed that addiction represents a spiritual hunger for wholeness. As others describe in *Alcoholics Anonymous: The Big Book*, Jung suspected that only a conversion to something equally satisfying to the individual at a deep level can promote recovery. Jung believed the solution to addiction is a vital spiritual experience, a re-arrangement of emotions, ideas, and attitudes, allowing for a completely new set of conceptions and motives. He detailed the shame, secrecy, and loneliness of addiction, which makes a person feel alienated from "the protective wall of human community." Jung delivered a series of lectures on the promise of kundalini yoga for ongoing psychic hygiene, which formed the basis of his book titled *The Psychology of Kundalini Yoga*.[61] As I mentioned in chapter 2, Jung found that kundalini provides a model of the developmental phases of higher consciousness, something that was almost entirely lacking in Western psychology; I agree. It won't surprise you to learn that many of the most prominent kundalini yoga teachers, including Tommy Rosen, Ramdesh Kaur, and Belinda Carlisle, are in recovery from addiction.

Yes, life is painful. But at a certain point, we have a choice. Will we let our emotions drive us to compulsion or obsession, or terminate them before they escalate? Brain scientist Jill Bolte Taylor says that emotions are meant to last ninety seconds; beyond that we're indulging them and rewiring our brain for negativity, like with anxious thoughts. When we choose to hang on beyond ninety seconds to negative emotions—when we indulge, even binge on those emotions—we may form destructive habits and armor around those emotions.

Digging Up the Roots

Healing is not just about giving up smoking, vomiting, or compulsive daily weigh-ins. Nor is it only about losing your drinking privileges or sticking to a budget. Healing is about the way your life expands when your brain gets healthier, when you stop numbing yourself against the inevitable pain of life.

To heal, the key is to develop better rituals and change the neural pathways. About 80 percent of my patients struggle with alcohol but are not chemically addicted. They are not falling-down drunks but enjoy partying and venting steam. (I did the same with brownies and nachos.) But when they stop drinking as a misguided attempt to cope with stress, they notice something extraordinary: giving up the drug (alcohol) isn't a bad experience, but a freedom. It creates an integrity loop. Instead of pouring themselves another glass of wine and lamenting how it harms sleep, liver, mood, and relationships, they chose not to drink. It's easier than they think it will be when they stop grasping for the thing that harms them. Deciding not to drink, then reinforcing the loop of integrity by not drinking, changes the brain patterning. You'll be more present at dinner with your family. You'll be more resourceful when the inevitable conflict arises. You'll sleep better that night, and make better decisions tomorrow. You don't have to cling to the crutch of alcohol or any other drug, legal or not.

Actress and activist Jane Fonda understands the deeper psychological and spiritual issues of addiction. We're not meant to be perfect, she said; we're meant to be whole. For the first fifty years of my life, I sought greater and greater stimulation with age. I counted on increasing intensity to feel most alive. Not surprisingly, these things weren't fulfilling, because I was craving the sacred in everyday life and didn't know it. I learned that there's a deeper joy in counteracting the human tendency to want *more* in simplifying, in becoming still instead of moving toward a target that stays just out of reach. Now I think of the itch as divine unrest. We don't need a "fix" or the right doctor to fix us; we need to connect to a power beyond ourselves.

Eventually, I found meditation as the portal to make friends with quietness, uncomfortable emotions, my obsessive need to know, and my other uncomfortable and distressing sensations. Meditation helped me pause before the compulsive behavior: *just one more email to check, one more check of the bathroom scale, one more pair of jeans to buy.* I realized that there is more in the universe than what I see, and I connected in faith to divine help. After my brain injury and delving deep to heal my brain body, I learned something very helpful: surrender. Not the passive surrender of a weakling or acknowledgment of defeat as we think of it in the West, but the empowered and conscious letting go of the extreme need to control—the surrender of one's inner war, allowing the shoulders to relax, the jaw to become unclenched, the mind at ease, a refuge. For the first time in my life, I stopped trying to push harder and do it all myself. Natural things became more alive: seeing a beautiful madrone tree, feeling the warm breeze through the redwoods on my skin, melting into a warm hug with my daughter. Tuning into something greater than myself connected me to wholeness and helped me stop beating myself up with food and dieting. You'll learn more about the specific ways I handled cravings and compulsions—and how you can, too—in the protocol.

The Brain Body Protocol: Healing Reward Deficiency Syndrome and Addiction

Thankfully, we have the science and tools to reclaim balance in our lives—to bridge the dopamine gap, restore gut/brain balance, calm down hyperarousal, and fill the holes caused by high stress. Every day we're changing our brain, sometimes for the better but sometimes for the worse. If you're like Marni used to be and idle at an intense, high frequency—please get ready to deliberately change the brain for the better first by noticing hyperarousal in your own body, and second by keeping yourself in check throughout the day, one day at a time, and then throughout your life—so you don't go full tilt. That means stopping short of crossing the line into hyperarousal in the first place, where you crave addictive substances and activities. The purpose of the Brain Body Diet is to restore balance, including purposeful ways of resetting the dopamine pathway. As women, it also means we need to activate the "tend and befriend" pathway, starting with ourselves, as the best biological antidote to the fight-flight-freeze response.

For those of you with socially acceptable addictions (accumulating wealth, shopping, exercise) or soft addictions (being right, arguing, leaving relationships, speeding, running late, and the like), we'll address them too. Overall, the gentle goal is to slowly exit the pleasure trap by taking baby steps. I've found that small actions, performed consistently and strategically, lead to the most profound change. We'll start with the physical—what you eat and how you move ("once I start, I can't stop"), then move on to the mind, a function of the brain ("once I stop, I can't stay stopped"), and finally, the spiritual aspect (the uncomfortable, whack-a-mole unmanageability of life). The aim is to replace the pleasure trap and old ways of jerking dopamine around with new, healthier ways of filling your tank.

We're going to build a shield to addiction by breaking its grasp on the mind, a function of the brain body. Instead of *morefulness,* we will fill the neurobiological gaps with mindfulness and a discovery of the gift of *lessfulness.* When it feels overwhelming or scary—and it will—take it one step at a time. My colleague Holly Whitaker describes it this way: "I don't just want to be a person who doesn't drink. I want to create a life that I don't want to escape from."

Much like the way I make a choice to stay in a difficult conversation with my husband or choose to dwell in and even enjoy the release into a challenging yoga pose, I give daily consent through prayer, meditation, and action to stay on the slow and obstacle-strewn path of healing my addictions.

In this protocol, you will:

- eliminate cravings and enjoy the foods that are right for your body.

- cut out the most addictive foods, allowing you to rewire and heal the reward center of the brain.

- be able to put down the fork by resetting leptin.

- fill the gaps that commonly occur prior to addiction, like with B vitamins, minerals, and fatty acids.

- evaluate any addictive tendencies with exercise, money, work, or pills.

- develop a habit of mindfulness—better awareness, consciousness, and potential.

- rewrite your model of wholeness: not a model of perfectionism or what you learned from your parents, but what might work for you going forward.

- build upon the protocols of previous chapters that help you escape the pleasure trap, including supporting your liver, balancing your hormones, and eating nourishing, whole, organic food.

Try it for forty days, and spend longer—in some cases eight or twelve weeks—to escape the pleasure trap and reset the reward pathways.

BASIC PROTOCOL

Step 1: Eat to cut cravings.

I'll start with the obvious: eat real, organic, unprocessed food that agrees with you and doesn't cause stress due to food intolerances. You've already removed the foods that spike your reward center (flour, gluten, grains, sugar, dairy) at the beginning of the Brain Body Diet, back in chapter 2. You've also been intermittently fasting, perhaps for twelve to fourteen hours, or even sixteen, which is the minimum for mild ketosis and what I think of as the molecular form of absolving the sins of your past—the broken DNA, the damaged proteins, the oxidative stress of a modern, addictive lifestyle. To help reduce hyperarousal and your faulty dopamine pathway, add at least three new items to your meals from the following list in order to absorb more of the precursors to dopamine—amino acids named tyrosine and phenylalanine: the focus in this part of the protocol is to eat more tyrosine- and phenylalanine-rich foods.[62] Does eating these foods truly raise your dopamine? Yes, some more than others.

- avocado
- banana
- garlic

- beets
- chicken, duck
- eggs
- leafy greens like arugula, kale, mustard greens, endive, watercress
- sea vegetables
- legumes, particularly fava beans, butter green beans, Dutch string beans
- pumpkin and sesame seeds
- turmeric
- almonds
- dark chocolate, 85 percent cacao or higher (yes, one ounce per day is probably good for you)
- green tea
- coffee, but use certain types to limit mold exposure
- nutritional yeast

What to avoid:
- animal-based saturated fat[63]
- sugar, period (Nothing about it is good for you. Same for artificial or natural sweeteners.)
- gluten and casein (milk protein)[64]
- snacking

Step 2: Rewrite your model for wholeness.

Most of us learned our model of wholeness, good or not, from our parents, usually most strongly from the parent of the same gender. Now it's time to question whether that model is serving you. Take space for this step ideally in the morning, when you are not in a hyperarousal state and have your wits about you.

1. Sit down and take a few deep abdominal breaths.
2. Jot down the perfectionistic or critical thoughts that drive you to drink, shop, or do other things that cause harm. Write down everything as if it were okay to feel whatever you're feeling and you won't be judged as bad or wrong ("I can do it all!"; "Just need to work

harder!"; "No time!"; "I can't say no to that offer even though some part of me wants to!"; "I'm a bad ____ [wife, mom, sister, daughter, friend]!"). It's important to write down exactly what your mind says to you, to get the language in your own words.

3. Then answer the question: *What kind of relief am I seeking?*
4. Next, think of what changes would make you feel whole (at peace, less driven, without obsession)—again, what would you do if there were no judgment, obstacles, or consequences? Think big, extravagant, audacious. Write those down. Trip to Costa Rica for a month? Yes, please. Quit your job? Get divorced?
5. Finally, write about what keeps you from implementing those ideas, strategies, and changes (hint: usually it's fear—scarcity, not good enough, etc.).
6. As an alternative, think of someone you know who is a model of wholeness and why. What keeps you from living that way? Fear? A sometimes harmful drive for achievement?

DR. BETHANY HAYS'S MODEL FOR WHOLENESS

Dr. Bethany Hays is a physician and Institute for Functional Medicine faculty member. Her model of wholeness includes "being and helping others *be* in ways that are coherent with our amazing physiology and our connection to and need to be in relationship with each other and the physical world. And understanding that we are hard-wired to be in connection with the energy that has been described as omnipotent, omniscient, and omnipresent and is the repository of life . . . that organizing principle which works in opposition to the tendency toward randomness and disorganization."

Step 3: Add supplements that reduce and repair hyperarousal.

If green tea and turmeric aren't hitting the mark after a one-week trial, choose one new supplement from the following list and try it for the rest of the protocol.[65] I recommend taking only one reward supplement or medication at a time; too much dopamine can be dangerous. If you are taking methyldopa, antidepressants, or antipsychotic

MEDITATION FOR HABITUATION

This practice will ease hyperarousal so you don't need a glass of wine to unwind. My friend and kundalini yoga teacher Guru Jagat recommends this kriya to demagnetize habitual tendencies so you gain freedom of choice.[66] You'll squeeze your molars together with each sound, which she believes helps to create a new pattern in the hypothalamus and pineal gland, the origin of habits and cravings. In her experience, this practice, when performed for three to eleven minutes per day, will break habitual patterns, including emotional binges, drinking, cigarette smoking, drug use, obsessive-compulsive disorder, and relationship sabotage.

Posture: Sit with legs crossed on the floor, spine lifted. With both hands, curl your fingers into the pads of your hands—not into fists, just down so that the fingertips are resting right on top of the pads at the base of each finger. Leave your thumbs extended, and place them on your temples.

Breath and mantra: Breathe normally in and out. Mentally repeat the sounds *Sa-Ta-Na-Ma*. On each sound, press your back molars together. You should feel something move underneath your thumbs. Keep going.

Time: three to eleven minutes

To End: Inhale, focus on the center of the forehead through closed eyes, set the frequency, exhale, and relax.

drugs, consult first with your prescribing clinician. Avoid combining supplements unless you've consulted with your health care professional. These supplements are not usually recommended for pregnant or lactating women. Start with the one choice from the list below that seems like the best fix, and then add another if you don't notice a benefit after one to two weeks.

- **Vitamin D, magnesium, omega-3s, zinc,** or **multivitamin/mineral.** If you're low in any of these basics, you may be at greater risk of dopamine deficiency and addictive behaviors—including binge eating chocolate![67] Take a high-potency multivitamin from a supplement manufacturer with good manufacturing practices (GMP, a minimal standard for supplements). Standard doses:

— vitamin D 1,000 to 2,000 IU per day
— magnesium 200 to 400 mg at night
— omega-3 2,000 mg per day
— zinc picolinate 25 to 50 mg per day

Ideally, work with a functional medicine doctor who can assess and follow your micronutrient levels over time and adjust the dose as needed.

- **N-acetyl cysteine.** NAC is a neuroprotectant that reduces craving, desire to use, and relapse.[68] NAC works by improving cognitive control in the brain, presumably by improving glutamate balance.[69] Yes, this is the same supplement used in hospitals that helps with liver detoxification and production of glutathione, and NAC has an excellent safety record. Dose: 600 mg two to four times per day (max 2,400 mg/day).[70]

- **Ashwagandha.** This is the primary herb of Ayurveda because it acts as a brain tonic and reduces perceived stress, which tends to be high and/or dysregulated in addiction.[71] Dose: 300 mg once or twice per day.

ADVANCED PROTOCOL

Follow the steps of the Basic Protocol, and add one or more of the following advanced techniques if you're still in a state of hyperarousal and/or reward deficiency.

Step 4: Perform activities that reset dopamine.

Since hyperarousal is at the root of the slippery slope of addiction, let's get your brain body back into homeostasis, which feels like a chilled-out, resilient, happy calm. No more hyperarousal—or the other extreme, hypoarousal. Allow space and time to breathe deeply, to rest the brain body, so you don't cross the line. Focus on activities that make you feel relaxed, like your needs are met. Choose one of the following to perform regularly for the remainder of the protocol:

- Altruism and service raise dopamine the same way as alcohol or heroin. So look for opportunities to step up and serve—for a neighbor, at your kid's school, at your church or synagogue, at a local march for justice, for any cause you believe in.

- Getting a massage may boost dopamine by 30 percent or more, while lowering cortisol.[72] (Remember, dysregulated HPA axis and high cortisol are associated with addiction.[73])

- Moderate- to high-intensity physical exercise is good for addiction—it raises dopamine, increases abstinence rate by 69 percent, eases withdrawal symptoms, reduces anxiety by 31 percent, and lowers depression by 47 percent.[74] People who exercise regularly are less likely to develop addiction, though not always in problem drinkers.[75] I measure my heart rate variability every morning to determine my brain/body connection and capacity for training

DO LESS BETTER

Mindfulness is a tool, not a master. Let's keep it in perspective. The point is the disciplined pursuit of less, and doing it intentionally. It's the counterbalance to what corporate researcher Jim Collins calls the "undisciplined pursuit of more," which I believe is the fallout of low dopamine. But be wary of the special kind of self-improvement hell that a long list of new habits like mindfulness can create.

My dear friend Jo helped me laser in on a practice that feels easier than mindfulness. It's called *essentialism*, which loosely translates as "do less better." I love that it can mean "do less well," for my inner overachiever, or it can mean "do less, and keep trying to get better at it."

For me, this is a better defense against the exigencies of modern life. I still do less, then obsess—but I obsess about the priorities in my life. I obsess about adding value but not in a perfectionistic way. I created a "stop-doing list." I spend a lot of time with my dog, shaping this beautiful sentient being so that we can really enjoy each other (as opposed to us circling each other with resentment and fury, like feral animals). I go on simpler vacations and focus on what's most important: spend time with my family and friends, read a good book, and walk outdoors. I do less, be more.

each day—and risk for hyperarousal from exercise. See Appendix B for recommended apps and devices.

- Activities that promote mindfulness for *you*, like knitting (yes!), gardening, painting, or home repair, help rewire your brain in more productive and balanced ways so you're less likely to be driven by cravings. Herbert Benson, MD, a pioneer in mind-body medicine, explains that the repeated actions of needlework—knitting, crocheting, needlepoint—induce a relaxed state similar to yoga and meditation. Once you learn how to do it, needlework can lower your blood pressure and heart rate, and reduce the harmful effects of the stress hormone cortisol.[76]

- Yoga is the twenty-five-hundred-year-old model of wholeness. One of my teachers, Ana Forrest, calls the twelve parts of the sun salutations her preferred twelve-step system for overcoming addiction, along with an intentional practice to attain a meditative state and enhance the spiritual aspects of yoga. I consider yoga a call to the Divine that awakens the soul, and is proven to help with smoking cessation and heroin addiction.[77]

- Listen to music or chanting (or play music) that you enjoy. In a recent kundalini yoga class, I listened to the Guru Gayatri mantra (Gobinday Mukanday), which is believed to eliminate karmic blocks and past errors, balance the left and right brain hemispheres, and cultivate compassion and patience. See Appendix B for specific suggestions.

- Activate the right hemisphere of your brain with left nostril breathing (see the sidebar on page 132). I recommended left nostril breathing for three to eleven minutes in the body weight set point chapter because it interrupts overeating. Add it to your hyperarousal toolbox now to activate the parasympathetic nervous system and unwind purposefully.

Step 5: Bathe in a forest.

Yes, you can keep your clothes on. Sometimes I wonder if nature deficiency is at the root of addiction. In Japan, spending time in the forest is a serious activity and has led to the development of forest medicine.

They call it Shinrin-yoku, which translates as experiencing the forest atmosphere or forest bathing. In one study, walking in a forest environment altered dopamine activity, lowered blood pressure, and increased blood level of DHEAS (a growth and repair hormone, made in your adrenal glands) and adiponectin, that hormone that burns fat—compared with an urban walk next to a freeway.[78] (City dwellers, find a park with trees, away from the freeway.) Another study showed that forest bathing for twenty minutes lowered cortisol levels.[79] A total of twenty trials show the benefit of Shinrin-yoku on blood pressure, a measure of sympathetic tone, so why not try it?[80]

Step 6: Shift your mind-set.

Part of making appropriate lifestyle changes to increase your dopamine levels involves recognizing the distortions in your thinking that may be contributing to addictive tendencies. You can even think of them as *addictions of thought*. I have a PhD in negative thinking, criticism, fault finding, and seeing the differences everywhere I look—and it contributes to my old pattern of working myself into hyperarousal. Maybe you do the same. These are tendencies of left-hemisphere-dominated thought.

One promising area of research is *interoceptive awareness*: the ability to sense internal states such as satiety, hunger, pain, thirst. People with addiction have a deficit of interoceptive awareness. Yoga and mindfulness may improve interoceptive awareness or bring it back,[81] as long as one is careful not to swap one addiction for another and develop yogarexia—practicing excessively to bypass uncomfortable feelings, going to multiple yoga classes in a day, and becoming unhealthily obsessed about the length and intensity of daily practice.

So there are a few things you'll stop doing. You'll stop relying on willpower, a scarce resource, and build in habits and tools to prevent use of addictive substances, activities, and behaviors. You'll wean off constant hustle and image management, the drug of overworking or overproviding. You'll loosen your death grip on the thing you mistakenly believe you can't live without. You'll release some of those old resentments that are erosive and harmful, make you feel beleaguered, and block you from the sunshine of the spirit. In this portion of the Brain Body Diet, you'll take steps to heal the stress-response system and the HPA axis, and balance the sympathetic (fight-flight-freeze) and parasympathetic (rest-and-digest) nervous systems. You'll learn to transmute that feeling of "idling high"—which is how I experience the dominance of my left brain—with true energy from within. Here's what has helped me: getting a puppy, training our puppy, weighing myself only once per week (no exceptions), clearing out and simplifying my wardrobe, drinking more water (and no alcohol), giving up chocolate (because I can't be moderate), and asking myself what it will take to feel whole. Spend some time thinking about what you can do to ground yourself. Most essential of all: ask yourself what is your model of wholeness and integration, independent of other people's expectations and advice.

The following three tenets strongly support healing of the three aspects of addiction. Today, see how you can embrace these aspects of character in order to overcome addiction and be content with less.

Humility

I used to think of myself as humble. I'm from Alaska, where arrogance can get you killed. But the truth is that before my fainting episode where I hit my head, I was left-brain dominant: ego-driven, high-achieving, full of anger, resentment, and—I hate admitting this one—superiority. Maybe there's something about medical training that takes people who have a tendency toward arrogance and narcissism and turns them into creatures who think they are God-like. To survive medical training, particularly the surgical training to become an OB/GYN, you have to grow the ego strength to deal with life-and-death situations, which can occur with only a moment's notice. The problem is that the lack of humility blocks compassion, grace, and the connection to inner divinity. Humility is about being open-minded and willing, and seeing various situations with objective clarity. It's not perfectionistic, but it's being curious. So for you, humility may begin with the recognition and acceptance of your dopamine-challenged state and even your soft addictions. One simple practice that helps me is that when I'm starting to feel superior with someone, I will stop and look for similarities. It's a way of quieting the left brain and activating the right brain. James Baraz, who leads a course called Awakening Joy in Berkeley and wrote a book by the same name, suggests trying to see in each person you meet the desire to be safe, accepted, and loved—the same desire you have. Activate your right brain to see similarities, not differences.

Service

When I was a burned-out working mom turning thirty-five, if you told me to serve others, I might have punched you. But paradoxically, serving others gets me out of the self-centered fear at the root of my problem behaviors. Some of the fear dissolves simply by resetting my dopamine, but the truth is that I need not only a physical solution, but also a spiritual and mental solution. Humility gets me started on the path of healing, and service helps me get out of my own stuck wiring. It can be as simple as serving your family or friends, or broader by serving community or folks you don't know. It can be offering a kind word to your neighbor while walking your dog. Again from Baraz: Our joy practice is a gift we give to everyone we meet.

Structure

Most of us don't like to be hemmed in. We want freedom while simultaneously wanting security. Nevertheless, more structure is strangely freeing. For me, that means a daily hike in nature, ideally a forest, no matter the weather. It means that I call a friend or three every single day, even though I hate to talk on the phone. It means I meditate every morning for about thirty minutes, no matter what. I perform a kundalini kriya to regulate my neurohormonal dashboard. I eat regular meals, four to six hours apart, and that's nonnegotiable. The structure creates new and healthier habits in my brain that it starts to crave.

Step 7: Take time to muse.

Try meditation, such as with the Muse brain-sensing headband that gamifies your quiet time. Take it from me, addicts love games! We want to win! You can start like I did with Deepak Chopra's guidance, followed by ocean sounds that get louder if you're distracted and quieter when you're calm. When you maintain a calm mind, you hear bird sounds. Start with ten to twenty minutes, and slowly build up to thirty.

(No surprise, I get very competitive about how many birds I get in thirty minutes.)

Step 8: Add additional supplements that may help ease addictive behavior.

Now that you are creating a day that doesn't wind you up to the point where you need extreme measures to unwind again, you may consider adding one or more supplements from the list below. (If you are on prescription medications, talk to your pharmacist about any drug interactions first.)

- **A combination of amino acids,** including 5-HTP (5 mg), phenylalanine (300 mg), and glutamine (150 mg), reduced alcohol withdrawal symptoms in people undergoing hospital-based detoxification.[82] Anecdotally, others have found benefit in taking amino acid supplementation for other addictive behaviors.[83] More prospective clinical research is needed.

- **Huperzine A** increases dopamine and acetylcholine in animals, and may be helpful in treating drug addiction.[84] Dose: 200 to 400 mcg twice per day.

- **Progesterone** has been shown to reduce cravings in addiction, particularly in cocaine-addicted and food-addicted women. Progesterone may raise dopamine activity, at least in animals.[85] Doses of 400 mg per day for seven days helped women experience less negative emotion and a more relaxed mood when provoked by stress.[86] Dose: 200 to 400 mg at night, available by prescription, or you can start with a smaller dose as a progesterone transdermal cream, available online and at health food stores.

Last Word

A few years ago, my husband and I went on a double date with my friend Jo and her husband. They ordered most of the food on the menu and, together with my husband, drank two bottles of wine. I ordered a simple salad, steamed fish and vegetables, and sparkling water. As we left the restaurant afterward, I turned to Jo and said: "See, I'm just as fun off of flour, sugar, and alcohol!"

Jo didn't miss a beat. "Actually, you're not."

Sigh. It's okay, even amusing. My new model of wholeness isn't meant to satisfy anyone but me. It reveals my truth, not my mother's, my husband's, or even my friend's. I love the feeling of avoiding the extremes of hyperarousal and hypoarousal, the feeling of dopamine in balance—and I was able to recover from my addictive behaviors with the functional medicine protocol in this chapter. Like many of my patients, I could work around my genetic tendencies and the molecular adaptation that has occurred in my brain from past addictive behaviors with food and work. The amount of stress and tension that I used to carry in my body—in an effort to be perfect at work, and then perfect at home with my husband and kids—was eroding my life force. I sought solace in chocolate, wine, and overwork, similar to Marni. Now I can focus, but with clean energy—not idling high in hyperarousal, being pushy and snarky, running hard and fast on adrenaline and cortisol. I do less than five or ten years ago, and perform more service. My left and right hemispheres are in better balance. I no longer have that feeling that something's not quite right, that I'm unfulfilled. I am pleading with you to take a fresh look at what you may be medicating in your own life.

Marni is better too. After admitting she had a problem with alcohol, overexercising, and chocolate, she quit. She stopped trying to figure out how to drink less. She can't drink. She tried Alcoholics Anonymous, but it didn't speak to her, so instead she worked the Brain Body Diet. She realized the secret of addictive behaviors: address the hyperarousal. When you address the root cause and create a model of wholeness for yourself, steeped in tools to cope with hyperarousal so it rarely occurs, it's no longer defeat to give up the substance. It's freedom. Now she's been sober for two years; sleeps better; exercises one hour per day, four days per week; and no longer craves chocolate. She tells me, "I know I can't drink. There's no back door." She found freedom.

I suspect you will similarly love feeling liberated from obsession, despair, and resentment. You may be less fun, but prefer the loop of integrity: I eat what I say I will and go to bed whole, not fragmented and running debates incessantly in my head about what I ate, how much, and when I should have stopped. (Substitute your drug of choice: alcohol, pot, exercise, shopping.) My issues with addiction are no longer hidden behind a veneer of normalcy or even what others may perceive as success. I am open and honest about being in recovery, and now consider my addiction to be an important initiation into spiritual growth. Now that I've restored homeostasis in my reward circuit, I have much healthier ways to tame the tension and have stopped using substances (food, alcohol) and activities (spending, exercise) to fill the spiritual hole.

The power of the human brain is extraordinary when it's freed from addiction in any form. The brain thrives on breaking out of compulsion, obsession, and addiction cycles. You become more stress resilient. You're more fun to be with, and healthier people are attracted to you, my friend notwithstanding. You're present to the pain and suffering of others. You are of service, so that you're no longer part of the problem, but part of the solution. That's the power of escaping the pleasure trap—the power of the addictive mind once it's recovered. Extraordinary things can happen. We have an untapped potential in terms of awareness and consciousness. This isn't a path of deprivation and despair, but a path toward light and freedom.

6

Anxiety

How to Calm Down Overactive Wiring, Manage Stressful Thoughts, and Turn On the Brain/Body Healing System

What gives you angst? Turbulence on a flight, bills you can't afford, a visit from your in-laws, your kid learning to drive? Anxiety has been considered a medical disorder since the time of Hippocrates. Ancient Greek physicians didn't believe anxiety was purely psychological, though philosophers like the Epicureans and Stoics offered techniques to reach an anxiety-free state of mind by directing thought and limiting pleasure in order to attain a state of tranquility, free of fear and absent of bodily pain.

While I agree with Hippocrates that anxiety is a medical—that is, brain/body—condition, I don't agree with what strikes me as a masculine, brain-down approach to solving it merely by controlling thought and reducing pleasure. For a woman with anxiety, that's just not enough—or even possible! Act-right, think-right (i.e., calm down enough to philosophize objectively about one's anxious brain body)? No, thanks. Not helpful.

As you may understand by now, I believe in a broader, food-centered, lifestyle-driven brain/body solution. Taken further, food is the greatest lever, the most important environmental factor, when it comes to repairing the brain/body disconnection that results in anxiety and the other issues we address in previous and upcoming chapters. Unfortunately, the word *diet* has lost the richness that it had during Hippocrates's time. As I mentioned in the introduction, the Greeks defined diet (*diaita*) as a "manner of living" that's prescribed by a physician—signifying not only a personal dietary regimen but also other daily habits that help you lead, govern, and arbitrate your life—a day's journey for the health of your brain body.

In this chapter, I want you to immerse yourself in a prescribed way of living that will get your brain and body back into peaceful alignment, free of the suffering that results from anxious thoughts and feelings, no longer clinging to things beyond your control and creating an unnecessary orgy of stress. That's the lifestyle medicine of the Brain Body Diet, to create a balanced state of body, mind, and spirit—starting first with simple additions of food and lifestyle tools to your daily regimen.

Anxiety is like a radio that's not tuned to a strong frequency. There's no clear connection to a strong signal; instead, the radio projects a lot of noise and overlapping messages—and a clear, calm, enduring picture in your mind is your birthright, a true sign of healthy homeostasis. Homeostasis includes diet-driven neurogenesis,[1] new brain cell growth that increases happy brain chemicals like serotonin and improves mood, and synaptogenesis,[2] new connections between brain cells that keep you calm and resourceful. If your brain body is gently nudged back into congruence, you will no longer have to accept worry as an inescapable fact of life.

What creates the noise, the inability to tune the radio of the brain to the proper channel? What I didn't learn in medical school is that the noise of anxiety often starts in the body, such as from food intolerances that create unnecessary stress and high cortisol levels, hijacking the gut/brain connection and sending your neurohormonal system into overdrive. Or maybe it starts from toxic exposure like glyphosate (the main ingredient in the most common herbicide), or from an infection like Lyme disease or gastroenteritis (a stomach bug), or from the excess use of antibiotics.

My level of anxiety ratcheted up several notches in the past year when I discovered new brain/body concerns. First, I was diagnosed with fresh food intolerances because of my leaky gut. I had known for years about gluten and dairy and avoided them, but now I had intolerances to other delicious foods: beer, wine, coffee, grains (even gluten-free), quinoa, certain vegetables that were high in oxalates (kale, spinach, chard, beets, etc.), nuts, white meat, tempeh, beans, tubers like potatoes and yams, all sweeteners, chocolate(!), and many fruits. What's left to eat? Cucumbers and salmon? Second, I was prescribed several long courses of wide-spectrum antibiotics for multiple surgeries in 2017. Antibiotics wipe out the bad bacteria, but they also kill the good bugs that can keep you calm and content. Repeated courses of antibiotics are associated with a 17 to 44 percent increased risk of anxiety, and 23 to 56 percent greater rate of depression.[3] Not only that, but antibiotics increase the risk of obesity, diabetes, autoimmune disease, and learning and memory problems.[4]

Like Hippocrates, I believe disease begins in the gut, and anxiety is no exception. He was thousands of years ahead of his time, but now cutting-edge research shows that gut bugs can change the actions of your amygdala (the brain's center of fear), hippocampus (the center of emotional regulation and memory), and prefrontal cortex (the CEO of your brain).[5] So if we assume that anxiety begins in the gut, then *it must be healed in the gut first,* as well as by directing thought as suggested by the Stoic philosophers about twenty-two hundred years ago. Brain/body breakdown must be healed with a brain/body solution.

Unfortunately, anxiety is a conventional medicine label, which on its own means very little. It doesn't tell you why you have it—why your brain body broke down and the radio signal is fuzzy—and fails to offer a complete solution. Everything you do in a day affects your brain and risk of anxiety: what you (and what you don't) put on your fork, how you move, how you sleep, how you expose yourself to toxins in the environment, how you host microbes in your gut, and yes, how you think. Likewise, when you feel anxious or have been diagnosed with anxiety (and perhaps offered a pill), these are the very same ways to reset the brain body so you feel calm, pill-free.

Even if you don't relate to the term *anxiety,* you may feel the same underlying current of dread in other ways: inner turmoil; frenzy, like you're too rattled to calm down; churning; feeling overwhelmed; constant fight-flight-freeze (especially freeze) response; inability to cope;

irritability; uneasiness; restlessness; déjà vu; or a blank mind. These are all symptoms of anxiety that create the same physiological and bio-chemical states in the brain and body. It can feel automatic, beyond your conscious control. For me last year, anxiety showed up as a fear of dying during surgery that I couldn't get out of my mind—more than I imagine is normal, particularly for someone who had been on the other side of the knife for thousands of surgeries.

Take Karen as an example. We all fret from time to time, but some of us worry beyond what is helpful or adaptive. While stress combined with anxiety is inevitable, how we deal with it is not. Karen was forty-five when she first came to see me. She was warm and friendly, but I could sense that she felt tired and wired. She was highly successful as a professional journalist and professor at a local college, but three main worries occupied her thoughts:

1. my type 1 diabetic son won't wake up in the morning,
2. my children will die before me, and
3. all of the doctors I've been seeing are wrong and I have some awful diagnosis that they are missing.

Karen was so busy between work and taking care of her children and husband that she rarely had time for herself. Exercise and other ways to de-stress were a distant memory, and her jeans kept getting tighter. Symptoms worsened in the second half of her menstrual cycle from ovulation until her period began: "Doomed. I literally feel doomed." She had a prescription for alprazolam (Xanax) on hand for her worst moments, and was reluctant to try the antidepressant paroxetine (Paxil) that had just been prescribed by another doctor. (Meta-analysis shows that paroxetine has a modest if any effect on anxiety.[6]) She explained, "The Xanax numbs me out but doesn't solve any problems." Her stress, anxiety, and fitful sleep were affecting her work and relationships, even though her symptoms didn't cross a line into serious mental illness.

You may feel anxious just reading about Karen, so focus instead on the story of how we unraveled the underlying dietary, medical, emo-tional, and psychological roots of her sense of doom, and what we did to get her to the point she's at today, almost entirely free of anxiety.

Anxiety is the emotional experience of a fight-flight-freeze physio-

logical state. Consistent across all feelings that fall under the heading
of anxiety is an overreactive set of thoughts, a mind that cultivates
counterproductive responses to a given situation. The thoughts are felt
emotionally (dread, overwhelm, panic, etc.) *and* physically (breathless-
ness, heart racing, sweating, chest pain or discomfort, etc.). Similar to
the reward deficiency syndrome that we addressed in the last chapter
on addiction, anxiety shows us that the control system for emotions,
thoughts, and behaviors can get out of whack. Evolution has primed us
to be this way—and it takes a new level of awareness and discernment
to bring the brain and body back into balance.

It took peeling back the layers of my own anxiety and that of my patients to befriend and ultimately heal that anxious feeling, which has
been thought to originate in the brain's amygdala, but may actually
start in the gut (as has been found in mice). Emerging data suggest that
communication between the gut and brain plays a key role in the development of anxiety, depression, and cognition—meaning that you need
healthy and diverse microbiota in order to develop healthy and diverse
feelings, thoughts, and habits.[7] For instance, normal lab mice that have
their microbiota removed and then receive fecal transplants from mice
bred to be anxious become anxious mice.[8] For them, and perhaps humans, anxiety didn't *begin* in the brain; it began in the body but led to
too much excitation in the brain. Parts of their brain then change phys-
iologically, including the amygdala and hippocampus, and the problem
is now a brain/body imbalance with anxious behavior.[9] As another example, glyphosate, the key ingredient in the most common herbicide
used worldwide (Roundup), can induce leaky gut, anxiety, depression,
and cognitive changes in mice.[10] The same may be happening to you.

Once again, the gut affects the brain, and then the brain affects the
gut. The way we fix it starts with food—removing the foods that tend
to overexcite the gut and brain, and adding more of the foods that calm
the gut and brain.

Anxiety can be a waste of valuable resources, usually over something
you cannot control. It is like a trance that is accompanied by tight muscles, chaos, and missing out on life, all of which originate in a stress-
response system that is inappropriately heightened. Nevertheless, it is
within your power to grow more calm, de-stress, and restore an appro-

priate stress response. Given a smart protocol and your commitment, the trance can be broken.

Do You Have Anxiety?

Do you have now or have you had in the past six months any of the following symptoms or conditions?

☐ Did you have significant early life stress as a child or as an adult, including abuse or maltreatment? Did you worry about financial security while growing up, or now?

☐ Do you have trouble with sleep, such as falling asleep, staying asleep, and/or nightmares?

☐ Are you experiencing more shyness, introversion, or desire to avoid social gatherings than you used to?

☐ Do you have a parent (or another close relative) who is anxious or frequently worried? Do you have family members with trauma?

☐ Have you experienced any *physical* symptoms of stress, such as startling easily, upset stomach, diarrhea, constipation, dry mouth, tiring easily, shortness of breath, vertigo, sweating, palpitations, tinnitus, frequent urination, increased muscle aches or soreness or tension (such as an eye twitch or needing to tap your feet), bruxism (excessive grinding or clenching of teeth), pain at the temporomandibular junction (TMJ), or difficulty when trying to relax?

☐ Have you experienced any *cognitive* symptoms of stress, such as impaired concentration, feeling the mind go blank, irritability, edginess, restlessness, perseveration, or restlessness?

☐ Do you have "nervous" energy—too much to do, too far behind, hard to wind down, frenetic?

☐ Do you have worry that is out of proportion to actual risk?

☐ Have you undergone perimenopause or menopause (usually age forty-plus)? Do you have hot flashes or night sweats?

☐ Do you have severe fears that affect your quality of life—such as a fear of being alone, of the dark, or of strangers?

☐ Do you have the need for reassurance and soothing from others about your worry?

☐ Do you suffer from persistent negative thoughts you can't seem to stop?

☐ Do you feel overwhelmed, like you have insufficient coping skills for the tasks you face?

☐ Do you have elevated blood sugar or afternoon cortisol levels?

INTERPRETATION

If you answered yes to five or more of the questions above, you may have a tendency toward anxiety. It's easy to reverse anxious symptoms if you get help early. Excessive and disproportionate worry about a variety of topics for six months or more that is very difficult to control *and* combined with three or more cognitive or physical symptoms means it's time to talk to a licensed mental health professional or doctor about whether you have an anxiety disorder. Another clue that you should see a clinician is if you feel like you're worrying too much and it's interfering with relationships, work, or other aspects of your life. Some people with anxiety also feel depressed, have difficulty with alcohol or drug use (addiction), or have other mental health concerns—again, see a collaborative clinician. Read on to learn more about anxiety, the root cause, and how to calm down and reset your brain pathways.

State or Trait?

Occasional worry is adaptive, a temporary feeling that is proportionate to the stressor and resolves after you deal with the stressor. It's triggered by the amygdala for survival. However, there's a point when the anxious feeling becomes something less benign: the unconscious anxiety habit.

Anxiety can be a state or trait. As a *state*, it's an unpleasant emotional hyperarousal in the face of a threat. As a *trait*, it's a personality construct or the tendency to respond in anticipation of a threat. It's a poor habit of thinking you may develop without awareness that "reinforces and facilitates the 'worry pathways' between the prefrontal cortex, the anterior cingulate gyrus, the amygdala and other midbrain structures involved in the emotional and stress responses to a feared outcome," according to my friend and colleague Martin Rossman, MD, author of *The Worry Solution*.

For example, my husband was anxious driving in a parking garage while his favorite road bike was on the roof rack—his *state* of anxiety was rare for him and temporary. His cognitive appraisal of the situation— low ceiling, tall bike—prompted his state of anxiety. The anxiousness was warranted; we hit a cement barrier on the ceiling and broke his bike frame. Fortunately, he has a high level of self-efficacy, and his anxiety resolved when we exited the garage, although it was replaced by frustration and the immediate need to fix the bike.

On the other hand, my patient Laurie has anxiety as a *trait*. When she receives news, good or bad, she wants to immediately process everything wrong that could happen and needs reassurance and validation, a feature of anxiety. Although Laurie is a strong woman, she often doesn't feel competent to cope with challenging demands—and tries to control things beyond her control—so she worries and becomes *more* anxious.

As a trait, anxiety doesn't resolve when you make a decision or when a big presentation is over. The anxious feelings may impair school performance, your job or career, or relationships. It may even get worse over time.

Whether a state or trait, anxiety robs you of mental health. According to the National Institute of Mental Health, anxiety disorders affect at least forty million adults in the United States, with a prevalence of 18 percent of the adult population.[11] As the mother of a fourteen-year-old daughter, I'm horrified to learn that 38 percent of girls ages thirteen to seventeen, and 26 percent of boys, struggle with an anxiety disorder. The average age of onset is eleven.[12]

There are a few types of anxiety disorders: generalized anxiety disorder, panic disorder, social anxiety disorder, and post-traumatic stress disorder (PTSD).

Perhaps most ominous is the fact that psychiatrists consider anxiety to be a "gateway" condition that can lead to deeper issues such as depression, suicide, addiction, and fibromyalgia. Not only are body and brain health interdependent, but mental health also reflects brain health and vice versa. It's bidirectional. That's why I encourage anyone with anxiety symptoms to see a clinician for a complete evaluation that includes a workup for medical causes.

The Anxious Sex

As with depression, women have higher rates of anxiety compared with men, including a 33 percent lifetime risk of experiencing anxiety. (By comparison, a woman's lifetime risk of breast cancer is 12 percent.) Experts blame the difference on brain chemistry, hormones, gender inequalities (i.e., less pay for equal work, more chores at home, more childcare), response to stress, and sociocultural conditioning, meaning women tend to feel responsible for the happiness of others, such as a spouse or kids.[13] Women ruminate more over life stressors, whereas men generally engage in more active, problem-focused coping. Women have a greater probability of being victims of physical and mental abuse than men, leading to brain changes such as lower blood flow to the emotional regulation center (the hippocampus) and the development of anxiety disorders. Cigarette smoking and alcohol are also associated with greater anxiety, especially in women.[14]

In my research and clinical experience, women are more likely to have a problem with the control system for their sex hormones (the HPA axis), and this may make us more vulnerable to anxiety and depression. (Because the HPA is a feedback loop by which signals from the brain trigger the release of hormones needed to respond to stress, the HPA axis is also sometimes called the stress circuit.) Women with anxiety or depression have a blunted or dampened cortisol stress response, meaning they've become more numb to threat and the normal production of cortisol—they have a "burned-out" HPA axis—whereas men are the opposite: they have an increased cortisol response to stress.[15] (As noted later in this chapter, toxins can cause problems with the HPA, too.) Post-traumatic stress disorder, which is twice as common in women, involves a failure to reinstate physiological homeostasis after a traumatic event.[16]

Anxiety can also occur during different life transitions for women, such as while pregnant (perinatal anxiety) or after menopause. Approximately 20 percent of pregnant women experience anxiety and depression.[17] (Note that anxiety is *a response to perceived threat*, whereas depression is a *response to perceived harm or loss*.[18] Of course, there's overlap between them; depression is more prevalent in anxious people, and anxiety is more prevalent in depressed people, but I still find the distinction to be helpful.)

What Causes Anxiety

Freud believed anxiety reflected inner emotional conflict. Now we have a more biological understanding of anxiety, but the truth is that anxiety results from the interplay of many genetic, biochemical, trau-

UNITED STATES OF ATIVAN

Most people think of anxiety as a personality type or a medical or psychological condition, but increasingly I wonder if it's also a sociological condition—"a shared cultural experience that feeds on alarmist CNN graphics and metastasizes through social media."[19] Every time you open a tab on the web or turn on the news, you get assaulted with crime, shootings, terrorism, beheadings, and all sorts of dramatic human rights violations. It can mess with your head. Yet news organizations sometimes seem to leverage intrusive and emotionally charged images so you watch and click. Get this: rates of PTSD and depression increased 5 to 20 percent for adults and children after the news coverage of the 9/11 terrorist attacks.[20] Women had double the risk.[21] Research demonstrates that exposure to war trauma before age ten increases one's risk of developing internalizing disorders later, including a 17 percent risk of anxiety and 13 percent risk of mood disorders.[22]

Then there's social media: studies show that Facebook and similar outlets may make certain vulnerable people feel inadequate, excessively worried, disconnected, lonely, fearful, and stressed. Anxiety-inducing, perhaps? I think so. Having a large number of followers or "friends" is associated with higher cortisol, which is then linked with chronic stress, worry, burnout, and depression.[23] More American teenagers than ever are suffering from severe anxiety, simultaneously with unprecedented use and overuse of smartphones and social media.[24]

Given the stressors that we all face, the new normal is to pop a pharmaceutical drug like Xanax or Ativan when you feel freaked, but that is not normal at all.

matic, social, emotional, and psychological factors. Importantly, frequent anxiety can rewire the brain to produce *more* anxiety because the body and the brain feed off each other. Think of it like a callus, or thickened skin, that develops when you repeat certain activities. If you keep repeating the activity, the callus just grows bigger and tougher. You have to change the activity to heal the callus and return your skin to normal. So our goal is to rewire anxious pathways toward balance and health.

We still don't completely understand all of the causes of anxiety, but here are the consistent risk factors:

- female sex
- heredity/genetics
- childhood maltreatment or abuse
- traumatic events, from car accidents to natural disasters
- accumulated stress, including financial[25] and occupational (health care workers, teachers, police officers, attorneys)[26]
- toxins such as BPA, which can disrupt the function of the HPA axis,[27] and glyphosate, which can disrupt gut wall integrity[28]
- certain microbiota that can affect the anxiety regions of the brain and can be reversed by eating probiotic food as mentioned in the Brain Body Diet[29]
- drug withdrawal, including from substances such as alcohol[30]
- certain internalizing personalities, which are more prone to anxiety than others
- medical issues, such as blood sugar problems (prediabetes and diabetes), heart disease, thyroid dysfunction, respiratory disorders (asthma, chronic obstructive pulmonary disease or COPD), chronic pain, irritable bowel syndrome, and rare tumors like pheochromocytoma that produce "fight-flight-freeze" hormones
- other mental health conditions, such as depression

The downstream consequences of anxiety include substance use disorder (particularly drugs that temporarily allay anxiety, like benzodiazepines, alcohol, or opioids), sleeping problems, digestive issues, headaches, chronic pain, social isolation, difficulty functioning at work or school, poor quality of life, increased inflammation, depression, and even suicide.

HORMONAL CAUSES OF ANXIETY SYMPTOMS

If you suffer from anxiety, consider this list of hormonal imbalances that can cause symptoms of anxiety. Sex hormones and neurotransmitters in the brain interact, contributing to imbalances. Always address the root cause before resorting to medication.[31]

1. Dysregulated cortisol—high or low, or both within the same day

2. Insulin resistance—high insulin and high blood sugar

3. Thyroid dysfunction—usually high, but low thyroid function can also mimic anxiety symptoms

4. Low estrogen

5. Low progesterone

Women in perimenopause and menopause with hot flashes and night sweats are more likely to develop anxiety, more fears, decreased memory and concentration, poor sleep, and somatic complaints (like muscle pain) when they are experiencing symptoms of low estrogen and low progesterone.[32] Poor sleep can then exacerbate other hormonal problems, such as dysregulated cortisol and insulin resistance. Additionally, anxiety can make a woman three times more likely to have hot flashes.[33] On the other hand, evaluation of anxiety and depression during the menopausal transition is tricky because of the overlap between symptoms of anxiety and depression and symptoms of menopause.[34] Certainly lifestyle-based approaches like removing caffeine, eliminating foods that may trigger a stress response (gluten, dairy), exercise, and cognitive behavioral therapy are warranted, and if not helpful, a trial of estrogen and/or progesterone may help (see the protocol and discuss with your clinician). Overall, the evidence is not yet clear that supplemental estrogen[35] and/or progesterone[36] directly improve anxiety in women, although depressed women seem to benefit. The estrogen receptors have differential effects on anxiety. Estrogen receptor alpha is mostly anxiogenic (increases anxiety), and estrogen receptor beta is anxiolytic (lessens anxiety). Siberian rhubarb (*Rheum rhaponticum L.*) stimulates estrogen receptor beta preferentially and is shown in multiple clinical trials to reduce anxiety in perimenopause and menopause.[37]

Treatment: The Downside of Downers

We've come a long way in the past fifty years with how we treat heart disease and cancer, but not anxiety. In 1998, when I first took over the practice of a retiring physician, it seemed that almost all of his patients were taking diazepam, a tranquilizer that goes by the brand name Valium (often identified as the "little yellow pill" from the song "Mother's Little Helper" by the Rolling Stones) and one of the earliest benzodiazepines, a drug used to treat anxiety. (Valium was launched in 1963.) I was not taught as a gynecologist to medicate away my patients' existential worries with pharmaceuticals, so I rebelled and refused to carry on the tradition. What's the big deal? A lot, apparently. First, "benzos" are addictive, so I began the rather unpopular campaign of getting many hundreds of these unsuspecting but addicted women off benzos. Second, when you take an anti-anxiety pill like diazepam (Valium) for three to six months, you raise the risk of developing Alzheimer's disease by 32 percent. Take it for more than six months, and your risk goes up 84 percent.[38] Third, women who are diagnosed with breast cancer who are taking medication for anxiety are 48 percent more likely to develop heart disease, although it's not clear whether this increased risk is from taking the drug, having anxiety, or both.[39] Finally, diazepam can cause paranoid or suicidal ideation; impair memory, judgment, and coordination; and, when combined with alcohol, may slow breathing and kill you.

Just like in the practice I inherited, women are dismissed with a prescription for drugs rather than receiving a more nuanced and integrated approach that includes targeted diet and lifestyle changes first. The prescription drugs most commonly used to relieve anxiety are as follows:

- specific antidepressants, such as escitalopram (known by brand names Lexapro and Cipralex). These are primarily SSRIs.
- an anti-anxiety medication called buspirone (brand name BuSpar)
- sedatives called benzodiazepines (mentioned earlier)

So if you are taking a benzo, talk to your prescribing clinician about another approach, such as the functional medicine protocol in this chap-

ter. Several studies confirm that people who are on a long-acting benzodiazepine like diazepam (Valium) or flurazepam (Dalmane) are at
greater risk than those on a short-acting one like triazolam (Halcion),
lorazepam (Ativan), alprazolam (Xanax), or temazepam (Restoril).[40]
Correlation is not causation, but there is sufficient concern to warrant
trying other methods. In fact, for people sixty-five and older, downers
can make you more likely to suffer a fall, injury, or accidental overdose.
Maybe it's time to consider benzos inappropriate for anxiety.

Are SSRIs instead of benzos a good idea? No. SSRIs have their own
risks. While they help some severe cases, about one in three people
with anxiety disorders don't respond to SSRIs, and many others can't
tolerate the side effects, such as diminished sexual function, birth defects, or possibly cancer (although data are mixed).[41] The most common
SSRIs—fluoxetine, sertraline, and paroxetine—interact with the estrogen receptor.[42] So taking an antidepressant like an SSRI can hinder the
normal function of estrogen in the body (whether that contributes to
an increased risk of breast cancer is doubtful,[43] but limited data suggest
that if you develop cancer while on an SSRI, your outcome might be
worse[44]). Post-SSRI sexual dysfunctions—including altered libido, difficulty with orgasm, vaginal dryness, and ejaculatory disorders—occur
frequently, do not always resolve when you stop the SSRI, and may persist indefinitely.[45]

I need to add that there is a time and place for medical treatment of
anxiety. As Kendrick Lamar, one of my favorite songwriters and rap-
pers, states in his song "HUMBLE": "Watch my soul speak, you let the
meds talk, ay." No question, some of us need to let the meds talk, and we
also need a better way. Let's no longer accept being numbed out for our
emotional upheavals. Anxiety is not only a waste of valuable time, brain
resources, and body resources (i.e., unnecessarily sweating, upsetting
the stomach, racing the heart, tensing and guarding, etc.), but it worsens your brain function over time—further contributing to anxiety via
worsening brain/body balance. Fortunately, the anxious pathways can
be blocked off and new healthier grooves can be made with yoga, cognitive behavioral training, and meditation, but not with pharmaceuticals.
Let's determine the root cause and treat it with a functional medicine
protocol, which may include psychotherapy.

The Science of Anxiety

If reading more about the science makes you feel overwhelmed or anxious, skip this section and head straight to the protocol.

If you feel tense, overwhelmed, or anxious but don't pass the strict tests that clinicians use for generalized anxiety disorder, panic disorder, or social phobia, this content is especially for you.

Note that this chapter is intended to educate you about anxiety and to offer root cause analysis for those of you who meet criteria based on the questionnaire at the beginning.

THE AMYGDALA

Remember the last time you freaked out? For me, it was last summer when a vacation house we rented had mice in the kitchen. Eww!

Freak-outs and breakdowns start in the amygdala, the pair of almond-shaped structures deep in the temporal lobe, and belonging to the oldest part of your brain (sometimes called the reptilian or ancient brain) that constantly surveys your environment for threat. When you're chronically stressed out, feeling the ceaseless frenzy that something is wrong (e.g., you need to be somewhere else, doing something else), *your amygdala grows in size,* similar to how a muscle grows and reshapes when you work it hard at the gym. This kind of workout, though, is *not* a good thing. Even worse, as your threat center expands, your resourceful, thinking brain—the prefrontal cortex—shrinks.

CORTISOL: HIGH, LOW, OR BOTH?

Robert Sapolsky, a professor of biology, neurology, and neuroscience at Stanford University, wrote several groundbreaking books about stress and the risk of the ongoing, persistent release of stress hormones. Among animals, dominant animals like lions fare better than subordinate animals like mice, because being lower in the social hierarchy is associated with excess stress, which translates biochemically into increased corticotropin-releasing hormone (CRH), the precursor to cortisol. Over time, subordinate animals develop a less sensitive and nimble control system (i.e., the HPA axis—the ultimate brain/body loop—becomes numb). The problem is similar in humans, but a little more complex:

- Chronic stress leads to several physical and functional brain problems that increase the risk of anxiety.[46] Pathological features are diminished neurogenesis and loss of behavioral flexibility,[47] becoming overweight, and sexual dysfunction.[48]

- Anxiety is a manifestation, along with depression and addiction, of an impaired stress response. Think of anxiety as a restriction stress response. Over time, cortisol levels are lowered by 17 percent in anxiety disorders such as PTSD, probably due to the preceding period of hyperactivity, and now reflect an exhausted phase.

- Most studies suggest that the imbalance of CRH and cortisol that makes the HPA axis hyperactive occurs in people with anxiety, depression, or PTSD. Even more interesting, the heightened stress response predates the mental diagnosis and may be associated with certain genetic variations of the key stress genes (FKBP5, CYP1A2, FAAH, WWC1, MR, TH). Being aware of this issue presents health care providers and citizen scientists with a golden opportunity to intervene before all the bad stuff takes over. Another anxiety gene is the regulator of G protein signaling 2 (RGS2), associated with generalized anxiety disorder, panic disorder, PTSD, suicide, and overall intermediate levels of anxiety.[49]

- The biggest problem in dysregulation of the HPA axis is that you keep feeling stressed even when the threat is gone. The state becomes a habitual trait while the brain and the body continue to hype each other up. What happens is the HPA axis fails to suppress certain control hormones—including CRH and adrenocorticotropic hormone (ACTH, the hormone that signals your adrenals to produce more cortisol), meaning that the stress response doesn't get turned off properly.

Basically, when you're under too much stress for too long, you make too much CRH and therefore too much cortisol, and then your feedback loop becomes toast. It's like when you watch a violent movie, and at first you're shocked by the swearing, high-speed car chases, and brutal shootings. But by the end of the film, you're inured to and barely notice the violence. That's what happens to your HPA: it gets overactivated, and then as the HPA feedback system compensates, it barely reacts to the same images. Homeostasis is broken. Then you don't make the appropriate amounts of the control hormones when you actually need them.

Not only that, but the combination of heightened stress and high cortisol also shrinks your brain, damages your hippocampus, decreases brain activity, causes cognitive impairment, and increases your risk of other medical conditions, including anxiety disorders, inflammation, cardiovascular disease, depression, obesity, prediabetes and diabetes, autoimmune disorders, Alzheimer's disease, certain cancers, and other diseases of aging—an unhealthy feedback loop between your brain and your body.[50] Plenty of good reasons to calm your life down! Thankfully, in his work, Sapolsky discerned what helps: a sense of control and autonomic flexibility—basically, your ability to roll with the punches of life (or more technically, the ability to respond to stress with a broader range of adaptation, both biologically and behaviorally—which we'll address in the protocol).

SLEEP DISTURBANCE

Lack of sleep activates the sympathetic nervous system (fight-flight-freeze) via the HPA, again leading to an overactive stress response, anxiety symptoms, and underactivity of the parasympathetic nervous system (rest-and-digest).[51] So you lose your ability to rest and digest—a rather crucial feature of stress recovery and reversal of anxiety! As with other root causes of anxiety, the effect is bidirectional: anxiety can interfere with a restful night of sleep, and chronic sleep deprivation can trigger anxiety disorders and, as you'll read in the next chapter, depression.

GUT/BRAIN AXIS IN ANXIETY

The foundation of the brain/body connection is the gut/brain axis. Your microbiome is the DNA belonging to the three to five pounds of microbes, mostly bacteria, located in your gastrointestinal tract. That's a lot of DNA; the DNA of your body's microbes outnumber your own host cells a hundred to one. Not long ago, scientists observed that the gut microbes and their DNA may strongly affect our behavior, and alterations in the composition of your gut microbes (or their metabolic products) could be at the root of psychiatric and somatic complaints and disease in humans, including anxiety, depression, pain response, and irritable bowel syndrome.[52]

When your gut microbes digest your food, the nutrients or toxins you've consumed enter your bloodstream and go straight to your brain through the blood-brain barrier. People who eat more processed foods and carbohydrates are more likely to experience anxiety because it messes with the health of the microbiome. On the other hand, a good microbiome, rich in lactobacillus (found in yogurt, kefir, sauerkraut, microalgae, and miso, as long as they are not pasteurized or subjected to high heat) and bifidobacteria (also found in yogurt and fermented vegetables, like kimchi, sauerkraut, and pickled vegetables), may increase BDNF, the growth factor that acts like fertilizer for the brain—allowing you to focus and perform executive functions—and BDNF is more likely to prevent depression.[53] In animals, the gut microbes are intimately involved in brain development, anxiety, other emotional behaviors, how the HPA axis responds to stress and pain, and the interaction of brain chemicals.[54]

Here's further evidence of the connection between gut and anxiety: food intolerances increase psychological distress—but in women, not men.[55] Food intolerances (common in adults) and food allergies (common in babies and children) are increasing in prevalence at rates of up to 20 percent, although determination of true prevalence is challenging.[56] Food allergies are associated with greater internalization of emotions, lower quality of life, and more mental health problems.[57] In a study of 1,641 outpatients with gastrointestinal disorders, 84 percent had state anxiety and 67 percent had trait anxiety—furthermore, 27 percent had depression. Rates were higher—as expected—in women. The state anxiety was associated with food allergies, small intestinal bacterial overgrowth (SIBO), *Helicobacter pylori* (Hp) infection, and ulcerative colitis in active phase. Trait anxiety was linked to food allergies, small intestinal bacterial overgrowth (SIBO), irritable bowel syndrome, and Hp infection.[58]

That brings us to potential solutions. Could shifting your microbes and their DNA lessen anxiety? In a small study of twelve healthy adult women at UCLA, eating a type of yogurt that contained four different types of bacteria twice per day for a month was associated with a change in the brain activity (specifically, in the midbrain), as measured by imaging the areas involved in anxiety, irritable bowel syndrome, and pain.[59]

Because problems with the microbiome are associated with both anxiety and depression, if you follow the protocol outlined in the toxin chapter—rich in vegetables, fruits, fish, anti-inflammatory meats, and probiotic foods—you may prevent your microbiome from creating anxiety. The main takeaway is that altering your microbiota with the right food and lifestyle may improve your brain function.[60]

OVERTAXING THE NERVOUS SYSTEM

When you're highly stressed, the chemical load is more than you can bear, and you lose homeostasis. Your balance between the sympathetic nervous system and the parasympathetic nervous system falls out of whack. Chronic stress overactivates the sympathetic nervous system and underactivates the parasympathetic nervous system. You also make less GABA, nature's benzodiazepine. You may be more vulnerable to overtaxing the nervous system and losing homeostasis because of your genetics (including variations in the NPSR1 gene, BDNF, CLOCK, or oxytocin receptor gene, OXTR),[61] inheriting an epigenetic change from your mother (such as in the gene FK506 binding protein 5, or FKBP5, a gene involved in the stress-response system),[62] previous experiences including your trauma survival,[63] even your own experiences in utero.[64] Microbiota shifts may increase your risk, as I've just described. In the protocol, we will reset the stress-response system, the balance between the sympathetic and parasympathetic nervous systems, microbiome, and other ways that your body is in conversation with your brain. That's what I did with my patient Karen.

Back to Karen's Anxiety

When I first met Karen, she was waking up between 2 and 4 a.m., ruminating on her to-do list, her son's diabetes, and her classroom demands. Her labs showed probable insulin resistance with a high fasting glucose, borderline high blood sugar for the past three months based on hemoglobin A1C, and low vitamin D (see Notes for details[65]). Her anxiety raised her blood sugar because her stress-response system wasn't working properly. Higher blood sugar led to more belly fat, a risk factor for metabolic syndrome.

Here's what I recommended:

- Remove alcohol, caffeine, flour, sugar, artificial sweeteners, and processed foods since they may increase anxiety, especially premenstrual anxiety.

- Begin taking a softgel containing lavender oil, which has been used for its calming properties as aromatherapy, although we used a special formulation orally for anxiety and to improve her sleep. In the brain, lavender essential oil and its main components act on the activity that impacts anxiety, including the glutamate receptor (NMDA), serotonin-1A receptor, serotonin transporter, and calcium channels in the brain.[66] She took it as needed for relief of worry instead of the Xanax because it is highly effective against anxiety in clinical trials, non-habit-forming, and well tolerated.[67] Additionally, the preparation is helpful in people with mixed anxiety and depression.[68]

- Start magnesium and B vitamins, especially B_6 since it reduces PMS-related anxiety.[69] Vitamin B_6 is involved in the production of many neurotransmitters, including serotonin, which controls mood, sleep, and appetite, and dopamine, which is involved in pleasure, reward, learning, and satisfaction. Be cautious: higher-than-recommended doses of B_6 can cause nerve toxicity. She began a dose of 50 mg of vitamin B_6 plus 200 mg of magnesium, as recommended in a clinical trial to help premenstrual anxiety.

- Begin 5,000 IU of vitamin D_3 per day, with a plan to recheck levels in six weeks.

- Add fish to her diet. Low dietary and blood levels of omega-3 fatty acids are associated with anxiety.[70] Omega-3 fatty acids have been shown to reduce anxiety and to modulate cortisol levels.[71] Karen began a dose of 2,000 to 4,000 mg per day.

- Start craniosacral therapy to calm the overdrive in her sympathetic nervous system. "I think craniosacral therapy is above everything else for my parasympathetic nervous system," Karen says. "All my anxiety symptoms go away temporarily. It's subtle but profound." Just be certain to find someone who is properly trained and certified by the Osteopathic Cranial Academy.[72]

- Make a "stop-doing list" in the office and begin a to-do list for her own body's needs, like for sleep, joy, relaxation, and exercise. Exercise for a minimum of thirty minutes, alternating high intensity for sixty seconds with a one- to two-minute recovery. Karen likes to walk near her home in Berkeley, and would alternate a rapid, full-effort brisk walk with a more moderate walk. This helped improve her autonomic flexibility.

Within one week, Karen's anxiety began to calm down. She lost four pounds the first week, probably due to reduced inflammation, and two pounds the second week, and then one pound per week after that. Exercise seemed to help her respond to stress more adaptively. After three weeks, she had lost three inches off her waist, so she no longer was at risk for metabolic syndrome. Karen barely noticed her next period and no longer ruminated about kids or career.

The Brain Body Protocol: Calming Down Anxiety

In Sylvia Plath's poem "The Colossus," she writes, "Thirty years now I have labored / To dredge the silt from your throat." Silt is a fine type of soil, between sand and clay in texture, that accumulates in all rivers. Accumulation of silt in one's throat is a good metaphor for the accumulated traumas and indignities of modern life that can clog the spirit and disrupt the proper workings of the brain, such that your synapses can't fire, no matter how hard you try, leading to anxiety. My job is to help you periodically remove the silt from the channel of your brain/body connection so that silt doesn't make you feel anxiety-ridden, subjugated to living a smaller, more contracted life than you were meant to have. I've never seen the usual pharmaceutical treatments for anxiety provide this type of service. Instead of reaching for another drug, clean the channel with a comprehensive and integrative approach. Your daily choices and actions have a direct and measurable impact on anxiety—on the genetic, cellular, and regulatory level (homeostasis). Make the right choices, and you can restore balance, peace, and calm.

Now it's time for a sigh of relief. I mean it literally: a heavy sigh or noisy exhale helps lower brain tension, particularly in anxiety-sensitive people like me.[73] This protocol is designed to calm your amygdala, reduce your heightened stress response (which researchers call autonomic flexibility), and improve your sleep—all of which will reduce your anxiety.

You'll notice that food is the core once again of this chapter's Brain Body Protocol. I explained earlier in the chapter how I think of *diet* in the ancient Greek sense—as a prescriptive way of life, encompassing what and how you eat, as well as the way you live. There are common metabolic processes in the body that exist within every cell. If you take a medicine, like a pill for anxiety, you're targeting just one metabolic process, whereas if you make a change in the food you eat, you can influence a broad variety of systems like the brain, gut, liver, pancreas, muscle cells, blood vessels—all with one intervention.

When it comes to anxiety, the truth is that stress will bombard you throughout life in various forms. But you can work with stress more skillfully by slowing down, actively hitting the pause button, and bolstering your rest-and-digest pathways. In a short amount of time (eight weeks, according to one study), you can counter the shrinkage of the thinking brain (the gray matter) so that the threat center in your amygdala contracts back to its proper size.

That's the goal of this protocol: to make your thinking brain bigger—with rapidly firing, efficient, and connected neurons working on your behalf—and to make your amygdala smaller. It requires awareness, acceptance of what you can't control, developing a sense of control over what you can, and contemplation. As ambiguous as that may sound, I'll walk you through how to do it. Spend a minimum of forty days on this protocol if you qualify for anxiety (or longer, depending on your level of anxiety). Remember that slow, consistent practice is the special sauce to cease anxiety patterns and foster new, calm wiring.

BASIC PROTOCOL

Step 1: Eat for calm.

What you put on your fork can increase or decrease your risk of anxiety.[74] Your food is how your body provides the brain with what it needs to make neurotransmitters, many of which are implicated in anxiety when out of balance. Specifically, the typical American diet sets you up for chronic low-grade inflammation that often leads to anxiety—refined flours, sugars, distorted fats, preservatives, pesticides, herbicides, alcohol, and other chemical toxins.[75] These fake and adulterated foods can increase intestinal permeability, disturb the microbiome, cause physical stress, overexcite the brain, and create hyperarousal, leading to a greater susceptibility to anxiety.

On the other hand, the ideal diet for mental health is one that consists of the nutrients you need to make outstanding neurotransmitters: whole organic foods like vegetables, fruits, healthy fats, nuts, seeds, and fish—and eating a diverse range within each food group. These foods actually help calm your brain and promote restful sleep.[76]

Many people need to avoid *lectins*—the type of protein found in raw legumes and grains that can bind to cell membranes—because they may increase your chance of leaky gut.[77] Choose foods that balance blood sugar, aiming for 35 to 50 grams of fiber per day. Be sure to include prebiotic and probiotic foods to tighten the junctions in your gut.[78] The caveat here is that if you eat a diet high in prebiotics in order to feed the good bugs in your gut and you have an existing bacterial imbalance (for instance, small intestinal bacterial overgrowth, or SIBO), you may feel worse. Most prebiotic foods are high in FODMAPs (short-chain carbohydrates found in everyday foods; the acronym stands for fermentable oligosaccharides, disaccharides, monosaccharides, and polyols) and could trigger leaky gut, histamine release, and inflammation. For more on SIBO, see Notes.[79]

Eat these:

- **bone broth,** which helps to seal leaky gut and simply feels soothing
- **magnesium-rich foods,** like almonds, cashews, spinach, pumpkin seeds, and avocados
- **foods rich in B vitamins,** as deficiencies in B_9 (folate) and B_{12} may be linked to anxiety.[80] Great sources of B vitamins include oysters, mussels, mackerel, and organ meats (liver and kidney). Excellent sources of folate are asparagus, spinach, and liver. (If you have an MTHFR genetic variation, you will want to supplement with the right amount of methylfolate.)
- **clean protein,** like oily fish and pastured poultry, to build up calming neurotransmitters
- **probiotic foods,** which have been shown to tighten junctions between cells[81] in the intestinal wall and to reduce social anxiety.[82] Focus on the choices we've covered in previous chapters: sauerkraut, kimchi, coconut kefir.
- **healthy fats** like avocado, nuts, seeds, oily fish (salmon, herring, sardines), olives, and coconut, which help to stabilize blood sugar so your brain can have a steady supply of glucose that's not too high and not too low. Additionally, fat helps neurotransmitters move rapidly from neuron to neuron. Healthy omega-3s and omega-6s play a vital role in reducing neuroinflammation and anxiety.[83]

Avoid these:

- **caffeine,** as it raises cortisol and amplifies the fight-flight-freeze response, and can rob you of restful sleep if you metabolize it slowly
- **sugar and refined carbohydrates,** as they set you up for a roller coaster of anxiety-triggering blood sugar spikes. Instead, eat one square of extra dark chocolate (85 percent cacao or higher).
- **processed and packaged foods,** which are high in refined sources of inflammatory omega-6
- **alcohol**
- **lectins,** particularly wheat, rice, spelt, legumes, and soy
- **genetically modified foods** (eat organic)
- **conventional cow milk**

Step 2: Avoid other common adverse reactions to food.

Beyond the calm foods, you may want to avoid the foods that crank up the worry. That includes the foods that increase cortisol, dysbiosis, and leaky gut by causing an overzealous immune reaction in the gut—that is, food allergy. The most common food allergens are **wheat, cow milk, eggs, peanuts, tree nuts, shellfish,** and **soy.**[84] Allergic responses are most common in children and tend to diminish in adults. Food intolerances are reactions to food that are not mediated by the immune system, like caffeine intolerance, tyramine intolerance, lactose intolerance, fructose intolerance, irritable bowel syndrome, and malabsorption. Furthermore, foods loaded with sugar, saturated fat, inflammatory polyunsaturated fats, and high cholesterol can be associated with impaired glucose tolerance and rising blood sugar.[85]

Step 3: Go analog.

Given the role of smartphone and social media use and overuse, it makes sense to take a break. Get off all screens at least one hour before bedtime. My curfew is 9 p.m. Once per week, try a twenty-four-hour digital detox where you do old-fashioned things like read a good book, talk to your loved ones, go for a picnic, or throw a Frisbee. If taking a break from digital feels impossible, try the habituation kriya on page 210.

Step 4: Improve your sleep.

When you don't sleep enough, your brain makes more cortisol, and you now know all about that wretched cycle and how it makes you prone to anxiety. Correcting your sleep patterns will help you get anxiety under control. One study of thirty sedentary women with anxiety found that resistance exercise was superior to aerobic exercise in improving sleep, including time spent in bed, sleep efficiency, and anxiety symptom severity.[86] (See more in the Advanced Protocol on resistance exercise for anxiety.) To improve your sleep hygiene, go to bed consistently at the same time each night. Make it to bed early enough to sleep seven to eight and a half hours per night to stabilize your blood sugar. Consider taking one of the chill-out brain botanicals and nutrients mentioned on pages 248 to 250 to help you stay asleep. Don't fret—they are all safe!

Two options to help you sleep: *magnesium* and *melatonin*. Magnesium plays a role in more than three hundred biochemical reactions in your cells and can help you feel more rested.[87] Foods high in fiber are more likely to be high in magnesium, including legumes, vegetables (principally broccoli, squash, and green leafy vegetables), seeds, and nuts. Women tend to be lower in magnesium than men, putting us at a greater risk of osteoporosis and stroke,[88] and body levels generally decline with age. Dose: Magnesium 250 to 500 mg at night.

Melatonin is a hormone made in the brain by the pineal gland, and it has actions on the brain and body. When you're short on sleep, your sleep/wake cycle is disrupted, or your circadian clock is off, taking extra melatonin beyond what your body makes can help you fall asleep faster, increase total sleep time, and improve overall sleep quality.[89] Additionally, melatonin may help seal the blood-brain barrier—the key barrier to keep out toxins and other blood components that may disturb the brain—and reduces inflammation.[90] Perhaps as a result, melatonin helps ease anxiety associated with surgery in adults and children, and in adults it may be superior to midazolam (Versed), a benzodiazepine, because it does not cause amnesia or impairment of cognitive or psychomotor function.[91] Dose: Melatonin 0.3 to 3 mg at night for forty days. (Most studies look at use for up to three months, so I do not recommend a longer duration.)

Step 5: Improve flexibility.

People with anxiety have a stuck nervous system—also known as autonomic nervous system inflexibility—whether stressed or unstressed.[92] They have a higher heart rate, less slowing of heart rate with deep abdominal breathing, and lower heart rate variability. When stressed, they fail to increase their heart rate, and they recover more slowly when the stress has passed.[93] So one of our goals is to improve autonomic flexibility using one or more of the research-based techniques below. Pick one and stick with it at least four times per week for forty days.

- **Guided imagery.** When you worry, the body enters its fight-flight-freeze response, setting off a cascade of physiological effects like high blood pressure, elevated heart rate, and sweating. You can reverse this state with the relaxation response of guided imagery.

YOGA FOR ANXIETY:
STANDING FORWARD BEND AT A WALL

1. Stand in mountain pose, or Tadasana, with your back against a wall, the backs of your heels about six to eight inches from the wall, and hands on your hips.
2. Exhale, and bend forward from the hips toward your feet. Allow your sit bones to rest against the wall. (Grounding against the wall can be very soothing when you feel anxious.)
3. Lengthen the front of your body as you reach for your knees, shins, or feet.
4. Cross your forearms and hold onto your elbows.
5. Turn the top thighs inward without moving your feet.
6. Lift the sitting bones toward the ceiling or sky.
7. Take five slow, deep abdominal breaths.

I first learned these techniques from Herbert Benson and Alice Domar at Harvard Medical School. Now I recommend the excellent guided visualizations of Martin Rossman, MD. Not enough physicians are aware of the benefits of guided imagery, relaxation, and meditation, but these tools can be extremely helpful, especially in stressful situations such as medical procedures.

- **Yoga.** I practice yoga every morning to guide my nervous system in the right direction: calmness. Yoga and meditation have been shown to correct imbalances in the autonomic nervous system and GABA.[94] Consequently it's not surprising to learn that yoga reduces anxiety and depression in as little as ten days.[95] Calming forward bends (see example above) are the best for anxiety, whereas back bends and inversions are ideal for depression (see example on page 274). For pregnant women, a combination of tai chi and yoga reduces anxiety and depression and improves sleep. Yoga is my preferred way to promote neurospirituality.

- **Mindfulness-based stress reduction (MBSR).** In a randomized trial, a group of ninety-three adults with generalized anxiety disorder learned MBSR and improved their anxiety scores, stress reactivity, and coping.[96] In another trial involving 103 older adults with stress disorders and neurocognitive difficulties, MBSR improved anxiety, depression, and memory.[97]

- **Other methods:** Emotional Freedom Technique[98] and Yoga combined with CBT (Y-CBT)[99] are described in the Notes.

ADVANCED PROTOCOL

Once you have the Basic Protocol in action, add one or more of these advanced options if you're still feeling anxious.

Step 6: Try chill-out brain/body botanicals and nutrients.

If you are on prescription medications, talk to your pharmacist about any drug interactions first.

- **Lavender.** In multiple clinical trials, lavender taken orally as a softgel reduces anxiety. You can also inhale essential oils, including lavender, rose geranium, Roman chamomile, clary sage, and bergamot. Unfortunately, not many large-scale studies involve essential oils as a treatment for anxiety, but essential oils are inexpensive and relatively harmless.[100] Dose: Lavender oil in a softgel 80 mg once to twice per day, or when anxiety hits.

- **Cannabis.** There's a reason that cannabis has become a $7 billion industry. Cannabis, or marijuana, can be used for medicinal purposes to relieve anxiety and pain—in fact, relief for anxiety symptoms is the most frequent reason cited for using cannabis.[101] The two main constituents in cannabis are the primary psychoactive ingredient, delta-9-tetrahydrocannabinol (THC), which reduces amygdala reactivity,[102] and cannabidiol (CBD), which reduces chronic unpredictable stress, fear, and inflammation.[103] After a single oral dose, THC may increase anxiety, whereas CBD does not, and in other studies CBD seems to block some of THC's adverse effects.[104] In fact, CBD seems to calm down the limbic system and shows benefit in social anxiety.[105] From a brain perspective, I agree with the editors of the *New York Times* that cannabis should be legalized.[106]

For cannabis, the rate of addiction as well as other adverse effects is lower than for alcohol, but risk factors are early onset of use and weekly or daily use.[107] (If you are concerned that you are misusing cannabis and crave it daily or weekly, contact your health care professional for help.)

If you suffer from anxiety, I'd prefer you take medical marijuana (versus recreational), ideally in tincture form extracted with carbon dioxide (instead of solvents) and only organic, so that you avoid toxic chemicals, including pesticides and herbicides, used especially when marijuana is grown indoors.[108] The content of edible marijuana products and the timing of the drug's effect can vary so widely that I don't recommend edibles for anxiety—stick to oral use, such as a tincture that you can carefully dose for your situation. Do not smoke cannabis because it is associated with chronic inflammatory and precancerous changes in the airways, putting you at greater risk of lung damage and cancer—and in some people, smoked cannabis can compromise information processing and memory.[109] Of course, do not drive after taking medical marijuana, as it can increase the risk of a motor vehicle accident for up to eight hours after use.[110] Doses vary depending on species.

- **Lemon balm.** An extract of the medicinal plant lemon balm reduced anxiety symptoms in patients with anxiety disorders. More research is needed, but this lemon-scented herb is safe to try. Dose: 300 mg twice daily for fifteen days.[111]

- **Passion flower.** Taking an extract of passion flower reduces anxiety.[112] Two trials of passion flower compared to benzodiazepines (oxazepam or Serax, and mexazolam or Sedoxil) showed that they are similar in efficacy.[113] Passion flower has been used to reduce anxiety before surgery and as a sleeping aid.[114] Dose: 200 mg of a dried, alcoholic extract of passion flower taken in a dose of two capsules twice daily for two to eight weeks, or liquid extract forty-five drops once daily for four weeks.

- **Rhodiola.** In a small study of patients with generalized anxiety disorder, rhodiola decreased anxiety and depression.[115] It may also help patients with high perceived stress, anger, and confusion.[116] Dose: 170 to 200 mg twice daily for two to ten weeks.

- **Magnesium with vitamin B$_6$.** For premenstrual anxiety, take 50 mg of vitamin B$_6$ with 200 mg of magnesium. With my patients, I found that for those with the short allele of SLC6A4, taking the bioactive form of vitamin B$_6$, called Pyridoxine-5-Phosphate (P5P), can be helpful. P5P levels can be low in patients with inflammation.[117] Dose of P5P: 50 mg per day.
- **Other options** for supplements are mentioned in the Notes.[118]

Step 7: Perform resistance training.

You can perform resistance training in several ways: lifting weights (even using small barbells, like I do, of two to five pounds), swinging a kettlebell, or using your body weight as resistance, such as with the plank pose or boat pose. One review of randomized trials found that resistance training lowers anxiety by 29 percent[119] and has other brain/body benefits, including better cognitive function, better memory, and less fatigue. In another randomized trial of thirty sedentary women ages eighteen to thirty-seven, resistance training twice per week for six weeks caused remission of anxiety in 60 percent of patients, compared with 40 percent remission with aerobic exercise.[120] It turns out that aerobic exercise may not help anxiety.[121] I recommend resistance training for ten to thirty minutes twice a week. Start with an easy regimen, like the *New York Times'* Scientific 7-Minute Workout, and build up to thirty minutes by performing each exercise for longer.[122]

Step 8: Develop a sense of control.

Cognitive behavioral therapy (CBT) is a form of practical therapy aimed at helping you manage your thoughts and behavior to address specific problems. CBT is commonly used for anxiety and depression. Traditionally, CBT was performed by mental health professionals one-on-one with a patient, but increasingly CBT is taught in a live group class or an online format. About half the people with anxiety disorders who do a course of CBT—about twelve to fifteen sessions with a therapist—get clinically significant relief.[123]

CBT is based on the concept that poor thinking habits trigger anxiety and stress and that learning healthier ways to think about things can change your habitual emotional and behavioral responses. (Note that CBT also has been used successfully to treat insomnia.)

Step 9: Test yourself.

The test that I find to be most helpful in people with anxiety is to measure daily heart rate variability (see Appendix B for details). Other helpful tests include cortisol, estrogen, progesterone, 25-hydroxy vitamin D, red blood cell magnesium, homocysteine, and SLC6A4 and MTHFR genetic mutations.

Last Word

Mental health reflects both brain *and* body health, and vice versa. As I discovered with Karen, anxiety impacts the brain in such a way that other biological functions, like blood sugar regulation and vitamin absorption, take a hit. Once you're anxious, the crazy spiral downward can begin, and one factor, like stress, can feed another, like disrupted sleep. When your sleep, amygdala, or cortisol—or maybe all three—is off track your brain is vulnerable to anxiety and a lack of discernment about real versus perceived threats. This creates a vicious cycle of worry, but you can get it under control by rebalancing your delicate nervous system so worry occurs only as an occasional state, not a trait, under warranted threats.

Faith helps—in yourself, in science, in God, or in some power greater than yourself. Spiritual contemplation creates a healthier brain body, but it must become a daily practice for healing. It helps to remain open to your own spiritual unfolding, exposing yourself to new ideas about your own spirit, or the divine spirit, in various ways and as deeply as you can. Calmness can become the new norm. Ultimately, your brain and body will be able to distinguish the difference between a true threat and an overreaction. Your brain and your body will complement each other and help you to face daily challenges with a healthier outlook, flexible nervous system, and peaceful mind.

7

Depression

How to Climb Out of the Hole, Kick the Pills, and Bring Joy Back into Your Life

While on a hike with me, a friend mentioned feeling depressed. I jumped into doctor mode: "How's your diet? How's your gut?" My friend did a double take. "What does my gut have to do with my bad mood?"

Plenty.

After thinking it over, she added: "Do not take my chocolate away from me. It's the only thing that makes me happy!"

When most people think of depression, they don't think of the body and its role in creating a depressed mood. They think of a chemical imbalance in the brain—maybe low serotonin—and how a prescription might help. But what if depression is a symptom of something else, like inflammation? That is, what if depression is actually an inflammation disorder in the body that begins in the gut and then seeps into the brain, not a disease? Yes, depression is like other brain/body complaints like anxiety, foggy thinking, weight gain, memory loss—a symptom of inflammation from a brain body out of balance.

According to the National Institute of Mental Health, 16.1 million adult Americans, or 7 percent of the adult population, and 300 million people worldwide have at least one episode of major depression each year. Over your lifetime, your risk of developing depression is approximately 21 to 45 percent for women and 10 to 30 percent for men.[1] Rates are highest in the United States and lowest in Asian countries, with the median age of onset around thirty-two years. Depression is the leading cause of disability for US adults ages fifteen to forty-four, the leading cause of disability worldwide, and one of the top global health issues.[2] Across the globe, prevalence of depression ranges from 3 to 21 percent.[3]

As with anxiety, your brain hits a failure state that can lead to depression. When your brain is tired, weary, overtaxed, and overstressed, there's a downward spiral, but many of the reasons your brain gets overtaxed in the first place are under your control. Various physical, psychological, spiritual, and sociocultural factors are involved in the root cause of depression. Like anxiety, the effect is bidirectional: eating too much sugar and processed food, drinking alcohol to excess, and not exercising lead to a greater risk of depression; and depression triggers a downward spiral of unhealthy lifestyle choices and other chronic diseases.

When I have a patient who tells me she feels run down, overwhelmed, or depressed, I inquire about the body's inputs and outputs, starting first with food. "How many cups of vegetables are you eating each day?" I ask, because consuming more than five to eight servings is associated with happiness and better sleep, whereas caffeine and sugar are not.[4] (In fact, more joy is an immediate benefit of eating more veggies![5]) I probe about perceived stress, because even if you don't *feel* emotionally traumatized or acutely stressed, you could be depleting your stress reserves by not sleeping enough, overexercising and underrecovering, eating too many of the wrong carbohydrates or fats, skipping meals, or getting exposed to (known or unknown) toxins. Of course we all know that not all stress is bad, but if your perceived stress is chronically elevated, it may be associated with leaky gut, dysbiosis, hormone imbalances, leaky brain, burnout, and depression. I know because I've been there in the past and have written three books about it.

After I take a history of inputs and outputs in a patient who may have depression, we look at the gut. Did you know that you produce four hundred times more serotonin in the gut compared to the brain?[6] That your gut makes other feel-good hormones like melatonin and estrogen (recall that estrogen is the master regulator of the female body)?[7] Or that imbalances in your gut flora can cause altered thyroid function?[8] So you can start to see how problems in the gut can be contributing to the symptoms of depression. The key is to look upstream of the depressed symptoms for the root cause—but first let's see if depression is a problem for you.

Are You Depressed?

This questionnaire is different from the previous ones; it's called the PHQ-9, a series of nine questions validated to be very reliable at diagnosing depression, as accurate as a structured interview with a mental health professional.[9] The best way to use it is to assign a relative weight to your answer for each question as follows:

0 for not at all

1 for several days in the past two weeks

2 for more than half the days

3 for nearly every day

Fill in your score for each question, then tally each score at the end.

Over the last two weeks, how often have you been bothered by any of the following problems:

☐ Little interest or pleasure in doing things?
☐ Feeling down, depressed, or hopeless?
☐ Trouble falling or staying asleep, or sleeping too much?
☐ Feeling tired or having little energy?
☐ Poor appetite or overeating?
☐ Feeling bad about yourself—or that you are a failure or have let yourself or your family down?
☐ Trouble concentrating on things, such as reading the newspaper or watching television?
☐ Moving or speaking so slowly that other people could have noticed?
☐ Or the opposite—being so fidgety or restless that you have been moving around a lot more than usual?
☐ Thoughts of hurting yourself in some way or that you would be better off dead?

INTERPRETATION

The first two questions are the most important in screening for depression, but the entire questionnaire can inform you about depression severity and whether you should consider seeing a clinician (and inform your health care professional). Here's how to interpret your results.

- 0–4 points, minimal or no depression

- 5–9 points, mild depression: consider discussing symptoms with a primary care doctor or mental health professional.

- 10–14 points, moderate depression (10 or more points classify you as having *major depression,* which includes moderate and severe categories): definitely time to see your health care professional.

- 15–19 points, moderately severe depression: see a clinician to discuss your symptoms.

- 20–27 points, severe depression: similarly, see a clinician to discuss.

A Case of Depression?

We all feel blue at times, but depression—clinically, major depression—is different. It persists, depleting life force, isolating you from friends and family, and causing you to lose heart and hope.

Case in point: Gretchen, a thirty-nine-year-old lawyer, came to see me to alleviate her symptoms of depression. At age thirty-seven, she had started on venlafaxine (Effexor) for depression by her primary care doctor, which she found "incredible but horrible." It helped even out her mood, but she couldn't tolerate the numerous side effects: inability to orgasm, night sweats, bruising all over her body, and profuse sweating with exercise. She stopped after one year and tried nutritional neurochemistry, taking mountains of marginally proven amino acids (including 5-HTP and GABA), but still felt muted, with a thrum of anxious depression and irritability, like she had nothing to look forward to. She still felt emotionally exhausted. She worked long hours at her demanding law firm, tried to navigate a nearly impossible workload by fueling with candy in the break room, ate many of her meals out with clients, and then headed home to binge watch television with a glass of wine and takeout for company. She was on a partner track at the law firm but not sure she had what it takes, nor did she desire the depleting lifestyle.

As I listened to Gretchen, I wondered if her label of "depression" was accurate. Perhaps her emotional exhaustion, high-demand job, and lack of future job security were creating burnout. She looked puffy and inflamed, the root cause of depression and other mental health concerns, including anxiety. Of course, there is overlap between the diagnosis of burnout and depression. When I told Gretchen that I thought a more accurate diagnosis was burnout, she was pleased because she felt like burnout had less stigma—that she was less of a moral failure. In the end, the label mattered less than helping Gretchen feel better. Next she asked why the venlafaxine would be helpful if she didn't have depression as a diagnosis. I explained that it was a prescription drug called a "selective serotonin-norepinephrine reuptake inhibitor" (SNRI), but that it was also proven to help reduce inflammation.[10] So taking the SNRI reduced inflammation, helping her symptoms, but didn't address the root cause.

The first sign of a problem was that Gretchen's lab tests revealed piles of brain trash. She was in the toxic range for mercury and high in homocysteine, a blood marker of inflammation. A urine test was high in glyphosate, associated with gut dysbiosis and depression in animal studies and possibly humans.[11] Her stool showed another sign of inflammation: high lactoferrin, an iron-binding protein released from inflamed immune cells. The delicate checks and balances between the feedback loops in her brain and body were disrupted because her brain was inflamed. One region of her brain was overactive whereas another region of her brain was underactive. One of her sex hormones, dehydroepiandrosterone (DHEA), was low-normal, hinting at a burned-out HPA axis.[12] Her salivary cortisol pattern was flat, meaning that it didn't fluctuate throughout the day as it should, from a peak upon awakening to slowly downhill throughout the day. Fortunately, her thyroid function was normal.

What we learned together is that Gretchen is vulnerable to accumulating brain trash for three reasons: her toxin-coping genes are poor, her stress-coping genes are marginal, and her DNA repair genes are

not great. Taken together, these genes determine your ability to revitalize your brain and body, from metabolism to mood. (Gretchen's dirty
genes—see chapter 2—affected her mood, but mine affect my metabolism and weight.)

What helped Gretchen? Detoxification, cooling her inflammation,
and yoga, which allowed us to restore the feedback loops in her brain. As
I marveled at her recovery from depression with a few simple changes,
I performed an exhaustive search of the scientific literature and was
stunned to find that yoga is actually better than standard care, aerobic exercise, and relaxation exercise for depression. It helps to reset the
HPA axis, cortisol, and sleep—providing an integrative approach to the
root cause of depression. Yoga has been one of the most transformative
anti-inflammatories in my life. You'll learn the details in this chapter.

As mentioned in chapter 6, depression is a *response to perceived loss*.[13]
Depression can be low-grade or major, or anything in between. Either way, depression can drain your energy, turn off the birth of new
brain cells (neurogenesis), cloud your brain, and cut you off from joy.
Sometimes relating to the experience of depression more directly and
compassionately—along with addressing the brain/body breakdown
resulting in inflammation and immune system overactivation—can
help you prevent, treat, or reverse the symptoms.

My Own Experience with Depression

My first episode of depression occurred at age twenty-nine, when I
was in my intern year of obstetrics and gynecology residency. I was
the "night float" at work, meaning that I worked every night from
7 p.m. to 7 a.m. Then a renovation began in the apartment next to
mine, and I stopped sleeping because of jackhammers and shouting
construction workers. I began psychotherapy with a kindly sixty-
something social worker, who told me to eat well and to find another
place to sleep. It worked.

My second episode of depression happened at thirty-two, when I was
postpartum and working at my first job as an obstetrician/gynecolo-
gist. My baby was ten months old, and I hadn't slept soundly since early

---

LAWYERING, ANOTHER DEPRESSION-PRONE JOB

It turns out that depression is most common in lawyers, not doctors: 28 percent of lawyers have mild or more serious depression; overall, lawyers are three and a half times more likely to be depressed than those in other occupations. As my husband put it, being a lawyer raises cortisol because you're always in a fight. What's interesting to me is that law students don't start out that way. Before law school, they have *less* depression and hostility, drink less, and use drugs less often compared to the general population. But something happens during law school: they experience a marked increase in depression, physical symptoms, and negativity, along with a decrease in positive mood and life satisfaction. What makes lawyers depressed and negative? The killer combination of stress, convenience and packaged food, caffeine, alcohol, sleep deprivation, and, yes, conflict. That means environment has a strong effect on your health, as you'll see in the science section of this chapter.

---

in pregnancy. (Notice the pattern of sleep deprivation and working too hard.) Climbing out of this hole took much longer, about six months. That's when I discovered that those in the helping professions—like teachers, nurses, physicians, and physician trainees—are more inclined to burnout, with rates for physicians at 25 to 60 percent.[14] In subsequent years, as I learned more about functional medicine and ways to prevent another recurrence of depression, I found that I have a genetic proclivity to be depressed and inflamed. My predisposition was always in the back of my mind, so I set about preventing those genes from dragging down my brain body based on environmental inputs. It worked.

The Science of Depression

We used to think of depression as a problem of brain chemistry, like not enough serotonin, or norepinephrine, or both. This line of thinking made pharmaceutical companies rich as the public bought into the idea that we need to take drugs to deal with the ups and downs of daily life, both serious and banal. Meanwhile, SSRIs, the treatment for moderate to severe depression, became the most commonly prescribed drug in the United States for adults ages eighteen to forty-four.

Depression can be one episode, chronic, or recurrent. Sometimes depression doesn't resolve and leads to persistent depressive disorder (PDD), a type of depression that lingers for at least two years (previously termed *dysthymia*). Treatment-resistant depression is very common: 20 to 50 percent of patients don't respond to treatment.[15] Fifty percent! That tells me that our current approach is failing. It's worth noting that the placebo effect is strong in depression: 30 to 40 percent of depressed patients respond to a placebo, and there's evidence that the mechanism involves the HPA axis—simply altering expectations can alter brain/body chemistry.[16]

Now we know that depression is a brain/body issue. We used to think that depression was simply an imbalance of brain chemicals like serotonin, norepinephrine, and dopamine that needed to be adjusted individually in isolation, but now we know this concept is oversimplified and outdated. When brain chemicals are off, it is the result of a brain/body failure state, and the cause is a combination of genetic vulnerabilities interacting with environmental factors and, as a downstream result, a shrinking brain and hippocampus. Hello, excess brain trash.

So what's the risky combination? There's not one specific brain problem associated with depression, but several biological, environmental, spiritual, psychological, and sociocultural factors that in combination put you at risk. I think about depression as a trilogy:

- You have a gene that makes you vulnerable to depression.
- You encounter a trigger (a major stressor—say, a divorce or car crash or other trauma).
- Then you develop pathogenic intestinal permeability from environmental factors (examples: excess alcohol, excess stress, or glyphosate pokes holes in your gut wall, leading to leaky gut, and then inflammation).

Some people with depression have no family history of or genetic predisposition to it, so the triggers and environmental factors are playing a larger role.

DEPRESSION GENES

Having a family history of depression increases your risk. If one iden-
tical twin is diagnosed with depression, the other twin has a 70 percent chance of developing it. The gene-environment interaction was
the topic of my previous book *Younger*, but I'll review what we know
about the genetics of depression. The caveat is that a gene polymor-
phism (variation) does *not* mean a diagnosis of depression; it just
means that your genes may predispose you. So if you're exposed to
certain biological and environmental factors—such as maltreatment
as a child or specific toxins—your risk may be higher. Another caveat
is that we are still in the process of understanding which genes are
most important for which populations.[17] (See Appendix B for reliable
testing options.)

1. **Serotonin transporter** (SLC6A4).[18] Almost half of Caucasians
   have a genetic variant in the way serotonin is transported cell to cell
   in the brain, resulting in an increased susceptibility to depression,
   particularly under stress. The variants for this gene are classified
   as long (normal) or short (variant). Women who have one or two
   copies of the *short serotonin transporter gene* produce more cortisol,
   are less stress resilient, and have a diminished response to SSRI.[19]
   Women with short serotonin transporters show greater amygdala
   hypervigilance,[20] which may worsen when estrogen declines, as in
   late perimenopause or menopause.

2. **Brain-derived neurotrophic factor** (BDNF). If you inherit a variation from one parent, you have a three-fold greater risk of depression.[21] On the other hand, if you inherit the variation from both
   parents, you are more likely to be introverted and *resistant to depression* when faced with repeated defeat.[22] So inheriting a variation of
   this gene can work for or against your mental health.[23] Expression of
   the BDNF gene changes in response to work stress.[24]

3. **Glucocorticoid receptor** (nuclear receptor subfamily 3, group C,
   member 1, or NR3C1). Variations in the NR3C1 gene involving the
   glucocorticoid receptor are associated with major depression in women
   but not men, which points to the gene/environment vulnerability that
   may account for why women have higher rates of depression.[25]

ARE THOSE SHORT TELOMERES IN YOUR CELLS?

Telomeres are the caps on the ends of chromosomes that protect them from damage, and can shorten prematurely because of various lifestyle factors. They are a marker of accelerated aging, chronic exposure to toxins, inflammation, stress, and stress hormones. Studies show that short telomere length is a sign that may indicate depression and other chronic mental conditions, including suicidal ideation, anxiety, chronic stress, and even early mortality from rapid aging.[26] What's not yet known is which comes first: short telomeres or depression? In one study that followed patients for six years, a diagnosis of depression or anxiety was associated with shorter telomeres. Investigators found the short telomeres at the beginning of the study, but they didn't continue to shorten over time. That led investigators to hypothesize that short telomere length is either an underlying vulnerability or a long-term consequence of depression or anxiety disorders.[27] Other studies show short telomeres along with reduced hippocampus size in the following groups: men with internalizing disorders (depression, generalized anxiety disorder, and PTSD),[28] adolescents with unmedicated major depression, and young people with early-onset depression.[29] The bottom line: depression is a brain/body problem that ages the cells of the body too fast, shortens the telomeres, and can prematurely shrink and age the brain.

4. **Calcium channel** (also known as calcium channel, voltage-dependent, L type, alpha 1C subunit, or CACNA1C). This gene regulates the flow of calcium into cells and is crucial to normal brain development, plasticity, and function. When you inherit a variant, calcium flow gets dysregulated, which puts you at greater risk of major depression, as well as bipolar disorder, autism, attention deficit disorder, schizophrenia, and cocaine use disorder.[30]

5. **FK506 binding protein 5** (FKBP5). This gene is central to the HPA axis. In addition to being involved in PTSD and anxiety, FKBP5 is associated with lifetime major depressive disorder (MDD) diagnosis as well as structural changes in the brain.[31] Overall, variation may increase the risk of depression by 39 percent.[32]

6. **Methylenetetrahydrofolate reductase** (MTHFR). This gene has

an inconsistent or at best modest association with depression. The MTHFR gene controls the movement and use of folic acid and other B vitamins that help your neurotransmitters function normally. When you have a mutation of the MTHFR gene, it may impair folic acid metabolism so that the risk of depression, bipolar disorder, schizophrenia, and autism may increase, although genetic association studies are inconsistent.[33] If an association is present, it is most likely related to inflammation,[34] and may be more relevant to menopausal women.[35]

THE ROLE OF GUT BUGS IN DEPRESSION

The microbial ecosystem that resides within your intestinal tract isn't static—it changes with diet, age, stress, other environmental factors, and health status as well as medication exposures.[36] Some of these factors can shift your gut microbiome in the direction of depression. You may think your stress response is all in your head, but research shows the microbiome plays an important role in the programming of the HPA axis early in life and stress reactivity over the life span.[37]

Previously overlooked, the 100 trillion gut bugs of a healthy person, we now know, influence that person's well-being in substantial ways. Those trillions of bugs vary from one healthy person to another, and from one unhealthy person to another. All the conditions in this brain/body book are associated with an imbalance (dysbiosis) in the gut microbiome at some level. Depression is no exception. There is constant talk between the gut and brain: some of it travels along the vagus nerve and some of it travels in the blood, especially in nutrients, hormones, proteins, peptides (smaller versions of proteins), and inflammatory messengers like antibodies and cytokines. The good news is that while abnormal microbiota can lead to brain/body dysfunction and cause brain symptoms like anxiety, depression, brain fog, rising set point, and memory loss, correcting these disturbances is proven to reverse symptoms. Depression, like the other brain/body problems, is closely intertwined with a healthy balance in the gut. Maintaining and restoring the condition of the gut ecosystem can prevent and reverse brain symptoms like depression and burnout.

There are five key ways that your gut flora promote depression and anxiety: by making your gut wall leaky, by manipulating your stress response, by disrupting your immune response, by causing chronic inflammation, and by producing harmful peptides and other chemical messengers.[38]

It's beyond the scope of this book to solve each of these problems individually and comprehensively. In functional medicine, a simpler approach is to start with diet—to remove what's causing an imbalance and restore what brings balance. At a basic level, the best antidepression diet involves eating more vegetables, fruits, fermented foods, and other plants—the more varied the species, the better the microbial diversity and homeostasis. The worst food for depression is a typical American diet of sugar, fat, and inflammatory animal protein—a diet depleted of fiber—which leads to dysbiosis, reduced microbial diversity, and illness, including obesity, cardiovascular disease, hypertension, metabolic syndrome, cancer (especially colon and breast cancer), and even depression.[39]

The takeaway: eat for joy, not burnout and depression. Eat in a way that supports microbiome health, balance, and diversity. The protocol shows you how.

THE ROLE OF THE BRAIN IN DEPRESSION

Two areas of the brain are involved in depression: the HPA axis and the hippocampus. Remember how the cycle of depression is bidirectional? When a problem occurs in either of these areas, and a genetic predisposition exists, it's a recipe for the downward spiral. In the protocol, you'll learn some simple fixes to reverse this spiral, using supplements and, yes, even yoga.

HPA Axis

You've learned about how your HPA (hypothalamic-pituitary-adrenal) axis controls your hormones, mood, energy, and stress response. The brain/body failure state of HPA dysregulation contributes to depression—your mood drops, you don't have energy to combat the stress, and you just want to take a nap or sleep late so you don't have to cope.

Experts generally believe that depression is associated with hyper-activity of the HPA axis, resulting in higher cortisol levels.[40] You already know that when the HPA axis is overactivated, you are more vulnerable to anxiety (chapter 6). An overactive HPA axis in conjunction with other biological and environmental factors also affects the brain, setting you up for depression and a poor response to antidepressants.[41] The additional imbalance is with the sex hormone DHEA. A low DHEA (or DHEAS, or DHEA sulfate, which is how we measure DHEA in the blood) level can actually point to a problem with the HPA axis.

It turns out that the way you respond to stress—whether by choice or because of how your brain is wired—may make you more vulnerable to depression. Chronic stress and the stress hormone cortisol cause oxidative damage to mitochondria in the gut and can poke holes in the gut barrier and the blood-brain barrier.[42] You already know that the higher your cortisol is and the longer the elevation lasts, the more your HPA axis is affected. Unfortunately, results are inconsistent,[43] but clearly some level of HPA axis dysregulation is present in depression, particularly in women.

- Half of people with depression have high cortisol levels, or respond to stress with higher-than-normal cortisol levels, or don't recover to normal cortisol levels after a stressor has passed; in fact, high cortisol is a suicide marker.[44]

- Women with depression are more likely to have a flat cortisol pattern over the course of the day (i.e., it doesn't peak in the morning and stays high at night).[45]

- Patients with high cortisol have problems with emotion perception, processing, and regulation, similar to the mood symptoms found in depression.[46]

- Cortisol awakening response (CAR), which predicts depression and how long until there's a recurrence, is higher in people with depression and remitted (resolved) depression.[47]

Other hormonal factors in depression include low thyroid,[48] low estrogen or excess estrogen,[49] low and high androgens (both DHEA, mentioned earlier, and testosterone),[50] and low melatonin.[51]

More on the Shrinking Hippocampus

When you're depressed, especially with recurrent depression, there's a good chance your hippocampus has shrunk. The hippocampus is part of the limbic system, responsible for emotional regulation and moving information from short-term to long-term memory. So a smaller hippocampus may mean several things: more mood swings, memory loss (both forming new memories and long-term memory), and connecting emotions to those memories.

The hippocampus plays a primary role in depression. Recall that high perceived stress—the amount of stress load that exceeds reserves—can shrink the hippocampus, and this also occurs in depression.[52] Researchers found that hippocampal volume reductions generally occur after disease onset in patients with major depressive disorder. The more episodes of depression a person has, the greater the reduction in size of the hippocampus. This means that the brain environment in depression influences brain structure and function.

Before you lose heart, know that emerging research suggests the damage may be reversible because the hippocampus is one of the unique areas of the brain that is highly neuroplastic and makes rapid connections between nerve cells (synaptogenesis). What's lost in depression is the connections between cells, not the cells themselves. The possibility of reversing the hippocampal shrinkage makes early and complete treatment crucial, especially in teenagers and young adults. And as you'll learn, I don't mean simply popping a pharmaceutical. As with anxiety, we need a more integrative approach that incorporates mind-body tools, social connections, nutraceuticals, removal of toxins, and reduction of inflammation.

ENVIRONMENTAL FACTORS

While depression involves distinct genetic and brain factors, it also depends on lifestyle and environmental triggers that impact your gene expressions, HPA, and hippocampus. All told, environmental factors can worsen or improve your risk of depression. My favorite statistic is that exercising thirty minutes per day cuts your risk of depression by half.[53] Here are some major factors:

1. Air pollution[54]
2. Lead[55]
3. BPA[56]
4. Smoking[57]
5. Heavy alcohol use[58]
6. Lack of social support[59]
7. Lack of sleep[60]
8. Low physical activity[61]
9. Bad microbes, such as release of lipopolysaccharide (LPS)[62]

Dodge Depression with Diet

Changes in intestinal microbes may have a role in brain disorders such as anxiety, depression, and even obesity.[63] When you eat crap, you feel like crap. Seriously—evidence proves that what you put in your mouth modifies key biological factors linked to the development of depression. Fortunately, certain nutrients may help ameliorate the damage; these include omega-3 fatty acids, antioxidants (vitamin C and zinc), members of the vitamin B family (vitamin B_{12} and folic acid), and magnesium.[64]

When I help someone with depression or any other health problem, we start with nutrition because of the essential nature of the gut/brain conversations and microbiome in creating a healthy brain/body connection. And as I reassured my friend—no, I won't take away your dark chocolate.

What's bad for your mood? You're probably already guessing—the same foods that trigger anxiety. Eating higher on the glycemic index and/or eating added sugars is more likely to make a person feel depressed, at least in women.[65] The nonnegotiables are to give up flour, sugar, and alcohol (it turns into sugar in the body) because of their association with depression.[66] I think of flour and sugar as sludge—or silt—in the brain, preventing your synapses from firing.

In women, following a lacto-vegetarian diet may help, reducing the risk of depression by 35 percent.[67] This result is especially important since vegetarians are predominantly female, and women are more vulnerable to depression than men.[68] Another study found that women who

THE BLOOD SUGAR/DEPRESSION LINK

In the United Kingdom, adults consume double the recommended level of added sugar, and in the United States, the amount we consume is triple![69] High sugar intake is linked to a greater risk of depression.[70] The largest study to date to look at sugar intake (the Whitehall II study in the United Kingdom, involving 10,308 individuals) showed that consuming more sweet food and beverages is associated with a 23 percent greater risk of depression, independent of other health behaviors or sociodemographic factors.[71] What's the mechanism? Rodents fed high-fat and high-sugar diets, but not high-fat diets alone, have lower BDNF levels, which is associated with the shrinking hippocampus seen in depression.[72] Sugar is addictive, tying in the addictive and depression effects of dopamine.[73] Eating a diet high in refined sugar increases inflammation, which may lower mood and lead to exaggerated insulin responses, harming mood.[74] In addition to an inflammatory response that can trigger depression, a high-sugar diet may cause obesity and resulting psychological problems, such as having to cope with weight discrimination.[75] In short, sugar harms your body, then your brain.

Just as depression is twice as common in women, it's twice as common in people with diabetes, and blood sugar problems are worse in depressed people with diabetes. Depression and diabetes likely share the same mechanism of overactivation of the immune system, leading to a cytokine-driven inflammatory response, as well as overactivation of the HPA axis.[76] Other mutual mechanisms (meaning they are associated with both blood sugar problems and depression) are sleep disturbance, sedentary lifestyle, poor nutrition and eating habits, and other environmental and cultural risk factors.[77]

These same mechanisms result in different downstream effects: insulin resistance, diabetes, heart disease, depression, and early mortality. The cytokines are like bombs and gunfire that inflame the brain, causing depressive symptoms, poor stress coping, and blood sugar problems. In my opinion, we need to consider these shared origins of blood sugar problems, stress overload, and depression to improve the outcomes of both disorders simultaneously and, ideally, prevent and reverse disease.

It's interesting to note that depression often occurs for the first time in pregnancy or postpartum, which is when diabetes often gets unmasked for the first time.

are vegan experience less stress and are less likely to consume desserts.[78] Some studies confirm that following a plant-based food plan probably reduces depression,[79] in as little as one week.[80] Why is this? One reason may be that an omnivore's diet contains more arachidonic acid compared to vegetarian or vegan diets. A high intake of arachidonic acid fosters brain changes that increase inflammation and disturb mood, even among omnivores who consume more omega-3 fats (EPA and DHA, although when it comes to depression, EPA may be more important than DHA).[81] One randomized trial found something fascinating—omnivores were randomized to one of three groups: eating meat, fish, and poultry daily; eating fish three to four times weekly but avoiding meat and poultry; or eating a vegetarian diet. Only the omnivores who went vegetarian—restricting fish, meat, and poultry for two weeks—improved their mood.[82]

At the same time, vegetarians tend to be thinner, healthier, and more often single and urban; drink less alcohol; and exercise more compared to nonvegetarians.[83] Not all studies demonstrate that being vegetarian is protective against depression,[84] so my advice if you're vulnerable to depression is to try it and see if eating plant-based is a good fit for your body, brain, and genetics. I perform best when I eat about 95 percent plant-based, with the remainder consisting of fish and pastured meats (e.g., a lettuce-wrapped bison burger about once per month).

Further, a plant-based (or mostly plant-based, with limited fish and eggs and no dairy, gluten, caffeine, red meat, or alcohol) diet helps you detoxify: again, eating a plant-based food plan for one week reduced toxic load—as measured by dialkylphosphate metabolite (pesticide) residue in the urine before and after.[85]

Not All Is Lost

Many factors can collide to lead to depression. Sally was a forty-nine-year-old woman with longstanding depression. Her depression was intermittent, even paroxysmal—sometimes short and intense, then better. Genetic testing showed an MTHFR variation, so she started a multivitamin with methylated folate. Sally also had the CACNA1C

THE DOWNSIDE OF ANTIDEPRESSANTS:
THE EMPEROR HAS NO CLOTHES

It's a sad state of affairs when antidepressants are the most popular class of drugs in the United States. From 1990 to 2000, prescriptions for SSRIs increased 1,300 percent. Antidepressants supposedly work by correcting a chemical imbalance (specifically, a lack of serotonin in the brain), but that chemical imbalance theory has been proven to be flawed.

A breakthrough meta-analysis from Irving Kirsch, a psychology professor at the University of Hull in the United Kingdom, showed conclusively that in the best-case scenario, antidepressants have only a tiny advantage over a placebo, if any, and it's unlikely to be clinically meaningful, while in the worst-case scenario, given the side effects, antidepressants may be worse than a placebo.[86] Put another way, most if not all of the benefit of antidepressants is due to the placebo effect, proving false the serotonin theory of depression. More recent analysis suggests that "instead of curing depression, popular antidepressants may induce a biological vulnerability, making people more likely to become depressed in the future."[87] In short, antidepressants harm your brain and your body.

The dramatic increase in the use of antidepressants has been a profitable failure based on flawed experiments, in the words of one researcher.[88] Any measurable response to an antidepressant may relate more to a decreased placebo response as depression severity increases.[89] Perhaps worst of all, documents obtained from the US Food and Drug Administration demonstrated an explicit decision to keep this information from prescribing clinicians and the public[90] and showed that the agency has a policy of discounting negative data in psychiatric drug trials.[91]

As Gretchen found, antidepressants mute your range of thoughts, feelings, and experiences. They slow down your HPA axis and can rob you of orgasm. The best researchers, such as Kirsch, have concluded that other lifestyle approaches, such as exercise, hypnosis, and psychotherapy—and alternative therapies such as those described in Brain Body Diet—may be a better treatment choice for people with depression[92] because they do not incur drug risks and side effects.

variation, associated modestly with bipolar, so we tried lithium at a microdose of 400 mcg, which has been shown in a clinical trial to improve mood and happiness in former drug users.[93] She recently gave up drinking wine because it made her feel toxic and negative. Within six weeks, her depression lifted.

The Brain Body Protocol: Emerging from Depression

Certainly, depression is a complex issue, involving food, stress triggers, genes, and environmental factors. Yet you actually wield control over most of these factors. When you take action to address them, you'll address the root of depression and start to restore your joy, clarity, mood, and brain/heart connection. It's not an easy task, especially if you are in a depression or if your brain is already overtaxed. That's why social connections and help from others are so crucial to lifting yourself out of the dark. A supportive therapist, a kind friend, or an understanding relative can help encourage your gene expression to support a better mood.

Regarding the duration of the protocol: be guided by the severity of your symptoms as determined in the Interpretation section earlier in the chapter.

- For people with mild depression, follow the protocol for forty days.
- For moderate depression, perform the protocol for six to eight weeks.
- For moderately severe to severe depression, see a clinician and do the protocol for eight to twelve weeks, or longer until symptoms resolve.

BASIC PROTOCOL

Step 1: Eat for joy.

What's good for your mood? Consuming olive oil, fish, fruits, vegetables, nuts, legumes, poultry, and unprocessed, pastured meat—they are all associated with reduced depression risk and improved depression scores.[94] Another comprehensive review recommends several of the following strategies to lower the risk of depression, as reported in *Nutritional Neuroscience*; I modified them slightly:[95]

1. **Eat according to traditional diets,** such as the Mediterranean,[96] Norwegian,[97] Icelandic[98] (lots of fresh fish), or Japanese.[99]
2. **Make sure you get your dark leafy greens** or take a supplement for the B vitamins, such as methylfolate and P5P (see page 277).
3. **Consume more vegetables,** nuts (just one serving per day), and seeds. Continue to eat the rainbow.
4. Make sure to get foods rich in **omega-3 fats.**[100]
5. **Avoid sugar, processed foods, fast foods, commercial bakery goods, desserts, grains, alcohol,** and **caffeine.** Repeat after me: sugar is a depressant. Eating it most days of the week, especially if you have insulin block, can trigger depression. It only takes three weeks for an addictive pattern to kick in and trigger cravings. Postmenopausal women may be at the greatest risk for the tie between sugar and depression.[101]
6. **Eat prebiotic foods,** such as green bananas, potatoes, and crackers made from yuca.
7. **Taking probiotics** decreases a depression score by 30 percent on average and works best on people under age sixty. Prefer to eat yogurt? That works too.[102]

Step 2: Get bright light in the morning.

Sunlight (or bright light) works faster than prescription antidepressants to boost serotonin and mood, usually within one week, and with few side effects. Conversely, inadequate light in the morning is tied to circadian disruption and depression.[103] So in this part of the protocol, I want you to get bright light from the sun or a specially designed light fixture for fifteen to sixty minutes a day. On a sunny day, the brightness is approximately 10,000 to 100,000 lux. On a cloudy, rainy, or snowy day, it may not be comfortable or possible to get the morning light that you need, so it's helpful to have a high-intensity light box available at home.

Back in medical school in 1989, one of my roommates positioned a light box in our apartment to keep her mood upbeat through the grueling work of learning to be a doctor. Bright light therapy is the treatment of choice for seasonal affective disorder and has expanded into therapy for mood and sleep disorders.[104] It is a very safe way to get the mood-boosting benefits of a trip to a sunny beach.

1. Make sure your light box is 10,000 lux. (Most indoor lighting is 100 lux.) Typically the light source is a specialized fluorescent lamp, but low-intensity, shortwave blue light (750 lux) from LED bulbs also offers equal antidepressant benefit.[105]
2. Your light box should provide the full spectrum of bright white light, but block ultraviolet rays with a diffusing screen and filter.
3. Position the light box at eye level or higher, about two to three feet away from your eyes, but at a forty-five-degree angle, such as at two o'clock or ten o'clock.
4. Keep eyes open, but don't look directly into the light.
5. Use the light box in the morning for fifteen to sixty minutes, depending on your needs.

Many folks notice an immediate benefit of a brighter mood with light therapy, but expect it to take one to two weeks with daily use to notice a difference.

Step 3: Practice yoga.

As you learned in previous chapters, yoga and meditation have been shown to correct the imbalance in the autonomic nervous system, lower cortisol and inflammation, and raise serotonin, sometimes in as little as ten days.[106]

You can practice yoga in a way that reduces depression, and I highly recommend it along with the rest of the Basic Protocol for people with mild to moderate depression. I think of it as a great monotherapy when you feel depressed, as long as your score on the questionnaire earlier in this chapter is not in the severe range. (If it is, remember: see a clinician, and once your symptoms are improved, add yoga.) If you are already on an antidepressant, yoga can help. Infusing your body with fresh air with pranayama and, when warm, performing back bends and inversions are thought to be great remedies for depression (see example on page 274).

YOGA FOR DEPRESSION: SPHINX POSE

Back bends are notorious in yoga for releasing stored emotions. Sphinx pose (Salamba bhujangasana) is a great pose for beginners and experienced yogis alike because it gently warms up the low back and is thought to awaken kundalini energy at the base of the spine. Do not perform if you have a low back injury.

1. Start by lying on your belly, legs parallel and feet hip-width apart. Lengthen your tailbone toward your heels to engage the lower abdomen. Spiral the inner thighs toward your tailbone so that toes point inward and the outer thighs into the floor so that your heels point outward in order to broaden and protect the low back. This action helps to decompress the lumbar spine and sacrum.

2. Continue to reach through your toes behind you, keeping the feet active as you place your elbows below your shoulders with your forearms parallel on the floor. Gently press your pubic bone into the mat or floor. Notice if you are clenching your buttocks—ideally, they are firm but not tense.

3. Inhale as you bring your torso and head up into a gentle back bend, keeping your neck and brain in alignment with the thoracic spine. Lift your upper spine toward the crown of your head and away from the lower spine to create length and traction.

4. Finally, lift your belly to provide even engagement of the curvature of your back bend. Inhale and exhale slowly and smoothly for five to ten breaths (I like a four-second inhale, pause for seven seconds, and an eight-second exhale).

5. Release on an exhale. Repeat once or twice more.

Yoga is better than standard medical care, aerobic exercise, and relaxation exercise for depression.[107] Yes, you read that correctly. Yoga is better than standard care. Makes total sense to me, because I believe the standard care is failing people with depression. Do you need more proof? In men, yoga raises not only serotonin, but also dopamine and BDNF.[108] That's not all: yoga has been shown to raise other good brain/body chemicals like nitric oxide and antioxidants like glutathione (the most important one), bolster immunity, and reduce adrenaline and lipid peroxides, which are the ugly metabolites of fat breakdown that can damage cells.[109] So try yoga.

- If you struggle with depression, my recommendation is as follows:
  — Practice yoga three times per week for ninety minutes, ideally with a seasoned yoga teacher.
  — Include at least twenty minutes of breath work using a six-second inhale and a six-second exhale (i.e., five breaths per minute).
  — On the other four days of the week, practice your favorite postures at home for thirty minutes, with fifteen minutes of slow, deep breathing (five breaths per minute) after the asanas (physical postures).

As you may know, yoga refers to a range of practices especially in the Western world. One type is the more Westernized version, with an emphasis on physical exercise only. The other type, and the kind that I prefer and prescribe, is a more integrated and traditional form of yoga, with physical exercise combined with breathing practices called pranayama, meditation, and deep relaxation, and is the form of yoga that is proven to help depression, especially in pregnant and postpartum women.[110]

Remember from the last chapter that yoga helps anxiety, too. Yoga helps to reset the HPA better than any supplement or medication and provides clarity, insight, and equanimity.

ADVANCED PROTOCOL

If you are not getting better after two weeks, add one or both of the following Advanced Protocols and consider working with a functional medicine doctor.

Step 4: Treat yourself with brain/body uppers.

These treatments are designed to calm the HPA axis, grow the hippocampus, balance the microbiome, and favorably influence gene expression. Many are known to increase neurogenesis.[111] Choose one of the following uppers and stick to it for two weeks. Then add another supplement for two weeks. If unimproved, add a third for two weeks, and so on. (If you are on prescription medications, talk to your pharmacist about any drug interactions first.)

- **St. John's wort.** For mild to moderate depression, St. John's wort is better than paroxetine 20 mg—patients treated with it not only showed a reduction in depression severity score but also yielded greater response and remission rates compared with patients treated with paroxetine.[112] Other trials show it is as effective as selective serotonin reuptake inhibitors, including fluoxetine,[113] paroxetine,[114] and sertraline,[115] as well as tricyclic antidepressants, but with fewer side effects.[116] However, since St. John's wort causes many drug interactions, it might not be an appropriate choice for some patients, including those who take other conventional drugs. Dose: For mild to moderate depression, most trials have used St. John's wort extract standardized to 0.3 percent hypericin content, 300 mg three times daily for up to six weeks.

- **Omega-3 fatty acids.** While evidence concerning the effects of omega-3 fatty acids and depression are conflicting, low omega-3 levels are associated with depression.[117] Eating fish reduces one's risk of depression and suicide.[118] In a randomized trial of postmenopausal women with moderate to severe depression, 1.5 grams per day of omega-3 (1.05 grams EPA and 0.15 grams DHA) reduced depressive symptoms.[119] Dose: 1.5 to 2 grams per day.

- **Vitamin D.** The sunshine vitamin, when deficient, may be associated with an increased risk or severity of depression.[120] Dose: 600 to 2,000 IU per day, or enough to keep your serum vitamin D levels at 60 to 80.

- **Low-dose lithium.** Lithium has been used at standard doses for bipolar disorder dating back to 1870, but now trace and low doses have been found to be effective in depression, suicidal ideation, dementia, ADHD, and Parkinson's disease.[121] Lithium is a mood stabilizer and can be found in vegetables, mustard, kelp, thyme, pistachio nuts, and tap water. Dose: 0.4 to 2 mg a day for the long term helps some patients with depression.

- **Rhodiola.** Rhodiola decreases overall depressive symptoms, emotional instability, insomnia, and somatization in patients with mild to moderate depression, treated for six weeks.[122] Compared to sertraline (Zoloft) in mild to moderate depression, rhodiola has a better benefit-to-risk profile.[123] Finally, rhodiola helps burnout or stress-related fatigue.[124] Dose: 340 mg once or twice daily.

- **Saffron.** Based on six randomized trials, saffron effectively treats mild to moderate depression and appears to be as effective as the antidepressant imipramine.[125] Dose: 30 mg once per day for six or more weeks.

- **Vitamin B$_6$.** According to limited studies, taking vitamin B$_6$ may help reduce depression in premenopausal women, but not in the general population or older women.[126] Dose: 50 to 100 mg per day of vitamin B$_6$ or pyridoxine-5-phosphate (P5P).

- **Folate.** Women may be more vulnerable to depression when their folate level is low according to observational studies, which are considered lower-quality evidence compared with randomized trials. On the other hand, folic acid was not effective as a replacement for conventional antidepressant therapy (trazodone) in older adults with depression and dementia.[127] Dose: 200 mcg to 15 mg daily for up to six months.

You would think that taking DHEA would help mood, but in the largest meta-analysis, it didn't. However, it does help with low libido but can cause androgenic side effects like acne.[128] In my opinion, taking DHEA helps a subset of perimenopausal and menopausal women, but not everyone.

Step 5: Move for mood.

Depressed people often have something called psychomotor retardation, which means they don't want to move. Depression can make you sedentary, and being sedentary—watching TV, driving, using a computer—can make you depressed,[129] yet movement heals. Exercise increases blood flow to the brain, boosts neurogenesis, releases endorphins and BDNF—it's basically your body's very own antidepressant. It may be the last thing you feel like doing, but it should be the first thing you schedule in your day. Studies show that exercise is equally effective as psychotherapy or pharmacotherapy in treating depression.[130]

Physical activity includes both planned exercise and habitual, repetitive movements such as housework and gardening.[131] Long-term, prospective studies show that the more you move, the less likely you are to be depressed[132] or to develop burnout.[133] And once a person is depressed, physical activity is moderately effective at reducing symptoms.[134]

Overall, the best scientific evidence proves that exercise boosts your mood whether you're healthy, clinically depressed, or chronically ill.[135] When it comes to prevention, physically active people have a 45 percent lower chance of developing depression.[136] Taken further, in one randomized trial in 946 depressed outpatients, exercise outperformed the usual care for depression.[137] Even though aerobic exercise may not help with anxiety, aerobics helps depression. In fact, depressed women may get more of a response from aerobic exercise compared to men.[138]

What works:

- **Moderate exercise seems to be best**—such as walking on a treadmill or outdoors—at about 64 to 76 percent of maximal heart rate for thirty minutes. (Maximal heart rate is 220 beats per minute minus your age. For me at age fifty, that's 170, and 64 and 76 percent of 170 is 109 and 129, giving me a target heart rate range of 109 to 129 beats per minute.) BDNF seems to rise the most in response to exercise in women who are not currently taking antidepressant medications and those who have greater pre-exercise depression.[139]

- Another study in women only shows that exercise of **any intensity** helps with a depressed mood.[140]

- **For new moms,** light- to moderate-intensity aerobic exercise improves mild to moderate depressive symptoms.[141]

- **The optimal frequency** isn't as well defined, but five days per week is recommended.[142]

- **Invest now:** high levels of physical activity in middle age predict a lower chance of depression twenty-five years later.[143]

Step 6: Test yourself.

Beyond the salivary and urinary cortisol testing that I recommended in previous chapters, I suggest measuring your cortisol/DHEAS as an indicator of HPA responsiveness, and perhaps your cortisol awakening response. See Appendix B for recommended laboratories. I've found the following panels to be helpful.

- complete blood count
- complete metabolic panel with expanded lipid panel
- iron studies (to look at how well iron is transported in your blood: ferritin, iron, transferrin or total iron binding capacity)
- thyroid panels (TSH, free T3, free T4, reverse T3, thyroid antibodies)
- high-sensitivity C-reactive protein, homocysteine, possibly erythrocyte sedimentation rate
- vitamin B_{12}, folate, selenium, zinc
- 25-hydroxy vitamin D
- cortisol, DHEAS
- total and free testosterone
- iodine
- antinuclear antibody, rheumatoid factor
- red blood cell magnesium
- Lyme disease with coinfections
- Epstein-Barr virus antibodies
- gene mutations, including SLC6A4, BDNF, glucocorticoid receptor, calcium channel, FKBP5, and MTHFR

Last Word

Sure, you can try to treat depression with prescription drugs, but your brain and body will continue to suffer, and up to half the time, it won't work. The drugs may even cause harm by affecting your sex drive and your risk of future depression. Instead, when you address the many root causes that create mountains of brain trash, you reconnect cells in your hippocampus, and as a result, your clarity and joy grow. Focus instead on the low-tech interventions that have the greatest impact: fresh whole food that makes you happy, bright light, filling micronutrient gaps, yoga, and meditation. In my years of practice, I've found that these treatments are the most reparative and healing for people with mood issues. Or you can stay on your antidepressant if you have moderate to severe depression and discuss with your health care professional the option of adding the Basic Protocol for forty days. Once symptoms improve, talk over with your health care professional whether weaning off your medication is possible. The changes from using an integrated approach far exceed the limited benefits I've observed with prescription antidepressants—and there's little to no risk.

8

Recall

How to Take Care of Your Brain Body in Middle Age and Older to Keep It Young and Prevent Memory Loss

When most people walk into a room and can't remember the reason, they automatically think they're just getting older. They laugh it off and ask their friends if they're similarly at the are-we-losing-it stage, but internally, they freak out.

What if I told you that what you put on your fork could increase your brain volume and offset memory loss?

Symptoms like memory loss and diminished capacity for learning are the brain symptoms of a brain body out of balance. Instead of rushing to complete Sudoku or serial crossword puzzles, look at the root cause—which, as you know by now, is inflammation, usually originating in the gut, causing neurodegeneration (nerve cell breakdown) and ultimately leading to memory loss.[1] Sometimes the reason for the inflammation is simply eating too many of the wrong foods and not enough of the good foods. Add in chronic stress, insufficient exercise, and maybe antibiotics, and, over time, your gut becomes leaky, the bugs get out of balance, you become inflamed, the inflammation passes into your brain, and your synapses weaken. All *you* notice is that your memory declines.

Memory is no small issue after age forty. My patient Jane's experience with memory loss was no laughing matter: at age sixty, her short-term memory started to fade. She came to my office with her husband as her advocate, a look of serious concern on both of their faces. Jane explained that her symptoms began just a year or two before with some forgetfulness, like not recalling a word in conversation or sometimes repeating herself, as in asking her husband a question she had already asked. Together they had seen an Alzheimer's specialist who didn't think she had the disease (and she didn't have the so-called Alzheimer's gene, APOE4) but didn't know for sure and recommended that she consider hormone therapy to help her memory and cognitive function.

What I found was that for Jane, estrogen was no longer serving in its role as her master regulator of the female brain and body, as we discussed back in the introduction. Her brain was no longer adaptive and able to grow and respond to chemical and physical insults, and memory loss was just one of the symptoms of her brain/body breakdown. Her blood sugar was in the prediabetes range, setting her up for *type 3 diabetes*—a term that captures the overlap between type 2 diabetes and Alzheimer's disease, including a constellation of inflammation, oxidative stress, insulin resistance, increased glycation (a form of sugar-induced aging that occurs when chronically high blood glucose levels injure various proteins, making you look and feel old), and cognitive deficits.[2] Several blood tests of inflammation were elevated, putting her at yet greater risk for cognitive decline.[3] Her brain MRI showed mild to moderate cerebral atrophy (brain shrinkage), and that scared the daylights out of her.

"What can we do?" she asked plaintively. I felt for her, and I gave her my best recommendations, covered in this chapter. We needed to get estrogen back into its rightful role as the regulator of her brain/body health. You can do that too, if you're perimenopausal or postmenopausal and estrogen bioidentical hormone therapy is a smart option for you. I'll show you how to determine if it's the right choice.

Memory stitches together your inner life. The term *memory* refers to the complex interplay of multiple brain functions: nerves and chemical processes that govern the learning of new information, storage, and, finally, recall. Most important, memory is the main indicator of the balance in your brain between growth and repair (neurogenesis) versus wear and tear (neurodegeneration). Some of your memories are stored in the brain permanently and can be recalled as needed. Other memories are stored in the temporary memory bank, then discarded.

My memory has never been perfect, but I was better able to remember appointments in my twenties than I am now. My husband and I are similar in this regard. It turns out that after forty, it's the recall of recent life events, people, faces, names, and dates that starts to fade first. When memory begins to disappear, thoughts do not get properly encoded and stored, leading to a loss of cognitive function and quality of life. Hormone loss can amplify poor memory. The question is, does memory start to go because age is taking its natural course, or because of something we thought was harmless, such as drinking too much wine or not filtering fluoride from our tap water? Read on to find out.

Memory is an important indicator of your cognitive reserve, or your brain's resistance to damage, injury, decline, and neurodegeneration. A few memory glitches are normal as you age—after all, your brain works perpetually and is constantly interrupted. So how do you tell the difference between a little forgetfulness and early signs of dementia? Even if you have only normal age-related memory issues, there is good news about the malleability and plasticity of memory as you age.

Do You Have Memory Issues?

Do you have now or have you had in the past six months any of the following symptoms or conditions?

- ☐ Have you found that a word is "on the tip of your tongue," but you can't quite access it?
- ☐ Have you forgotten someone told you something and needed to be reminded, especially something you just heard? Or did you mix up the details of what somebody has told you?

☐ Have you forgotten what you just said, or repeated what you just told or asked someone?

☐ Have you developed facial blindness (i.e., difficulty recognizing faces)?

☐ Have you forgotten important details of what you did yesterday?

☐ Have you experienced less mental clarity or brain fog, particularly later in the day?

☐ Have you had difficulty remembering what you just read and have to start the page or article over again? Or have you observed that you have difficulty following the thread of complicated stories, conversations, or plots, such as in movies, or started to read something without realizing you had read it before?

☐ Have you experienced less interest in reading or other cognitive tasks that you previously enjoyed?

☐ Have you perceived a decrease or simplification in vocabulary?

☐ Have you forgotten to do things you said you would do or planned to do, or had to check whether you had done something? Can you not recall when something happened?

☐ Have you detected a decreased ability to communicate in a foreign language that you previously were able to speak and read readily?

☐ Have you experienced increased anxiety when driving or trying to find your way to familiar places?

☐ Have you forgotten to tell somebody something important?

☐ Have you forgotten where things are normally kept?

INTERPRETATION

If you said yes to three or more questions, you may have an issue with memory. Five or more, and it's highly probable that you have a problem with storing and retrieving information, tracking conversations and tasks, and performing routine activities. No need to freak out just yet—we need to cast a wide net when it comes to memory so that we can catch any loss as early as possible, when inflammation and breakdown might be occurring but before brain/body failure. Help is on the way! The protocol at the end of this chapter will strengthen your recall, reverse memory issues, and help prevent further decline.

How Memory Works

In medical school, I encountered several people with photographic memories. They didn't need to study for hours in the library like I did, trying to cram an impossible volume of facts into their brain. They saw a biochemical structure of a cholesterol or a diagram of a complicated mechanism in the immune system once and retained it. Similarly, both of my daughters remember lyrics to entire songs after hearing them only a few times, while I can barely jump in with a line from the chorus. But human memory is not designed to be perfect, regardless of age. Perhaps I should repeat that—for memory's sake: memory is not designed to be flawless.

Memory is complex, involving encoding and storage into short-term memory, and then sometimes long-term memory, and *then* retrieval of that information. Memory is what allows you to remember past experiences and recall frames of mind, education, impressions, circumstances, habits, and skills. Similar to how I delete emails on my laptop to make space in my inbox, you delete or prune old memories if they no longer seem relevant, like the phone number for your local nail salon that you need just once.

When it comes to memory, the creation of neurons matters less than maintaining the connections between them. We used to think that synapses were simply a transfer point between neurons; now we know that synaptic plasticity is the key capacity of connections between neurons to strengthen or weaken over time in response to higher or lower activity. Synaptic plasticity contributes greatly to learning and memory and may be the answer for older brains to adjust for lesser function as they age.

As the name implies, short-term memory is fleeting, whereas long-term memory is more hardy and enduring. Memories aren't stored like an image in one place but in fragments distributed across various parts of the brain (see Memory in the Brain, page 287). Upon recall, your brain reassembles the various pieces for an intact memory. Perhaps because of the fragmentation, our memory is subject to error, even under normal circumstances.

The Science of Memory

Functional brain-imaging techniques have allowed scientists to map how and where memories are made.

- **Hippocampus:** The hippocampus is the key part of the memory process. Recall from chapter 1 that acquiring and consolidating memories begins in this horseshoe-shaped structure found in both hemispheres in the brain. The hippocampus is the way station before memories are placed into long-term storage. An indexer catalogs memories so they can be reconstructed at a later time.
- **Amygdala:** The amygdala stores emotionally charged memories.
- **Prefrontal cortex (PFC):** The CEO of the brain is responsible for the short-term memory of any information that needs to be immediately processed (aka *working memory*), such as a pitcher who has to remember how many outs there are and where the runners are on base. These temporary and conscious memories are based on linguistics and perception and guide your reasoning, decisions, and behavior.
- **Cerebral cortex:** This large outer layer of the brain stores and maps long-term memories.
- **Striatum, or corpus striatum:** Any voluntary activity you do is triggered by the striatum. It receives information about a desired goal from the cerebral cortex and prompts your body to move, in a smooth and fluid manner, based on previous experience. The **nucleus accumbens,** your reward center, is part of the striatum.
- **Cerebellum:** As partner to the striatum to effortlessly perform procedures, the cerebellum is key for attention, language, emotional response, and timing based on prior experience, such as how to tie your shoes. The cerebellum helps you hone skills for daily tasks without having to consciously recall each step.

ENCODING

Encoding is the first step of memory-making. Sight, sounds, smells, touch, and words create our perception of something. That perception becomes a construct stored within the brain in either short- or long-term memory and may be recalled later. Sufficient sleep is crucial for memory encoding as well as later offline consolidation of memory. Our hormones—particularly estrogen, progesterone, and testosterone—may influence our ability to encode.[4] Not long ago, scientists thought that steroid hormones like these were produced only in the body, not the brain, which meant it would take a long time—hours to days—for them to affect a brain cell. Now we know that the brain itself produces these steroid hormones, called neurosteroids, that can impact brain cells in a very rapid timescale of seconds to minutes.[5] Low levels of sex hormones in women are linked to negative bias with memory encoding, meaning the women were more likely to remember negatively charged events.[6]

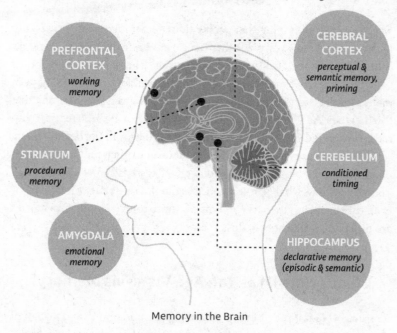

Memory in the Brain

SHORT-TERM MEMORY

Your short-term memories consist of information that you need to re-call only transiently for a few seconds or minutes, like the date and time of the dental appointment you just made or the price of your dinner entrée at a restaurant. One form of short-term memory is working memory, such as when you're shopping online and comparing the prices of different brands.

You have space for about seven bits of information at a time, which is why doctors try to get you to remember a seven-digit phone number as part of a test called the "mental status exam." New memories overwrite the old ones. Distraction also brings in new information that can overwrite what you just learned, requiring you to go back and look up information again, or retrace your steps as you try to remember what you were about to say.

LONG-TERM MEMORY

You know the old saying that people don't remember what you say, but they remember how you made them feel? Your brain discerns if a memory is important enough to store long-term, usually because of an emotional charge or personal meaningfulness (thank you, amygdala). Long-term memories are stored throughout the cortex as groups of neurons that fire together. As a whole, long-term memories are a gigantic reserve with rather unlimited space in the cerebral cortex, at least in the healthy brain.

There are two types of long-term memory: explicit and implicit. Explicit memories require a conscious effort to recall, including factual knowledge, like what you learned in school, the details of *Titanic,* or even that bachelorette party you may want to forget. Implicit memories are procedural, like how to floss.

What's Normal as You Age Vis-à-vis Memory?

As we age, we fall prey to momentary lapses in memory, and not all of them are due to aging or something more serious, like toxicity or dementia. Now, this is the part I know you're probably most concerned about. We all are! Remember, memory is imperfect for all of us at one time or another. Just think about children or teens in your life—how often do you have to instruct them before they really remember on their own? By age forty or fifty, we've all had issues with memory because of correctable problems like a stretch of poor sleep, acute stress, or an overwhelming workload.

However, as you age, mental capacity can get smaller, meaning there's more pruning. After turning fifty, I'd occasionally be mid-interview, about to make the last two points in response to a question, and my mind would go blank. I'd make the first point, then search for a beat or two for the missing point. This problem is thought to be a result of the frontal lobes briefly losing track of the next step in the brain process. Fortunately, brain exercise helps your frontal lobes stay sharp; consistent meditation and physical fitness improve this type of memory loss.

Not all forms of memory are equally affected by age. Procedural memory, such as how to ride a bike, remains intact. In general, the frontal lobes and hippocampus are more vulnerable than other parts of the body and thereby more susceptible to momentary memory lapses. Other types of declarative memory decline, such as semantic and episodic. Semantic memory is the recall of general facts, like state capitals, world population numbers, and carbon dioxide emissions. (These are the hot topics in our household right now.) Episodic memory is a recall of autobiographical events or episodes at a particular time and place—like a birthday celebration when you were forty. Moreover, spatial memory—such as the geography of your neighboring towns or how to find the bathroom in your friend's home—tends to decline with time. Lisa Genova's novel *Still Alice,* also made into a movie, tells the story of a professor who developed early Alzheimer's and chronicles painfully how she got lost in familiar territory.

Here's a summary of how aging affects memory:

- Slower processing speed, so you learn more slowly
- More effort to learn new information in the first place
- Reduced ability to perform tasks involving attention—less detail is taken in, such as where you put your wallet or keys
- Slower recall of memories

These behavioral changes reflect biochemical and structural changes, including a smaller hippocampus, loss of function and structure in the frontal lobes, loss of brain cells, and lower quantity and function of receptors.

Nevertheless, we have reasons to face growing older and its inevitable memory changes with optimism. It may take slightly longer to learn new information, but retention is the same as that of a younger person. Processing speed may be a little slower, but you can adjust and work around it: crack a joke as you wait for the right word to arrive or pick a second-choice word. As you learn, simply pay attention more closely. In my podcast, I used to have a time-out for the "sexy librarian moment" when I would recap what we just learned. I did it because it helps everyone's learning, including my own—revisit, review, and recap more after age forty to strengthen and reinforce the memory pathways.

The best news is that memory is malleable, meaning that much of your memory is under your control as you age. Your task is to understand the nefarious factors that increase neurodegeneration and replace them with the virtuous factors that enhance neurogenesis.

What Affects Memory

The most important levers that impact your memory are diet, physical activity, stress, sleep, gut function, social and mental engagement, toxins, and genes. Jane had problems with all of these: on the Perceived Stress scale, her level of perceived stress was high at 32. (Take the simple ten-question test and score yourself—the link as well as how to score it is in the Notes.[7]) She started wearing a fitness tracker and barely got seven thousand steps per day. Her gut tests showed leaky gut and dysbiosis. Heavy metals were high in her blood, and a gene test showed that she had a variant of the FKBP5 gene, making her potentially more vulnerable to stress.

DIET

I've mentioned previously that the brain is only 2 to 3 percent of body weight but consumes up to 25 percent of energy in the body; this mismatch means that the brain is especially hungry for the nutrients you eat compared with other body organs.[8] The enormous drive for energy means that brain cells are more vulnerable than the rest of the body to mitochondrial problems and oxidative stress, and once damage occurs, neurodegeneration and memory problems follow.[9] Food affects memory in many ways—it can lessen or worsen the stress response, increase or decrease nerve growth factors and neurogenesis, provide antioxidant defense or not, and trigger inflammation in the body that leaks into the brain.[10] Sugar is perhaps the best known offender when it comes to your ability to think, learn, and remember—and develop stroke and dementia, including Alzheimer's.[11] Eating more sugar doubles your risk of cognitive impairment.[12] For women in their forties, you need to know that perimenopause is when the brain's ability to regulate sugar in the brain begins to falter because of dropping estrogen levels.[13] Importantly, cognitive loss occurs even without a change in weight from excess sugar consumption.[14] So if you think your consumption of sugar is acceptable because your weight isn't going up, think again. Limited data from a small study in younger women ages twenty-five to forty-five suggest saturated fat may worsen memory, while fats found in oily fish (salmon, mackerel, herring, anchovies, sardines) improve it.[15] Trans fats: shocker, bad for word recall—avoid them.[16] Similarly, in a larger prospective study in older women, saturated fat again predicted worse cognition and verbal memory, whereas monounsaturated fat (think avocados, macadamia nuts, extra dark chocolate) was protective.[17] Not surprising, the worst combination for your memory is the high sugar/high saturated fat diet (i.e., the binge-on-a-pint-of-ice-cream diet).[18] That combo makes you fat, inflamed, and heading to a nursing home. *Forgetaboutit.*

GUT

As the foundation of the brain body, the gut/brain connection is critically important to your sound mind. Your gut contains 100 trillion bugs that influence your well-being in various ways, including your risk of anxiety and depression as described in the last two chapters. Microbes have their own memory.[19] The DNA belonging to these bugs, your microbiome, is involved in most if not all biological processes, including the messages of the brain, cognitive function and flexibility, and the ability to remember.[20] Taken further, when the microbiome of a healthy person is compared with that of a person with memory impairment, there are changes in the bacteria, including Bacteroidetes, Firmicutes, Proteobacteria, and Verrucomicrobia. These phyla of bacteria correlated with cognitive test performance.[21] In mice, fecal transplants improved memory and learning.[22] Why? When your gut wall is leaky, your blood-brain barrier becomes leaky. On a molecular level, the tight junctions between cells loosen, and the process of intestinal permeability is regulated by proteins (like zonulin and occludin) produced in the gut. Inflammation spreads from the body to the brain, and memory can suffer.

Overall, you're fighting an uphill battle as you age because the composition of the gut microbiota changes in the direction of less diversity and fewer good bacteria.[23] You harbor more gram-negative bacteria, which secrete the dreaded lipopolysaccharide (LPS) and create inflammation in the gut that can travel to the brain.[24] Changes in gut microbiota can alter blood-brain barrier permeability.[25] In sum, the gut microbiota's effect on inflammation and brain function in the hippocampus can rob you of memory and a sense of calm.[26]

PHYSICAL ACTIVITY

Regular exercise enhances memory and reduces dementia by 38 percent.[27] It increases the brain-derived neurotrophic factor (BDNF), which is like fertilizer for the soil of your brain.[28] It boosts neuroplasticity.[29] Whether you're a kid or an adult, being physically fit is linked to a bigger hippocampus and better memory.[30] What type of exercise? How much? Aerobic exercise seems to be the best at preserving brain volume and memory as you age, perhaps because it boosts BDNF, whereas strength training may not be as effective, particularly in women.[31] All types of exercise—aerobic, resistance, and multimodal—benefit executive functioning in women more than men.[32] Ideally, exercise four or more times per week, which is associated with halving the risk of dementia.[33] While it's never too early to exercise, middle age may reap the greatest benefits. That means *you*. Now. Today! And it's never too late—even physical activity in patients sixty-five and older with cognitive impairment and/or dementia can improve cognitive function.[34] Conversely, when you don't move much (like Jane, as documented with her fitness tracker), memory worsens and cognitive function declines.[35]

Yoga also prepares the body and mind for meditation, which also helps memory. Even inexperienced people improve their memory with yoga—as few as six sessions have been shown to enhance working memory.[36] Many other studies confirm that yoga boosts memory and cognitive performance.[37] Yoga increases melatonin production, which may improve sleep and indirectly promote better memory, as shown in multiple studies on different populations.[38] Specifically, kundalini yoga has been shown to improve memory and executive function in twelve weeks, and it boosts depressed mood and resilience among patients fifty-five and older with mild cognitive impairment.[39] In fact, the study showed that kundalini yoga is better than memory-enhancement exercises, which have been considered the gold standard for managing mild cognitive impairment. Yoga turns on the relaxation response and regulates the genes that help you calm down, produce more glutathione (the body's most important antioxidant) so you can detoxify better, sleep more soundly, and wake up refreshed, ready to remember.[40]

STRESS

By now you're probably feeling stressed from hearing about all the horrible things associated with stress. I'll keep this short. You've learned that excess cortisol is a brain/body toxin—it pokes holes in the gut wall, leading to leaky gut, and disrupts the gut/brain axis. Additionally, the hippocampus, the brain's memory center, is extremely vulnerable to stress.[41] When you have a high degree of perceived stress and, as a result, a high level of cortisol, the excess cortisol deactivates and hurts the hippocampus.[42] Over time, the hippocampus shrinks in volume in response to prolonged cortisol in the blood.[43] Metabolism of the brain in the hippocampus and prefrontal cortex decreases significantly, and connections between brain cells weaken.[44] Memory becomes impaired, especially retrieval.[45]

On the other hand, there are hormones that can protect your brain from the neurotoxic effects of cumulative cortisol. In women, estrogen plays an important role in buffering the effect of aging and stress, keeping the volume of the hippocampus larger before menopause compared with men, and growing the hippocampus after menopause in women receiving estrogen therapy.[46] In addition to estrogen, DHEA can protect the hippocampus, but not in everyone. In my opinion, preserve your memory: keep your cortisol, estrogen, and DHEA in the mid-range up to menopause, and possibly for up to ten years postmenopause. Scientific proof is lacking, so this is my opinion based on the literature and clinical experience.

Jane's cortisol was high on a dried urine test, and both estrogen and DHEA were low, so cortisol was running the show—raising blood sugar and blood pressure, increasing visceral fat at the waist, poking holes in her gut lining, fanning the fire of inflammation, decreasing lean body mass, lowering brain-derived growth factor production—making blood sticky and slowing down cognitive speed and memory. What helps your memory is to develop *stress plasticity* or resilience—the ability to cope with and adapt to a wide range of stressors over time.

SLEEP

Sleep is when your brain sorts and stores the day's information. Would you believe that the primary purpose of sleep is to form memories? So bedtime may be the most important time of the day for your brain's health and neuroplasticity. During sleep the brain restores neuron networks so they are ready for action once more when you awaken. The space between brain cells enlarges, making room for the flow of ions and debris, like amyloid.[47] It's called the glymphatic pathway, and it works best when you're sleeping on your right side. Additionally, sleep is the time of healing and repair, when growth hormone and melatonin are at their highest. Autophagy occurs, which is an important editing process that allows your body to remove damaged mitochondria and proteins. Overall, the clearance of metabolic by-products and toxins increases four-fold while sleeping.[48] Both REM and non-REM sleep enhance and strengthen long-term signal transmissions between neurons after repeated stimulation—another key requirement for memory and learning. All said, sleep is like hitting a refresh button on the hippocampus.

But how many of us sacrifice sleep for other life demands? When you don't get sufficient sleep, memories are misfiled or dropped. Sleep deprivation interrupts the movement of information from short-term into long-term memory banks by impairing function, encoding, and consolidation. Hence, memory performance suffers, like when my patients tell me they are experiencing "Mommy brain" and have trouble finding certain words.

Five hours of sleep deprivation in one night's cycle changes the connections between brain cells, at least temporarily, in mice.[49] Insomniacs show pathological thinning of the insulation called myelin around nerve cells; myelin's job is to enhance the ability of nerves to send signals to each other. Most of the thinning nerve tracks are on the right side of the brain, the seat of emotion, thought, and sensory information (sight, touch, smell), so the person who suffers from sleep deprivation may have more difficulty with proper vision and could be more left-brain activated.[50]

Lack of sleep affects neurogenesis, particularly in the hippocampus.[51] You can even develop false memories if you lose sleep.[52] Structurally, sleep deprivation blocks your synaptic plasticity and efficiency by changing the density and shape of neurons (the "dendritic spines" of neurons, to be exact—these are like sprouts on the branches of neurons) of the hippocampus.[53] One article called the problem the "tired hippocampus."[54] (Read more details in the Notes.[55])

Fortunately, recovery sleep (sleeping more to make up for a sleep deficit) restores memory, meaning that symptoms of poor memory from lack of sleep may be reversible, up to a point. Unfortunately, aging is associated with worsening quality of sleep, including shorter duration and more time awake after you fall asleep. People tend to awaken more frequently starting in middle age and to experience a profound decrease in the deepest stage of slow-wave sleep as they get older.[56] Homeostasis in the sleep regulation system and circadian rhythm declines with age. Overall, working memory and new episodic memories get worse. Even though poor sleep is associated with poor cognitive function, including memory, the good news is that older adults are more resilient around the cognitive hits of sleep deprivation and fragmentation compared with younger adults. Still, it's worth improving sleep in order to enhance cognition, performance, and memory, regardless of age.

TOXINS

By now, you're probably not surprised to see toxins on the list. Toxins can lead to loss of mental function, reduced brain size, and changes in the structure and function of brain cells, ultimately resulting in memory loss and the rest of the broken seven that we've covered.

Alcohol. Alcohol impairs memory, erodes mental function, reduces brain size, and causes brain cell dysfunction.[57] Makes you want to put down that glass of wine, doesn't it? Loss of brain volume is more likely to occur in women compared with men, according to the Framingham Study.[58] The more alcohol consumed, the greater the shrinkage. Both alcoholics and people with Alzheimer's disease demonstrate hippocampal atrophy.[59] It's like the hippocampus receives less blood flow and life energy and ultimately goes soft and decreases in size, like a neglected muscle. Alcohol (technically, ethyl alcohol or ethanol) and acetaldehyde (released as alcohol breaks down) kill brain cells.[60]

The frontal lobes are most affected by alcohol abuse.[61] Alcohol can degrade the prefrontal cortex (the brain's CEO), involving attention, inhibitory control, working memory, and cognitive flexibility.[62] Further, in a study from the University of California at San Diego of heavy and light drinkers, chronic consumption of alcohol interferes with balance and visual and spatial ability. Heavy drinkers compromise their short-term memory and working memory.[63] Granted, that's why many people drink—they want to forget what just happened at work or home, and alcohol makes forgetting possible. Alcohol also disrupts normal function of estrogen and cortisol, which can impact encoding of memory.

Chronic, dependent drinkers are at greater risk of alcoholic dementia and Korsakoff syndrome, a type of dementia that includes severe amnesia as a result of vitamin B_1 deficiency and alcohol toxicity. In a study of twenty-two female adolescents, nineteen of whom were abusing alcohol, results showed that the patients had less gray matter in the frontal lobes, resulting in poor control over behavior and decision-making, impairment in internal awareness, problems with error detection, and antisocial and drug-using behavior.[64]

Need more evidence relevant to you? When I was in medical school twenty-five years ago, a limit of one glass of wine per day was considered

WOMEN AND ALCOHOL

Women are more vulnerable to alcohol's adverse effects compared with men because we have more fat and less water. We also make less of the detoxifying enzyme called alcohol dehydrogenase, so that acetaldehyde, a possible carcinogen made from the breakdown of alcohol, can accumulate in our bodies. Since we metabolize alcohol differently, women have higher blood alcohol concentrations for the same serving, and the higher levels persist longer. So women are more likely to experience neurotoxicity, liver damage, heart disease, and cancer at lower drinking levels than men.[65] Alcohol is more likely to disturb a woman's sleep, but many women fail to notice.[66] Yet women are drinking now more than ever.[67] It's a growing problem. The *Washington Post* says that white middle-aged women are drinking themselves to death.[68] Indeed, more than 70 percent of white women drink, compared to 37 percent of Asian, 41 percent of Latina, and 49 percent of black women. Since 1992, the number of middle-aged women seeking rehab has tripled.

safe for women, two glasses for men. Then most of us thought moderate drinking was no problem—that is, about eight to twelve glasses of wine per week (one glass of wine is five ounces, which is typically about 12 percent alcohol, and contains 14 grams of alcohol). So over the years I began drinking more. Maybe it was an attempt to cope with small children, or just enjoying life near the wine country, but my occasional glass of wine on the weekend became one glass every night, and then two. As a recent *New York Times* article on the topic by a fellow mother from Berkeley describes: "We tell people to go ahead and have just a little bit of an addictive substance. Let's acknowledge that that's complicated."[69]

Over time, the data that seemed to promote moderate drinking have become less clear and robust. Imaging studies have failed to show that drinking offers any benefit to the brain.[70] Historically, the data varied or showed an adverse effect only with heavy consumption,[71] but moderate alcohol consumption can shrink the brain and its gray matter, too.[72] Evidence now suggests more conclusively that moderate drinking can have a deleterious effect on the brain, as shown by a recent study from Oxford that followed 550 people for thirty years with weekly alcohol counts, cognitive testing, and MRIs.[73] More alcohol was associated with atrophy of the hippocampus, even among moderate drinkers.

The upshot? Lay off the sauce to preserve your brain and memory.

Mercury. Mercury's effects on the brain have not been studied as extensively as other toxins. But a study from the University of South Denmark, Harvard School of Public Health, and the University of Copenhagen examined 923 children for mercury levels and neurobehavioral traits. The study found that mercury impairs visual, spatial, and working memory.[74] Mercury exposure can come from contaminated seafood, such as tuna and swordfish, and dental amalgams.

Mold. Mold exposure impairs memory, slows reaction time, disorders balance and cerebellar function, and decreases verbal recall, problem solving, and perceptual motor function. Whew! The most common contributors are from molds hiding under or behind appliances like your dishwasher, under drippy sinks, under leaky windows, inside wall cavities where plumbing leaks, on skylights, on air-conditioning coils, and in new buildings that were built in the rain or have water damage. Many molds in homes can impact the nervous system in the areas that control memory, attention, and other functions.[75] A study at the University of Southern California studied a group of about one hundred people exposed to mold toxins compared to a group of one hundred people exposed to toxic chemicals (e.g., diesel exhaust, formaldehyde, organophosphate insecticides, cleaning chemicals, carbon monoxide, chlorine). The impairments—such as forgetting the word *stroller* or *epiphany*—in the chemically exposed group were about the same as in the mold-exposed group.[76]

PCBs. PCBs were used widely in electrical appliances and other equipment. Exposure to PCBs is associated with poor visual recognition memory.[77] This form of memory begins in early infancy and is remarkably resistant to decay, unless you're exposed to PCBs. That means if PCBs have affected your memory, you could be staring at a friend at a party for ten minutes before her name comes to you. PCBs are no longer manufactured in the United States but can persist in the environment for decades. PCBs are still present in many products made before 1979, when their use was outlawed.

Aluminum. Excess intake of aluminum causes cognitive impairment, short-term memory dysfunction, and decreased learning.[78] Aluminum occurs in soil, air, and water. You may be exposed to aluminum in processed foods containing flour, baking powder, coloring, and anticaking agents. (But thankfully, you're not eating processed food by now.) The average US adult eats 7 to 9 mg of aluminum per day in their food, according to the Centers for Disease Control.[79] Beverage cans, personal care products like antiperspirants and cosmetics, and medicines are other common sources, including antacids (300 to 600 mg aluminum hydroxide per tablet or capsule), buffered aspirin, and vaccines.

Lead. Even though lead is no longer in household paints, it still lurks in some houses built before 1978, when the federal government banned consumer use of lead-based paint. It can occur in soil, and especially in drinking water, as we witnessed in Flint, Michigan. After the crisis in Flint, five people including the head of the state's health department were charged with involuntary manslaughter for ignoring a serious problem with lead pipes contaminating the water.[80] Lead can seriously harm your brain. Even at low to moderate levels previously considered safe for adults, lead exposure can impair short-term memory.[81] For children, there is no safe lower threshold for lead levels without hurting cognitive function, and pregnant women should avoid all exposure to lead.[82] Lead affects attention, processing speed, visuospatial ability, working memory, motor function, and general intellectual performance, resulting in lower IQ.[83] In animal models, lead creates inflammation and neurodegeneration.[84] So it's no wonder that lead exposure leads to elevated markers of Alzheimer's disease.[85]

I know, it seems like toxins are hiding everywhere. Unfortunately, they are. But I promise that we can mitigate their effects and protect our brains. Review the protocol in chapter 2 for specifics.

GENES

We are still identifying and trying to understand the genes most involved in memory. Here are a few of the important ones. (See Appendix B for help on whether to test and, if so, which labs to use.)

- **APOE4** (Apolipoprotein E4), the "Alzheimer's gene," can affect memory by early midlife (i.e., in your forties).[86]
- **FKBP5** (FK506 binding protein 5) is a gene involved in stress (glutocorticoid receptor sensitivity) and memory formation, including intrusive memories.[87]
- **KIBRA** (kidney and brain expressed protein) has certain variants that enhance memory.[88]
- **SCN1A** (encoding the α subunit of the type I voltage-gated sodium channel) provides instruction for sodium channels.[89]
- **NR2B** codes for part (subunit) of the glutamate (NMDA) receptor and is involved in working memory.[90]

Three Levels of Impaired Memory

Most of us think of brain damage as what happens when you hit your head on the football field and suffer a concussion or survive a car accident. But brain damage can result from seemingly innocuous things like eating too much sugar, or undergoing stress, or a tick bite. The brain tries to create balance in the face of competing demands, stressors, out-of-whack hormones, endocrine disruptors, and trauma. Memory impairment usually means there's been damage to brain structures involving storage, retention, and recollection of memories. Impairment can result from mild conditions such as dehydration and nutritional deficiencies to more serious problems like high blood pressure, PTSD, diabetes, small strokes, and dementia.

The three main categories of memory impairment are:

- **Age-related memory issues.** (See pages 288 to 290.)
- **Mild cognitive impairment (MCI).** MCI is an intermediate category between normal age-related memory loss and dementia. There are two subcategories: amnestic (impaired memory) and nonamnestic (decline of mental functioning such as language, attention, or processing).
- **Dementia.** Dementia is characterized by a marked impairment of memory and cognitive function that interferes with daily living,

sometimes accompanied by personality and behavioral changes like agitation and rage. Short-term memory fades first in dementia. Sixty to 80 percent of cases are Alzheimer's disease. The hippocampus, which turns perception into memory, is hit hard by Alzheimer's disease. Vascular dementia is the next most common and results from damage to the blood vessels that provide oxygen to the brain. Vessels can become narrowed or blocked and lead to silent or overt strokes as a result of high blood pressure or pathological cholesterol deposits. When blood flow is compromised, brain cells die.

THE QUESTION OF ESTROGEN THERAPY

The main estrogen you make during the reproductive years, **estradiol**, is neuroprotective, promotes synaptic plasticity in the hippocampus, and protects against cognitive decline associated with aging and neurodegenerative diseases.

When you have a sensory experience that provokes a memory, estrogen immediately sends signals in the service of improving your learning.[91] Estradiol (E2) is the main estrogen of interest when it comes to memory, and it is made in the ovaries, adrenal glands, and brain. After menopause, estrone (E1) is the dominant estrogen, and it's made primarily in the adrenals and fat tissues, plus a small amount in the ovaries.

Estradiol, both endogenous (the type made by you inside your body) and exogenous (i.e., estradiol therapy), benefits memory up to a certain point. There's a threshold that you reach with estrogen and memory, probably in the first ten years of menopause, when estrogen therapy stops being helpful. Based on the science, estrogen therapy may benefit healthy nerve cells, but weaker neurons may be compromised by long-term treatment. That is, once the memory loss and dementia process begins, treatment with estrogen is no longer effective and may even increase the risk of Alzheimer's disease.[92] So there is a window of opportunity to take estrogen for cognitive health and memory.[93]

While estrogen treatment in perimenopause and early menopause may postpone memory loss, it works in a bell-shaped dose-response. That means your best memory occurs when estrogen is midlevel—not too high and not too low.[94] Put another way, low levels of estradiol and high levels of estradiol are associated with poor memory, cognitive impairment, and declining brain function. However, the conventional approach at this time is *not* to treat women in menopause for the primary (before symptoms) or secondary (when symptoms start) prevention of dementia.[95]

So the debate rages on with many advocates for and against the use of estrogen for brain/body health as a woman ages, and specifically about the exact "midlevel" of estrogen that is optimal for the brain body.[96] The antiaging estradiol enthusiasts believe it is 80 pg/mL, while the more conservative epidemiologists concerned about prevention of osteoporosis believe it is somewhere between 5 and 20 pg/mL (as opposed to normal postmenopausal levels that are often less than 5 pg/mL).[97] After age forty-three or thereabouts, the ability of estradiol to improve cognition declines due to decreased estradiol levels and decreased expression of estrogen receptors.[98] Women who have their ovaries surgically removed and experience low levels of estradiol as a result show diminished cognitive function that is reversed by estrogen therapy, if it's begun immediately following surgery.[99] Menopausal women (mean age fifty-three) seem to experience mood benefits from estrogen therapy but not necessarily cognitive benefits.[100] Other studies of the benefits of exogenous estrogens for memory and executive function probably weren't large enough to achieve the power to prove they work or not.[101] So the appropriate next question is: if you want to start estrogen (estradiol) replacement to prevent or reverse memory decline, when is the best time to start?

Common sense says to start at the time of estradiol decline, which begins for most women in their forties, but it's a complex decision. The trick is to define your own window of opportunity to take estrogen for the maximum cognitive benefits, including memory, and it seems to be from about age forty-three to sixty-one.[102] From the Women's Health Initiative, the optimal period of estrogen therapy when considering heart disease and breast cancer is ages fifty to fifty-nine, but what about memory? It seems that earlier initiation may be better to protect against cognitive aging that occurs fifteen to twenty years later. Further, we may want to preserve estrogen levels instead of allowing them to drop in late perimenopause and early menopause and then try to play catch-up—the benefits of estradiol on the brain seem to decline if you take it after ovarian hormone deprivation, i.e., low estradiol levels.[103]

There are other factors to consider. On the positive side, estrogen preserves memory, brain function, vaginal lubrication, and bone strength and prevents hip fractures and colon cancer. Estradiol helps to preserve the blood-brain barrier, prevents neuroinflammation, refortifies weak mitochondria, and promotes neurogenesis in the hippocampus.[104] Therefore, you won't be surprised to learn that estradiol may help reverse the memory symptoms in Alzheimer's disease and might be helpful—we don't yet know definitively—in women at risk for dementia.[105] On the other hand, oral estradiol increases the risk of stroke and may increase the risk of cardiovascular problems in susceptible women. Transdermal estrogen is far safer than oral and is the only type of estrogen that I prescribe.[106] If you have a uterus, you will need to take progesterone or progestin (synthetic progesterone) to protect the uterine lining from cancer.

What I've done in my practice is to make a risk, benefit, and alternatives balance sheet for each patient based on her risk factors, genomics, and quality of life. It's not as simple as a yes/no answer of whether you should take estrogen. Rather, it's a question of whether it makes sense given your circumstances and whether it should be an in-between dose (like half a dose or three-quarters of the standard estradiol dose) and maybe even for a short period of three months (which can confer longer benefits[107] and can serve as an n=1 experiment for how estradiol works specifically for you). Fortunately, estradiol is available by prescription only, so there is a gatekeeper in place who can help you decide if taking estradiol is right for you.

Risks of Estrogen Therapy After Seven Years of Treatment		
Event	Risk without estrogen therapy	Risk with estrogen therapy
Venous thromboembolism (blood clot)	16/1,000	16–28/1,000
Stroke	24/1,000	25–40/1,000
Gallbladder disease	27/1,000	38–60/1,000
Breast cancer	25/1,000	15–25/1,000
Clinical fracture	141/1,000	92–113/1,000
Coronary events	No increased risk	No increased risk

The Brain Body Protocol: Restoring Memory

Our brains are remarkable because of their ability to bounce back—i.e., neuroplasticity! You can prevent decline or stop further decline up to a point, and it's important to start now during middle age. Many simple things can improve blood flow to the brain, heal body inflammation (which may reverse brain inflammation and damage), and rebuild the memory center. Overall, there's not one tip that solves the whole problem. Rather, we need to try several proven things at once.

So how do you put all this information into a doable plan that protects your brain? Most of this protocol includes simple changes that easily fit into any lifestyle, resulting in better neurogenesis, increased synaptic plasticity, and halting of neurodegeneration. Since memory is your main issue, perform this protocol for forty days and then incorporate your new habits for the rest of your life.

BASIC PROTOCOL

Step 1. Eat for memory.

The big idea is to eat more of the foods that strengthen the memory and avoid the foods that don't. That means we'll restore the brain/body axis with the way you eat.

- **Eat three meals per day,** no snacks in between, ideally following an eight-hour eating window and sixteen-hour overnight fast to promote mild ketosis, which can help prevent Alzheimer's disease, reduce inflammation, reset insulin, and improve cognitive function.[108] Ketones like beta-hydroxybutyrate are a more efficient fuel source and increase production of BDNF.[109]

- **Aim for one to two pounds per day of nonstarchy vegetables.** Set the goal to enjoy twenty to thirty different species, all colors of the rainbow, each week. There's no evidence that fruits or juices are effective in memory repair, so focus on the vegetables![110]

- **Eat protein at each meal,** ideally fish,[111] nuts, seeds, eggs, or anti-inflammatory animal protein.

- **Add in more plant-based fat.** The usual suspects: avocados, macadamia nuts, and coconut meat, milk, and cream. Cook with coconut oil, olive oil, or pastured ghee.[112]
- **Consume prebiotic foods** such as asparagus, fennel, garlic, leeks, and onions.
- **Add in probiotic food** like sauerkraut, miso, and tempeh.
- **Drink bone broth.**

Avoid:

- **Sugar.**
- **Processed food.**
- **Alcohol,** so you can keep estrogen and cortisol in balance and optimize sleep.
- **Grains** (wheat, rice, oats, corn) and pulses (beans, lentils).
- **Dairy**—I recommend an elimination diet for forty days, then add it back in to see if you react.
- **Advanced glycation end products** (AGEs)—AGEs can be made inside the body or consumed in the food you eat. Specific cooking methods can dramatically increase AGEs in your food. This means that in addition to keeping your blood sugar normalized (see Step 3), avoid fatty foods that are fried, barbecued, grilled, roasted, sautéed, broiled, seared, or toasted. Dry heat causes AGE formation to increase ten- to a hundred-fold. Foods highest in AGEs are red meat, fried eggs, butter, cream cheese and other particular cheeses, and highly processed products. So even if your diet seems healthy, you may unwittingly consume unhealthy amounts of AGEs because of how your food is cooked.

Step 2. Mind your eating atmosphere (and with whom you eat).

The sad fact is that 20 percent of Americans eat regularly in their cars. Twenty percent! Our genes are not designed for eating in the atmosphere of a toxin-filled vehicle. We were built and evolved to eat with people we love. In fact, science shows that as you get older, the people with whom you eat is just as important as what you eat. More social integration around meals protects you from losing your marbles as you get older.[113] The worst situation is older women eating alone with compromised nutrition. The takeaway: get the nutrition you need and eat your meals with people you enjoy.

Step 3. Normalize your blood sugar.

High blood sugar crashes your memory, processing speed, attention, and executive function. Even conventional scientists recommend earlier intervention in the prediabetes phase.[114] Most people with blood sugar problems like prediabetes have no idea, so start here with a blood test. If your hemoglobin A1C or fasting glucose are not in the optimal range, pay attention, because this is the biggest driver of current and future cognitive decline. Remember that if you control your blood sugar, you can prevent 60 percent of the cognitive decline that occurs as you age.[115] At the risk of sounding like a broken record, here's what you can do to improve blood sugar levels (note that many of these strategies are the same as the memory diet in Step 1):

- **Control your carb intake.** Carbohydrates are broken down into glucose, which raises blood sugar levels. Reducing carb intake can help normalize blood sugar. Define your carb threshold as described in chapter 3 and commit to staying under your threshold. Implement portion control.

- **Perform intermittent fasting,** ideally the 16/8 protocol as described on page 73, five to seven days per week.

- **Sleep seven to eight and a half hours every night.** One night of bad sleep will raise your blood sugar. See additional tactics in Step 4.

- **Increase your fiber intake,** such as by eating one to two pounds of vegetables per day.

- **Exercise regularly.**

- **Drink filtered water and stay hydrated.**

- **Monitor your stress levels.** Chronically high perceived stress raises cortisol and blood sugar.

- Discuss with and order from your clinician an **insulin/glucose challenge test.** In general, I suggest that if you have any memory issues (or weight or fat gain), you track your blood sugar level and aim for the optimal zone (see Notes for details[116]). It may take more than forty days to reset your blood sugar, depending on where you start and previous damage to metabolism.

- **Consider the use of supplements** such as berberine, chromium, cinnamon, and fenugreek.

Step 4. Make the other lifestyle changes that balance your hormones and improve metabolic flexibility.

- **Get a good night's sleep,** ideally seven to eight and a half hours per night, to store memories and think clearly the next day. This will help you make adequate hormones.

  —If you can't seem to sleep more, try camping or being out in nature. A study from the University of Colorado showed that one weekend of backcountry camping with natural light—sunlight, moonlight, firelight, and flashlights (no other artificial lights, including personal electronics, were allowed) helped reset melatonin so that sleep began earlier (by two and a half hours). It shifted the circadian rhythm by 69 percent. The camping itself probably has less of a benefit than being in nature and sleeping when the sun sets and waking with sunrise.

  —For women, sleep in a room at 64 degrees Fahrenheit or cooler. I've written about how temperature control helps women sleep better as they age, but often 64 degrees is too cold for their sleeping partners. Another strategy is to cool your bed on a local level using something like the ChiliPad, which can serve as a mattress pad on your side of the bed or under your pillowcase. It allows you to dial in the best temperature for your sleep, with a range from 55 to 110 degrees.

- **Napping** is another pathway to memory consolidation. A nap of twenty to ninety minutes appears to be ideal, according to one study—though medical opinions vary and naps seem to benefit younger more than older adults.[117] If you've read my previous books, you know that I'm a fan of the siesta because it reduces sleepiness, improves memory, prepares you for learning, enhances cognitive function, and boosts emotional stability, regardless of whether you obtained sufficient sleep the night before.[118] Duration matters: brief naps of fewer than fifteen minutes provide immediate benefits that last up to three hours, whereas naps of thirty minutes or longer can cause sleep inertia (grogginess) when you first awaken, and may interfere with deep (non-dream) sleep at night, but then provide cognitive improvement for longer, up to many hours.[119] One of the best ways to reap the brain/body benefits of naps is to sleep for up to thirty minutes, then exercise afterward to wake up.[120]

- **Detoxify your environment** from mold, mercury, aluminum, PCBs, and lead (see chapter 2).

Step 5. Exercise for memory.

- **Physical.** Strength or resistance training improves memory and cognition.[121] It raises testosterone and growth hormone to help you grow new nerve cells.[122] A single bout of high-intensity interval training improves memory in women.[123] Modest increases in physical activity in the range of 10 percent can significantly reduce the risk of dementia and Alzheimer's disease.[124] Multiple modalities are best, and women may benefit from the cognitive effects on executive function, including memory, more than men.[125] Exercise boosts the size of the brain, particularly the hippocampus, counteracting the shrinking effect of age. Additionally, exercise boosts BDNF, which promotes neurogenesis, synaptogenesis, and blood flow to the brain. Recommendation: a minimum of 150 minutes of moderate or HIIT exercise per week. That's just thirty minutes a day for five days a week!

- **Mental.** Bilingualism or multilingualism builds cognitive reserve and protects your brain from aging.[126]

- **Spiritual.** Meditation, yoga, and alternate nostril breathing all help memory.
  —Meditation can increase blood flow in the brain and improve memory, even in older folks with age-related memory loss, mild cognitive impairment, and early Alzheimer's disease.[127] A ten-day mindfulness retreat enhanced the capacity of working memory, improved attention, and lowered anxiety, negative mood, and depression of participants, and a four-day mindfulness retreat improved working memory for people who hadn't previously meditated.[128]
  —Kundalini yoga boosts executive function in people with mild

memory impairment. Yoga two to four times per week for thirty minutes or longer was very helpful to Jane, and I recommend that for you, along with several of the supplements mentioned in the next step of the Brain Body Diet. Add in the silent chanting of a mantra, usually part of kundalini but also simple to do on your own for a few minutes, to activate the hippocampus.[129]

—Left nostril breathing stimulates memory in the right brain hemisphere, and right nostril breathing seems to help with numerical data retrieval as a result of left-brain activation—and benefits occur after thirty minutes for four consecutive days.[130]

YOGA FOR MEMORY:
EASY POSE WITH THREE LOCKS

When I practice kundalini yoga, my final pose before Corpse pose (Sivasana) is Easy pose with application of the three energetic locks. I think of the locks as locking in memory, especially if it's leaky. Yogi Bhajan, the charismatic teacher from Pakistan who brought kundalini yoga to the West in 1968, taught this kriya as part of a practice for memory in 1969.[131]

The three locks together are called Maha Bandha: Mula Bandha (root lock) is where you pull up your pelvic floor, like you're trying to stop the flow of urine; Uddiyana Bandha (diaphragm lock) is where you keep lips closed and pull abdominal muscles and organs upward toward the thoracic spine; and Jalandhara Bandha (neck lock) is where you tuck your chin toward chest, pressing into the front of the neck.

1. Sit in Easy pose, with knees bent and legs crossed. Lengthen your spine from sit bones to crown.

2. Breathe long and deep for three minutes. Keep your eyes closed.

3. Deeply inhale, holding your breath at the top of the inhale, and apply the three locks, starting first with Mula Bandha, then Uddiyana Bandha, and then Jalandhara Bandha. Hold as long as is comfortable, trying ten seconds to longer.

4. Then release in the reverse sequence: Jalandhara Bandha, Uddiyana Bandha, and Mula Bandha.

5. Sit quietly and breathe before taking Sivasana.

Step 6. Supplement your memory.

Start with just one for two weeks, then add a second if your memory still needs help. If you are taking prescription medications, talk first with your pharmacist about any interactions.

- **Bacopa** has been used for thousands of years in Ayurvedic medicine to enhance memory, relieve pain, and treat epilepsy. Bacopa protects cells in the hippocampus, prefrontal cortex, and striatum against toxicity and DNA damage, which are commonly implicated in Alzheimer's disease.[132] Several studies show that it improves memory, verbal learning, retention, and information processing in healthy people.[133] Bacopa improves synaptic plasticity when taken for up to twelve weeks.[134] Dose: 250 to 500 mg, twice daily. Side effects include palpitations, dry mouth, nausea, thirst, and fatigue.

- **Citicoline** is the exogenous version of the natural intracellular precursor of phosphatidylcholine[135] and boosts neuroplasticity. Citicoline promotes neurogenesis and has been shown to help memory impairment, especially of vascular origin—such as from stroke or vascular dementia.[136] Initially developed for the treatment of stroke, it can be used to improve memory and even has the support of the Cochrane collaboration's systematic review.[137] There are limited data supporting citicoline in patients with Alzheimer's disease.[138] Dose: 500 to 2,000 mg per day.

- **Curcumin** improves memory in patients without dementia, according to a randomized trial lasting eighteen months.[139] This result confirms previous trials showing a benefit to working memory and attention within one hour of curcumin dose. Bioavailable curcumin can help working memory and attention within one hour.[140] Dose: 90 mg twice per day.

- **Huperzine A** seems to improve memory across the age span. It is an alkaloid isolated from Chinese club moss, *Huperzia serrata,* an inhibitor of acetylcholinesterase (an enzyme that breaks down the neurotransmitter acetylcholine) that is said to help both central and peripheral activity with the ability to protect cells against hydrogen peroxide, amyloid beta protein (or peptide), glutamate, and stroke. It has been shown to improve memory in healthy adolescents.[141] Multiple randomized trials suggest that Huperzine A is effective in improving memory and other outcomes in patients with Alzheimer's disease and vascular dementia.[142] Dose: 200 mcg per day.

- **Omega-3s.** More than twelve good-quality randomized trials have been published on the effect of omega-3 fats (DHA + EPA or DHA) on cognition and memory. Overall, participants with mild cognitive impairment gained a modest benefit from omega-3 supplements, especially for immediate recall, speed, and attention.[143] However, not all trials show a benefit.[144] DHA quells inflammation, improves memory, and prevents neurodegeneration in conditions such as Alzheimer's disease.[145] DHA increases production of BDNF, which helps enhance the structure and function of brain cells. Dose: 900 to 1,700 mg per day of DHA and EPA. The most proven form for memory is derived from marine algae. I suggest taking it for six months at a dose of at least 900 mg per day.

- **Phosphatidylserine** (PS) is one of my favorite memory supplements because it is like a cleanup crew. Multiple trials show that PS improves memory, attention, arousal, and verbal fluency in aging folks with cognitive decline.[146] It seems to work best in patients with good cognitive function at baseline. The majority of studies are positive, but not all.[147] Benefits seem to fade after sixteen weeks when combined with other treatments,[148] so think of it as a "pulse" to boost your memory. Dose: 300 to 800 mg per day.

- **Vitamin D** calms down neuroinflammation by reducing cytokines (the weapons of the immune system that cause damage in the brain body).[149] The ideal dose is based on your genetics and sun exposure, so the best strategy is to measure 25-hydroxy vitamin D in your blood after taking a consistent dose. Aim to get enough vitamin D to keep serum level at 60 to 90 ng/mL, associated with optimal sleep and the lowest risk of dementia. Dose: 2,000 to 5,000 IU/day, but the best strategy given the multiple genes involved in vitamin D metabolism is to track your blood level over time and to get out into the sun for thirty minutes per day.

- **DHEA** is an important sex hormone that is made in the brain and adrenal glands. It has many important jobs in the brain body, including antioxidant, anti-inflammatory, BDNF-raising, stress-buffering, and antiaging activities.[150] However, taking DHEA does not seem to improve memory in people over the age of fifty.[151] There may be a window of time during which taking DHEA is helpful, such as in younger women before the age of fifty, but the data are mixed.[152]

- **Other.** Additional supplements are found in the Notes, including acetyl-L-carnitine, cinnamon, magnesium L-threonate, and pyrroloquinoline quinone (PQQ).[153]

ADVANCED PROTOCOL

If your memory is not better within two weeks, add one or more of the steps of the Advanced Protocol.

Step 7: Initiate hormone therapy.

Since hormones decline in middle age, does it help memory and general cognitive ability to add back sex hormones as you lose them, such as estrogen in women and testosterone in men? The answer is, "It depends."

- **Estrogen** as bioidentical hormone replacement could be beneficial for some women (see the sidebar earlier in the chapter).

- **Testosterone** seems to enhance memory encoding in men but not women,[154] and though animal studies suggest that testosterone helps memory and cognition,[155] the data on the role of supplemental testosterone in men with mild cognitive impairment or Alzheimer's disease have been mixed.[156] However, one small trial suggested that testosterone therapy in women may improve postmenopausal verbal learning and memory.[157]

Test your hormones, including thyroid, estrogen, progesterone, and cortisol—and then work with your clinician to adjust in a way that makes sense for your situation.

Step 8: Perform computer-based cognitive training.

Computer-based cognitive training is growing in popularity and seems to be more effective than any pill. Evidence is moderate that cognitive training in adults with normal cognition improves memory, reasoning, and processing speed. In a meta-analysis of fifty-two studies, computer-based cognitive training improved nonverbal, verbal, and working memory.[158] The benefit seems to last two to five years, with the memory benefits fading by ten years post-training.[159]

There are many approaches to enhance memory with the help of a computer or app: brain training programs, working memory training programs, and video games.[160] The best tested are Elevate, Lumosity, Fit Brains, Brain HQ, and Brain Workshop. Many are effective in as little as ten to twenty minutes per day, five times per week, and four of the five (at time of publication) can be downloaded and used on your smartphone.

Last Word

It's time to rewrite the future of your brain body. Memory decline need not be in the cards for you. A little forgetfulness is normal, but in my case, the right diet, intermittent fasting (described in chapters 2 and 3), social eating, phosphatidylserine, plus high-dose vitamin D worked wonders on my own memory. Simple fixes like eating a diet rich in vegetables, nuts, and fish—along with making sure you get enough sleep and exercise—can go a long way toward making your brain bigger as you age and improving your cognitive function, whether you're middle-aged and just becoming aware of your forgetfulness, or you're older and fearing gradual decline.

Memory will never be perfect. But when consistent issues arise, take a closer look at the way you eat, move, think, and supplement—and, most important, make your brain/body relationship a priority. The challenge is to identify the brain/body issues that are causing neurodegeneration and memory loss. Once identified, they can be remedied with an integrated approach.

Conclusion

You did it. *Yes!* You solved a gigantic problem, one you may not have known you had. I am so happy for you because the work you've invested in healing the brain body will pay dividends for the rest of your life. Regardless of the symptoms you brought at the beginning of the book, you can now go forward with the brain body powerfully alive and the connection intact.

When the brain body is out of whack, life is hard and confusing, even brutal. It can turn us into zombies going through the motions of life. As you may recall from before you began the Brain Body Diet, the problem of brain/body dysfunction can feel daunting and scary, at times overwhelming—popping a prescription pill may seem like the right answer, or at least the easier answer. German philosopher and cultural critic Friedrich Nietzsche once wrote: "What doesn't kill you makes you stronger."[1] But Nietzsche was dying of syphilis, a terrible infection of the brain body.

Sometimes what doesn't kill you makes you weaker. The brain/body problems described in the book don't necessarily kill you, but they *will* weaken you—your health, resolve, clarity, joy, calm, energy to shop for and cook nourishing food, social ties, sense of purpose and meaning. By now you understand that the simple daily lifestyle choices outlined in the book, starting with diet, work better than any prescription.

Lifestyle medicine is the most effective solution to the brain/body dysfunction that we face as women. Your task as you go forward is to keep up the self-directed neuroplasticity—that is, the formation, growth, and development of new brain cells regulated by the behaviors under our own control. You can pick one of your favorite steps from the Brain Body Diet and keep going at it. The practices in this book are designed to activate self-directed neuroplasticity. Keep working your favorite practice and let it work you.

You are never too old for self-directed neurogenesis. As long as you practice it regularly each day, you can perform self-directed neuroplasticity until the day you die. For example, every day I go on a walking meditation with my dog (page 90). Before I go to bed, I perform a forward bend and hold it for about three minutes (page 247). I perform high-intensity interval training four times per week (page 308). These practices create a loop of integrity, of taking in the good, and are now habits. Over time, the emphasis you place on your favorite brain body practices will aggregate into a habit and, eventually, a durable brain/body union.

We all need help. This book is designed to help you reconnect the brain body so you feel whole, no longer at war, no longer full of toxins that cause the brain body to disengage, no longer feeling flabby and wondering why nothing works, no longer depleted after having kids (however long ago), no longer wondering if you're starting to get Alzheimer's. My hope is that this final chapter adds further motivation, like wind at your back, as you move forward on the path of healing. Over the years, I've learned that staying motivated is a process. Think of it as a hybrid car that goes far on a tank of gas. You don't need a full tank to keep driving the car; you simply need to watch the gauge and not run out of fuel. Similar to the hybrid, the process is regenerative— driving the vehicle generates more energy, just as the benefits of the Brain Body Diet will keep you motivated to stay on the path. The weight loss, clarity, peace, equanimity, happiness, and mental acuity will energize you and keep you motivated, even more so than when you began.

In this final chapter, I want you to take a moment to connect to your own drive for change. That drive can only come from you, not me. As you consider your own drive for changing the brain body, I want you to praise your success to date and accept any of your weaknesses, false starts, backslides, or plateaus—all in an atmosphere of collaboration rather than confrontation, judgment, or belittling.

Sometimes a difficult experience brings you to a book like *Brain Body Diet*: a scary diagnosis, a line you drew with your weight, feeling unable to get out of bed in the morning, forgetting a password or a child's name, stressing out over something you know is minor and *not worth it*, seeing your kid gain weight, a hospitalization, a family member with Alzheimer's disease. Whatever it is, there's one question to answer.

What Do You Want?

When it comes to the brain body, I know what I want. I want to be that woman who sings, gardens, skips with her grandchildren, loves deeply and without regret, causes trouble, protests inequities and injustices, writes books, stays at her ideal body weight set point, teaches yoga, and keeps expanding her soul. My memory sharp as a tack, mind clear and focused, eyes sparkling, energy buoyant. Until about age one hundred, maybe longer, similar to my great-grandmother Mud, who died peacefully in her sleep at age ninety-seven. Mud practiced most of the Brain Body Protocol before the term *functional medicine* was born.

I don't want to settle for the default. I see the default setting in Jane, one of my patients mentioned in the last chapter with poor short-term memory. She gets little exercise, drinks too much wine, and eats bread and pasta every day. Jane eats three meals per day with two snacks, starting at 6 a.m. with a mocha, and ending late with dinner around 7 p.m. High blood pressure and inflammation have caused severe cerebral atrophy, which showed up on an MRI of her brain. We are working to reverse these problems—with intermittent fasting, mild ketosis, yoga, supplements, and a low dose of bioidentical estrogen and progesterone, but it's easier to fix these issues ten or twenty years before symptoms begin.

I see the default in many women in their sixties and older when they are addicted to sugar, are anxious or depressed, and can't seem to hear or accept what would make them well—the realignment of brain body. They have shrinking brains, a result of brain/body breakdown over decades, and, consequently, shrinking personalities and personal power. In their seventies, they are at a time in life when I would hope they would be enlivening and expanding. They have more free time than ever to make a difference in the world, but they are literally shrinking before my eyes.

No one has to live this way. Certainly I want a different fate, and I hope by now that you do, too. It's actually a choice, a choice that you make starting in your thirties, forties, and fifties, with downstream effects in later middle age and beyond.

Now it's your turn. What do you want as you get older? Depressed with a vacant stare and foggy brain at a nursing home, chock-full of dysbiosis and inflammation? Or engaged, happy, calm, and sharp, well into your nineties?

Nietzsche wrote something more applicable to brain body: "If you know the **why,** you can live any **how.**" This quote is much more relevant to finishing the Brain Body Diet and moving on with life in a more balanced state. You too can live any how, including the sometimes difficult Advanced Protocols listed in the preceding chapters. Once you finish the Brain Body Diet, you know that this is a life plan—a prescription for the rest of your life to keep your brain body in balance. Repeat the protocol whenever symptoms arise, like a rising body weight, brain fog, addictive tendencies, worry, burnout or depression, or memory loss. Add in one or more steps from the Advanced list. You have the "how," and when you stay connected to your "why," you have an impeccable brain/body circuit for current and future health and homeostasis.

Your Choice Going Forward

You've learned in this book about the choices you have regarding the broken seven, the key conditions that result from brain/body breakdown, including toxin buildup and brain trash, a rising body weight set point, brain fog, addiction, anxiety, depression, and memory loss. The good news is that you can apply your brain to repair the broken seven and reconnect the brain and body into a cohesive whole. Hopefully, I've empowered you to apply your brain to solve these problems that are so prevalent in middle-aged women.

You are not stuck with the brain you have. The brain is malleable: it can keep growing, learning, storing new memories, and changing itself and the function of the body, often regardless of your age and previous deficits. That's the promise and benefit of neuroplasticity, which you can promote if you regularly remove brain trash, commit to the correct set point, and follow the other recommendations in this book. You want to keep your brain's synapses expanding and forming new connections throughout your whole life. That will keep you in your right mind.

Sometimes, the body and brain break down in their communication, leaving you with no choice but to pay attention, as I was forced to do after my concussion. The main problem we face is that the brain/body connection is extremely vulnerable to assaults from the environment— the sleep you skip, the sugar you eat, the metals stored in your bones, the wrong microbes you feed—and the inflammation that results. Out of the broken seven, toxins are the most influential when it comes to brain/body health. I used to think of the brain as a data processing machine, but now I think of it as a living entity, adapting and changing in response to the environment and improving with age and strategic environmental cues.

Whether your problem is brain trash, weight, brain fog, addiction, anxiety, depression, or memory loss, or some combination, as you've seen in the preceding pages, the Brain Body Diet can prevent and reverse harm to your brain body. We can even grow into the broken places with more wisdom. That's what I wish for you. When you heal the brain/body wounds, you become stronger than before. Jill Bolte Taylor is a great example.

Stroke of Insight

Let me tell you an interesting story about Jill Bolte Taylor, a neuroscientist performing research at Harvard University, who studied some of the issues regarding the brain/body connection.

At age thirty-seven, Jill had a research opportunity few people would want: a ringside seat to her own massive stroke in the left hemisphere of her brain.

On the morning of December 10, 1996, Jill woke up and felt pain behind her left eye, as if she had eaten an ice cream cone too quickly.[2] Then as she looked at her hands, she felt dissociated from them—like they were claws. She lost her balance and ability to process information. She later learned that a blood vessel in her brain had exploded. Over four hours, she watched as brain functions shut down one by one: motion, speech, memory, and self-awareness, until she could not walk, talk, read, write, or recall any of her life. She became an infant in a woman's body.

"How many brain scientists have been able to study the brain from the inside out? I've gotten as much out of this experience of losing my left mind as I have in my entire academic career," she described in her popular TED Talk. As her left hemisphere—the linear, methodical, categorizing, organizational side of the brain—shut down, her inner chatter ceased. Jill's right brain took over, and she could tell that she was no longer the choreographer of her own life. The right hemisphere is more Zen. It thinks in pictures and learns kinesthetically, through movement. It is rooted in the present moment, tunes into mystery, and operates in more abstract and mystical realms. Two weeks after the stroke, surgeons removed a golf ball–sized clot that resulted from her hemorrhage.

Perhaps Jill thought her life as she knew it was over, which would be even worse than the default setting of a shrinking brain. It took Jill eight years to recover her ability to think, walk, and talk, but she came back stronger and happier than ever before. The stroke, on the left side of her brain, unleashed a torrent of creative energy from the right side of her brain. Jill was able to choose to respond with her previously neglected, virtually unrecognized right brain—a place of deep inner peace and loving compassion.

Jill is now the most peaceful she has ever been. When the left half of her brain went silent, she experienced a great gift: a deeply different understanding of who she is and knowledge that the world is filled with beautiful, peaceful, compassionate, loving people—people who could choose to respond from their right hemispheres at any time and be masters of their own neuroplasticity and neurogenesis.

After my concussion on the left side of my brain, the noise of my left brain got turned down, my ego deflated, and my spirit grew. I felt the peace, joy, and connection that Jill describes. I began listening more to my heart and allowing it to tell my brain what to do. In yoga, we talk about the default setting, part of the human condition, as the illusion of the fabricated mind—called *maya* in Sanskrit. Much of the illusion is separateness, thinking we are alone and separate, perceiving differences in people compared to ourselves—a left-brain tendency, versus perceiving the similarities and features that unify us.

In my medical practice, I see this illusion at the root of the thought patterns of addiction, anxiety, depression, fear (of memory loss, fatigue, brain fog, or other chronic conditions), and even weight gain. According to the Vedic concept of maya, things that appear to be present are not what they seem, yet we perceive our own illusions as real.[3] Maya can lead to a distorted view of reality, and Jill's stroke pierced the veil of her own illusion, an illusion that I shared before my own traumatic head injury.

Both Jill and I actively promoted neurogenesis in the service of greater balance between the left hemisphere—the logical, factual, and scientific side—and the right hemisphere—the intuitive, imaginative, and holistic side. We both became stronger at the broken places. And having experienced this peace, we both choose to work at retaining it, moment by moment and day by day. Jill adds: "It is liberating to know that I have the ability to choose a peaceful and loving mind (my right mind), whatever my physical or mental circumstances, by deciding to step to the right and bring my thoughts back to the present moment."[4] You, too, can choose to rewire your brain by making the choices outlined in this book until they become habitual. You can even grow your neurospirituality circuits along with your gray matter and, along the way, activate your right brain. That's self-directed neuroplasticity at its best.

Of course, you don't have to suffer a concussion or stroke to become happy, peaceful, integrative, and healed. As I slowly recovered from my fall, I learned I had to actively turn off my left hemisphere to create a new way of being in the world. It was an essential part of my own brain/body rehab.

Moving Forward

For most of you, the Brain Body Diet will provide you with a renewed brain/body connection that allows you to reclaim your health, and even create a health metamorphosis in forty days. For others, the Brain Body Protocols will provide the first few steps in the larger journey of discovering the brain/body link, but you will need to continue the protocols until symptoms abate, usually for twelve weeks or sometimes longer, and ideally work with a collaborative functional medicine clinician. The duration depends on the severity of your symptoms: the greater the severity, the longer the duration. Never forget that small steps taken consistently are the most impactful. Repeat the protocols if and when symptoms recur, like when you begin having trouble again with language retrieval or you gain five pounds and don't know why.

Now that you're aware of toxins, you'll keep releasing them so they don't become brain trash. And you'll avoid future toxic exposures, since that's easier than removing them. Keep eating plants—and a lot of them. Eating one to two pounds per day of vegetables is what works best: cruciferous vegetables such as cauliflower, broccoli, and Brussels sprouts, as they support your liver; dark green leafy vegetables such as lettuce, spinach, and kale; sulfur-containing onions and garlic. Aim for lots of colors and 35 to 50 grams of fiber per day to absorb toxins in your gut. Sweat more: spin, walk in the forest, do hot or warm yoga, or visit a sauna. Foster friendships with people who eat and live cleanly, so your genomes can upgrade together. Repeat the Brain Body Toxin Protocol (chapter 2) at least twice per year. We can't rely on the old systems of our body to remove toxins behind the scenes because our bodies are overwhelmed. You've already made great progress in relieving your body burden; now you want to maintain your progress.

Let's not lose sight of what we've learned. Unfortunately, the brain body is sometimes vulnerable, prone to being pulled out of balance by modern lifestyle choices and exposures. The seven Brain Body Protocols help us live in a high-performance state where the brain and body are allies. That means there are ongoing, rich, deep conversations occurring between brain/heart, brain/gut (including liver, microbiome, microbiota, immune system), brain/fat, brain/mitochondria, brain/ muscles, and even brain/posture. Without those conversations, we can too easily fall back to that default setting that we agreed we're not settling for. Remember too that you now have a comprehensive diet in your back pocket, not a restrictive and short-term means to an end, but more the ancient Greek version (*diaita*), a doctor-prescribed program of living that includes a personalized dietary regimen that you've just tested on yourself, as well as the important daily habits that help you govern and arbitrate your life—in short, the broader functional medicine protocol that allows you to keep brain body in homeostasis for the win.

This book is about telling the truth, the sometimes difficult truths about being female, middle-aged (forty-plus) and older. The truth is that it's sometimes damn hard. Our hormones, like estrogen, drop, and our brains get overwhelmed. Metabolism slows down, yet appetite increases and weight climbs. We get more inflamed and feel beleaguered. If you chase the symptoms with medication, you are less likely to heal than if you chart a new path with the lifestyle medicine of the Brain Body Protocols.

Conventional medicine will keep prescribing a pill for every ill and tell you that lifestyle changes aren't enough. That's not what I've found as a leader in the functional medicine movement and practicing physician. Instead, it's our only hope of a comprehensive solution. Lifestyle choices, starting with food, play a huge role in brain health and, by extension, brain body health. Together we need to raise the bar. We have a long way to go—please help spread the message by talking to your doctor and other health care professionals about the topics and evidence-based protocols in this book. Tell your loved ones that there is another way to handle the symptoms of brain/body disconnection. Share your own story of challenge and success with me on social media. Help me spread the word. Service is good for the brain body. Please help me get the best information out to people who still suffer and need a change.

Ultimately, I hope you go beyond fixing the broken seven to create a balanced, soulful existence. Balance between the left and right hemispheres, the sympathetic (fight-flight-freeze) and parasympathetic (rest-and-digest) nervous systems, and the HPA axis and endocrine glands, and balance in favor of positive thoughts and feelings about the brain body—that's the restoration of homeostasis. The only way to achieve it is with comprehensive lifestyle medicine, not the next prescription pill or scientific breakthrough—but with the small daily choices that influence your ability to return to balance. Lifestyle factors powerfully affect brain body and vice versa. In fact, we can set ourselves free with the power of our brain/body connection and unleash that power to experience the peace and joy that Jill did. Leverage the malleability of your brain and become stronger at the broken places. Your body will be at one with itself. You will be healthier and feel more in sync with yourself. Your brain will learn to rewire itself to serve you and your highest purpose.

Recipes

Brain/Body Prebiotic Porridge

This is what I eat when I want something warm and comforting in the morning—or the occasional dinner!

Porridge:
- 1 cup warm unsweetened almond or cashew milk (or milk of your choice; volume will depend on desired consistency)
- 2 scoops vanilla or berry protein powder or medical food (look for one containing at least 20 grams of vegan protein)
- ½ scoop greens powder (look for one containing organic wheatgrass, spirulina, spinach, barley grass, alfalfa, chlorella, and kale)
- 1 scoop fiber powder
- Optional: ½ to 1 teaspoon each of fructooligosaccharides, inulin, or glucomannan (a prebiotic blend)

Toppings:
- 6 ounces berries
- 2 to 3 tablespoons soaked chia seeds
- 1 tablespoon hemp seeds
- Optional: 1 serving nuts of choice such as macadamia, walnuts, or almonds (one serving is 28 grams, a small handful, about 18–20 almonds)

Use a spoon to mix porridge powders with milk, using more or less milk to achieve the consistency you prefer. Add toppings and eat immediately.

Brain/Body Bowl

This is my meal of choice before or after a workout, when traveling, or when short on time.

    1 cup unsweetened almond or cashew milk (or milk of your choice; volume will depend on desired consistency)
    2 scoops vanilla or chocolate protein powder or medical food (look for one containing at least 20 grams of vegan protein)
    ½ scoop greens powder (look for one containing organic wheatgrass, spirulina, spinach, barley grass, alfalfa, chlorella, and kale)
    1 scoop fiber powder
    Optional: ½ tablespoon MCT oil

Toppings:
    1 banana, sliced
    1 serving (28 grams) nuts of choice, such as macadamia, walnuts, or almonds (28 grams is a small handful, about 18–20 almonds)
    1 tablespoon cacao nibs

Use a spoon to mix powders with milk, using more or less milk to achieve the consistency you prefer. Add toppings. Eat immediately.

Dr. Sara's Alternative Breakfast Bowl

Bottom layer:
    1 tablespoon sunflower seeds
    1 tablespoon sesame seeds
    1 to 3 tablespoons freshly ground flaxseeds (I adjust to help with regularity)
    1 tablespoon hemp seeds
    1 ounce raw macadamia nuts
    1 teaspoon or less moringa powder

Top layer:
    1 serving (6 to 8 ounces) coconut or cashew yogurt (dairy-free)
    1 tablespoon shredded coconut
    1 tablespoon chia seeds, soaked in filtered water
    4 to 6 ounces bananas, berries, apples, or other fruit

Mix each tier's ingredients together and layer in a pretty bowl.

Dr. Sara's Brain/Body Shake

1 cup unsweetened almond or cashew milk (or milk of your choice)
2 scoops vanilla or berry protein powder or medical food (look for one
  containing at least 20 grams of vegan protein)
1 scoop fiber powder
1 tablespoon MCT oil
2 tablespoons hemp seeds
1 tablespoon freshly ground flaxseeds
1 scoop greens powder (look for one containing organic wheatgrass,
  spirulina, spinach, barley grass, alfalfa, chlorella, and kale)
6 to 8 ice cubes
Optional: 1 to 2 teaspoons holy basil (also known as tulsi)

Whip all ingredients in a high-powered blender to desired consistency.

Mocha Shake

2 cups unsweetened almond or coconut milk (or milk of your choice)
2 scoops decaf cappuccino protein powder or medical food (look for
  one containing at least 20 grams of vegan protein)
1 scoop fiber powder
½ avocado
2 to 3 teaspoons cocoa or cacao powder
Coffee to taste and desired consistency
6 to 8 ice cubes

Whip all ingredients in a high-powered blender to desired consistency.

Red Velvet Shake

2 cups unsweetened almond or coconut milk (or milk of your choice)
2 scoops chocolate or vanilla protein powder or medical food (look for
  one containing at least 20 grams of vegan protein)
1 scoop fiber powder
½ avocado
½ small beet
¼ teaspoon vanilla

2 to 3 teaspoons cocoa or cacao powder
6 to 8 ice cubes

Whip all ingredients in a high-powered blender to desired consistency.

Berry Cobbler Shake

1 cup unsweetened almond milk (or milk of your choice)
2 scoops vanilla or berry protein powder or medical food (look for one
    containing at least 20 grams of vegan protein)
2 tablespoons freshly ground flaxseeds
½ teaspoon cinnamon
¼ teaspoon nutmeg
1 to 2 tablespoons chia seeds, measured dry
½ to 1 cup berries, fresh or frozen
6 to 8 ice cubes

Measure the chia seeds and add to the milk. Allow to soak for 10 to 30 minutes. Add all ingredients to a high-powered blender and whip to desired consistency.

Impeccable Pumpkin Shake

1 cup coconut milk (or milk of your choice)
2 scoops vanilla protein powder or medical food (look for one
    containing at least 20 grams of vegan protein)
½ cup frozen precooked pumpkin
½ cup frozen precooked butternut squash
1 cup frozen spinach
1 tablespoon chia seeds
¼ teaspoon pumpkin spice mix (recipe follows)
6 to 8 ice cubes

Whip all ingredients in a high-powered blender to desired consistency.

Pumpkin Spice Mix

This mix also makes a great seasoning for roasted vegetables, especially cauliflower.

3 tablespoons ground cinnamon
2 teaspoons ground ginger
2 teaspoons nutmeg
½ to 1 teaspoon ground allspice
½ to 1 teaspoon ground cloves

Mix well and store in a small glass jar for future uses.

Blueberry Green Smoothie

1 cup cashew milk (or milk of your choice)
½ to 1 cup frozen spinach
½ cup frozen blueberries
2 scoops berry protein powder or medical food (look for one
   containing at least 20 grams of vegan protein)
1 scoop greens powder (look for one containing organic wheatgrass,
   spirulina, spinach, barley grass, alfalfa, chlorella, and kale)
1 tablespoon flaxseeds
1 tablespoon nut butter of your choice (I prefer cashew or almond)
6 to 8 ice cubes

Whip all ingredients in a high-powered blender to desired consistency.

Ginger Spice Shake

1 cup unsweetened almond milk
2 scoops decaf cappuccino protein powder or medical food (look for
   one containing at least 20 grams of vegan protein)
2 tablespoons raw almond butter
2 teaspoons thoroughly minced ginger root*
1 teaspoon cinnamon
1 to 2 handfuls baby spinach, fresh or frozen
6 to 8 ice cubes

Whip all ingredients in a high-powered blender to desired consistency.

*The more you mince the ginger before adding it in, the fewer bits you'll
have to crunch on once it's all blended.

Green Coconut Shake

1 cup unsweetened coconut milk

1 cup baby spinach or kale

2 scoops vanilla protein powder or medical food (look for one
   containing at least 20 grams of vegan protein)

1 scoop greens powder (look for one containing organic wheatgrass,
   spirulina, spinach, barley grass, alfalfa, chlorella, and kale)

2 tablespoons chia, flax, or hemp seeds

6 to 8 ice cubes

Optional: dash of shredded coconut as a topping

Whip all ingredients in a high-powered blender to desired consistency.
Top with shredded coconut, if desired.

Ayurveda Soup

SERVES 4 TO 6

2 tablespoons MCT oil

2 teaspoons mustard seeds

1 cup onion, chopped

1 cup leek, chopped

2 cups carrots, chopped

1 cup sweet potato, diced

1 cup parsnip, chopped

1 cup burdock root, chopped

1 cup celery, chopped

6 to 8 cups chicken or fish bone broth

5 garlic cloves, chopped

½ teaspoon fresh ginger, ground

¼ cup fresh dill, chopped

½ teaspoon paprika

2 teaspoons cumin

Sea salt to taste

Pepper to taste

In a large pot, heat the oil. Toss in the mustard seeds until they toast
and pop open.

Add the onion, leek, carrots, sweet potato, parsnip, and burdock root,
and sauté until slightly softened.

Add the celery and bone broth. Bring to a boil over high heat.

Add the garlic, ginger, dill, paprika, and cumin. Stir well, and let the soup simmer over medium-low heat for about 30 minutes or until vegetables have softened.

Season with salt and pepper, if needed.

Chickpea, Greens, and Sweet Potato Soup

SERVES 4

1 yellow onion, peeled and chopped
3 to 4 garlic cloves, peeled and smashed with the side of a chef's knife
1 fennel bulb, thinly sliced
1 tablespoon oil (extra virgin olive oil, coconut oil, or pastured ghee)
6 to 8 cups bone broth
2 sweet potatoes, cubed
2 to 4 cups chopped greens (spinach, kale, chard, chard stems, beet greens, etc.)
1 can (15½ ounces) cooked chickpeas
1 cup cashews
1 lemon, juiced
Sea salt
Freshly ground black pepper
Optional: dollop of coconut or cashew yogurt (nondairy) for garnish

Sauté onion, garlic, and fennel in a large pot with oil.

After 5 to 10 minutes, add bone broth, sweet potatoes, chopped greens, chickpeas, and cashews. Bring to a boil, then simmer for 30 minutes or so.

Place in a high-speed blender and puree to desired consistency. Add fresh lemon juice, salt, and pepper to taste.

Garnish with yogurt if desired and serve immediately. Keeps in refrigerator up to 3 days.

French Onion Soup

SERVES 4 TO 6

1 tablespoon grapeseed oil
3 large yellow or white onions, quartered and thinly sliced

6 cups vegetable broth, or 4 cups water plus 2 cups chicken bone broth
2 cups greens (kale, chard, or spinach), thinly sliced
1 bay leaf
½ cup fresh thyme, chopped
Sea salt to taste
1 teaspoon fresh ground pepper
½ cup grated vegan cashew nut cheese or nutritional yeast flakes
¼ cup green onions, chopped (for garnish)

Heat the grapeseed oil in a large pot and cook the onions until they are soft and browned.

Add the broth, greens, and bay leaf. Season with thyme, salt, and pepper. Simmer over a low flame for 1 hour.

Garnish with cashew nut cheese or nutritional yeast flakes and green onions.

Cream of Broccoli Soup

SERVES 4 TO 6

6 cups vegetable or bone broth
1 large leek, chopped
2 cups broccoli, chopped
2 cups spinach, chopped
2 cups unsweetened coconut milk
1 parsnip, minced
2 teaspoons nutmeg
2 teaspoons pepper
Salt to taste

Bring the broth to a boil. Add the remaining ingredients and return to a boil.

Allow the soup to simmer for about 30 to 45 minutes until all the vegetables are soft. Turn off the heat and allow to cool slightly.

Blend the soup using an immersion blender or food processor. Taste and adjust the seasonings if necessary. Reheat to serve or enjoy cool.

Kimchi Shirataki Bok Choy Bowl

SERVES 2

2 packages (7 ounces each) thin vermicelli shirataki noodles
4 cups thinly sliced baby bok choy
2 Japanese eggplants, thinly sliced (about 2 cups)
1 tablespoon coconut oil, preferably unrefined and expeller-pressed
1 tablespoon sesame seeds
2 cups thinly sliced greens (kale, chard, or spinach)
Kimchi to taste
2 tablespoons sesame oil

Sauté one package of the shirataki noodles, baby bok choy, and Japanese eggplant in coconut oil, or steam. Sprinkle with sesame seeds.

Assemble all ingredients in a pretty bowl: greens and uncooked shirataki on the bottom, sautéed mixture in the middle, and kimchi on the top, all drizzled with sesame oil.

Sweet Potato Crunch Salad

SERVES 4

6 carrots, thinly sliced
2 fennel bulbs, thinly sliced
1 cucumber, seeded and thinly sliced
2 sweet potatoes, chopped and baked
1 cup fresh parsley, chopped
4 tablespoons freshly squeezed lemon juice
2 tablespoons avocado oil
Sea salt
Freshly ground black pepper
2 tablespoons sunflower seeds

Combine carrots, fennel, cucumber, sweet potatoes, and parsley in a large bowl.

Place lemon juice, oil, salt, and pepper in a sealable container. Cover and shake to make a dressing.

Dress the salad and toss gently. Top with sunflower seeds.

Crispy Cucumber Salad with Cilantro-Tahini Dressing

SERVES 2 TO 4

    3 Kirby cucumbers, thinly sliced
    2 kohlrabies, thinly sliced
    1 fennel bulb, thinly sliced
    1 jicama, thinly sliced
    ½ cup red onion, finely chopped
    1 cup fresh cilantro, chopped
    3 to 4 tablespoons homemade tahini dressing (recipe follows)
    1 tablespoon pumpkin seeds

Toss the cucumbers, kohlrabies, fennel, jicama, and onion together. Add the cilantro and toss well with the tahini dressing. Top with pumpkin seeds.

Heavenly Homemade Tahini Dressing

    1 cup 100% pure ground tahini (sesame paste)*
    ½ to 1 cup warm filtered water
    ¼ to ½ cup fresh lemon juice
    3 to 4 garlic cloves, crushed
    Dash of salt
    Dash of black pepper

Add the ingredients together in a sealable container and mix or shake well until fully combined. It should turn from a paste into a white sauce. Add more water or lemon juice based on your preferred consistency. Use as a salad dressing, a dipping sauce for grilled chicken, or a topping for roasted vegetables!

*Tahini is made from either hulled or unhulled sesame seeds. Unhulled seeds have a more distinct, bitter flavor, whereas hulled seeds are nuttier and make for creamier tahini. Unhulled whole sesame seeds have more calcium, yet hulled seeds are still packed with calcium and other nutrients. It's a question of personal preference.

Home-Style Middle Eastern Hummus

Traditionally, hummus is eaten on fresh bread. Instead, try it with chopped vegetables, yuca root crackers or cassava "flatbread" (see Appendix B), or on a salad.

2 cups cooked chickpeas, plus 1 to 2 tablespoons for garnish
1 lemon, juiced
3 to 4 garlic cloves
⅓ cup 100% pure ground tahini (sesame paste)
1 to 2 tablespoons filtered water, depending on your desired consistency
Dash of sea salt

Put the chickpeas, lemon juice, garlic, and tahini into a food processor. Pulse for about 5 minutes until a paste forms. Slowly add 1 to 2 tablespoons of water until you've reached an ideal creamy texture. Season lightly with sea salt.

Place hummus in a nice bowl or small plate. Garnish with a drizzle of olive oil and chickpeas.

For a more traditional style, use ground za'atar (hyssop), ground sumac, chopped parsley, sesame seeds, and/or pine nuts. For spicy, sprinkle hot pepper flakes, cayenne pepper, or straight-up hot red pepper. Experiment with different herbs mixed into the hummus or as a garnish.

Tzatziki Greek Dip

1 cup (8 ounces) plain yogurt
1 Kirby cucumber
½ cup fresh dill or green onions, finely chopped
3 to 4 cloves garlic, crushed
Pepper to taste
Sea salt to taste

Allow the yogurt to drain in a cheesecloth or muslin bag overnight.

Peel and chop the cucumber into small pieces. Salt them and place them in a colander for about an hour. Strain out the excess water from the cucumbers. Make sure to rinse them well and let them drain again. You may need to massage or squeeze the pieces.

Add the cucumbers, herbs, and garlic into the yogurt and stir well. Refrigerate for at least 30 minutes. Taste it and add sea salt or freshly ground pepper if needed. Delicious as a topping or dip for vegetables, chicken, or fish.

Tempting Tempeh Salad

SERVES 2 TO 4

1 Kirby cucumber, sliced
1 kohlrabi or jicama, julienned
½ cup steamed or baked tempeh, diced into chunks
½ cup grape tomatoes
¼ avocado, diced
¼ cup cooked beets, chopped
2 tablespoons kimchi
1 tablespoon hummus (homemade or preservative-free variety)
2 tablespoons grapeseed oil
Apple cider vinegar, to taste
3 cups arugula
2 tablespoons pumpkin seeds

Layer all ingredients except for the oil, vinegar, arugula, and pumpkin seeds at the bottom of a bowl or to-go container.

Drizzle with grapeseed oil and vinegar.

Top with arugula and pumpkin seeds, and toss when ready to eat. The hummus will blend nicely with the olive oil and vinegar to give the salad a creamy, flavorful coat.

Sassy Slaw

SERVES 2 TO 4

1 tablespoon grated ginger
3 tablespoons fresh lime juice
1 teaspoon coconut aminos
¼ teaspoon cracked black pepper, or to taste
Dash of sea salt
3 tablespoons grapeseed or MCT oil
2½ cups beets, peeled and julienned

1 large Granny Smith apple, julienned
1 small jicama, julienned
1 small kohlrabi, julienned
1 tablespoon sunflower seeds

Combine the ginger, lime juice, coconut aminos, black pepper, and salt in a small mixing bowl. Whisk in the oil and set aside.

In a large bowl, combine the beets, apple, jicama, and kohlrabi. Toss in the prepared dressing and refrigerate until ready to serve. Toss with sunflower seeds and serve.

Caribbean Shredded Salad

SERVES 2

¾ cup snow peas, trimmed
2 cups shredded red cabbage
1 cup shredded carrot
2 green onions, sliced thin
2 cups mizuna or other mixed greens
1 to 2 tablespoons miso mustard dressing (recipe follows)
1 cup chopped papaya
¾ cup macadamia nuts
¼ cup cilantro, chopped
Handful of plantain chips
Freshly ground black pepper

Toss the snow peas, cabbage, carrot, onions, and greens gently with dressing. Portion salad into two bowls. Add the papaya, macadamia nuts, and cilantro on top of the lettuce. Place the plantain chips around the edges of the bowls, then add ground black pepper to taste.

Miso Mustard Dressing

¼ cup avocado oil
3 tablespoons lemon juice
2 tablespoons mellow white miso
1 tablespoon Dijon mustard
1 garlic clove, minced

Whisk together all ingredients, add to a salad base, and toss thoroughly.

Greens Galore Salad

SERVES 2

2 cups dark greens (whichever ones you desire—go wild!)
½ cup purslane leaves, chopped
¼ cup parsley leaves, chopped
1 bunch scallions, chopped
1 medium carrot, grated
1 red bell pepper, chopped
½ jicama, grated
½ cup mushrooms of your choice, chopped
¼ cup chickpeas (if canned, use BPA-free)
1 tablespoon oil of your choice (avocado, olive, macadamia, etc.)
1 tablespoon apple cider vinegar
2 tablespoons walnuts, crushed

Mix together all ingredients except the oil, vinegar, and walnuts in a large bowl. Toss with the oil and vinegar. Top with the walnuts and serve.

Chef's Anchovy Salad

SERVES 2

3 cups mixed greens
½ cup red cabbage, shredded
½ red onion, sliced
1 cup cherry tomatoes, halved
1 kohlrabi, julienned
1 carrot, julienned
1 large hard-boiled pastured egg, peeled and julienned
4 ounces anchovies, sliced into thin pieces
2 tablespoons avocado oil
½ lemon, juiced
10 walnuts, halved
2 tablespoons pumpkin or sunflower seeds

Toss together the greens, cabbage, onion, cherry tomatoes, kohlrabi, and carrot. Place in a salad bowl and arrange the egg pieces and anchovies on top. Mix the avocado oil and lemon juice and toss with the salad. Top with walnuts and seeds.

Baked Onion Mackerel

SERVES 2

- 4 tablespoons extra virgin olive oil
- 1 shallot, minced
- 1 large Maui onion, minced
- 2 garlic cloves, minced
- 1 teaspoon lemon zest
- 1 lemon, juiced and separated
- 8 ounces mackerel
- Sea salt to taste
- Pepper to taste
- 1 to 2 tablespoons fresh dill, minced and separated

Preheat the oven to 450°F. Line a rimmed baking tray with aluminum foil or parchment paper.

In a skillet or small saucepan, heat the olive oil. Add the minced shallot and onion, cooking on medium heat for about 3 minutes, until softened.

Add the garlic and the lemon zest. Cook together for another minute. Once slightly cooled, squeeze in half of the lemon juice.

Place the fish on the prepared baking sheet. Season lightly with salt and pepper. Top with the oil mixture and add half of the dill.

Roast the fish in the oven for 10 to 15 minutes, depending on its thickness. The best way to check if it's cooked is to use a fork to gently prick the fish. If it flakes easily, it's ready.

Carefully remove the fish from the baking tray. Top with the remaining lemon juice and dill.

Grilled Salmon Steaks with Lemon-Herb Mojo

SERVES 2

- 8 ounces salmon steak
- 1 teaspoon sesame or MCT oil
- 1 cup lemon-herb mojo (recipe follows)

Grill salmon on a skillet or grill with a little oil until it's fully cooked. Plate with a generous serving of lemon-herb mojo.

Lemon-Herb Mojo

Mojo is Spanish for sauce. This mojo is great on salads, roasted vegetables, chicken, or fish.

    2 lemons, juiced
    2 tablespoons avocado or extra virgin olive oil
    2 to 3 garlic cloves
    ½ red onion
    ½ cup fresh cilantro or parsley
    Sea salt to taste

Place all the ingredients in a food processor. Chop to combine and pulse until you've created a fragrant, blended sauce.

Fully Loaded Shakshuka

This traditional Middle Eastern dish, pronounced "shaq-shoo-kah," is served for breakfast, but you can eat it anytime. It can be served with yogurt, kefir, or tahini.

SERVES 2

    1 tablespoon grapeseed oil
    1 large sweet onion, sliced
    1 red or green pepper, chopped
    1 small hot pepper, seeded and chopped
    4 garlic cloves
    3 to 4 cups very ripe tomatoes, chopped
    ⅔ cup chickpeas (if canned, use BPA-free)
    2 teaspoons cumin
    1 teaspoon salt
    1 teaspoon ground pepper
    2 tablespoons tomato paste
    2 cups spinach
    4 large pastured eggs
    ¼ cup fresh parsley, chopped

In a large deep pan, heat the oil over medium heat and sauté the onion until brown. Add the peppers and garlic.

Cook for about 5 minutes until soft, then add the tomatoes, chickpeas, cumin, salt, and pepper. Cover and cook on low heat for another 5 to 10 minutes, stirring often. Add the tomato paste and stir well.

Add the spinach and let the vegetables simmer for another 10 to 15 minutes until you've made a thick sauce. Feel free to taste and adjust the seasonings if needed.

Once the sauce has thickened, make four small wells in the pan. Carefully crack each egg and place one into each of the wells. It might be easier if you crack each egg individually into a glass and gently pour it into the sauce. Make sure that the yolks do not break. The egg whites should spread out over the sauce; use a fork to swirl the whites if needed.

Once you've added all the eggs, cover the shakshuka for 5 to 10 minutes until the egg whites have cooked. The yolks should remain slightly runny. Remove from the stove and top with fresh parsley.

Garnish with yogurt or kefir. Definitely experience this recipe while it's hot!

Slow Cooker Chicken

SERVES 4 TO 6

- 3 large onions, thinly sliced
- 2 to 4 cups chicken bone broth
- 1 organic pastured chicken
- 1 pound mushrooms

Assemble all the ingredients in a slow cooker. Cook on high for 4 to 6 hours or low for 6 to 8 hours.

Sweet Potato Burgers

SERVES 2 TO 4

- 1 small sweet potato, thinly sliced
- 2 tablespoons MCT, macadamia nut, or olive oil, separated
- Sea salt to taste
- ¼ teaspoon black pepper
- 2 cups mushrooms, cut into small slices
- 1 cup chopped onion or leek
- 1 to 2 garlic cloves
- ¼ cup walnuts or macadamia nuts, toasted
- ¾ cup almond flour
- 1 tablespoon fresh parsley, finely chopped

1 large pastured egg
1 teaspoon chia or flaxseeds
1 teaspoon fresh ginger, chopped
¼ teaspoon red pepper flakes
¼ teaspoon oregano
¼ teaspoon thyme

Preheat the oven to 400°F and line a baking tray with parchment paper.

Toss the sweet potato with 1 tablespoon oil and season lightly with salt and pepper. Roast for about 15 minutes, until tender.

In a large skillet, caramelize the mushrooms and onions together with the remaining 1 tablespoon oil. Cook until soft. Set aside to cool down.

Place the mushrooms, onions, 1 cup of the cooked sweet potato, garlic, nuts, almond flour, parsley, egg, and chia or flaxseeds in the food processor. Season with the ginger, red pepper flakes, oregano, and thyme, and pulse a few times just until combined.

Lower the oven temperature to 350°F and line the baking tray with a new sheet of parchment paper.

Form small patties of the mushroom/sweet potato mixture. You should get about 6 to 8 patties. Bake for about 30 minutes or until the patties are firm and slightly toasted.

Serve warm with a side salad.

Nut-Crusted Chicken Fingers

SERVES 2 ADULTS OR UP TO 4 CHILDREN

¾ cup ground almonds or walnuts
½ cup ground flax
¼ cup sesame seeds
1 large pastured egg
1 8-ounce boneless, skinless chicken breast, cut into strips

In a small bowl, combine the ground nuts, flax, and seeds. In a separate bowl, beat the egg. Place the chicken breast in the egg to marinate for 5 minutes, flipping the pieces to coat as needed.

Preheat the oven to 350°F. Cover a large baking tray with parchment paper.

Once the chicken is coated well in egg, carefully press the chicken tenders into the nut mixture, making sure they are well coated. Place the coated chicken on the baking tray. Do not crowd the tray.

Bake for about 20 minutes. Remove the chicken from the oven. Flip the chicken pieces and return them to the oven for another 15 to 20 minutes, until chicken is fully cooked and golden. Serve with a sauce or on top of a salad.

Garlic Mashed Yuca

Yuca is a root vegetable grown in subtropical climates, including Mexico and South America. Known also as cassava, yuca is rich in carbohydrates that burn more slowly and serves as an excellent prebiotic for healthy microbiota in the gut.

SERVES 2 TO 6

2 yucas
5 to 6 garlic cloves
2 tablespoons olive oil

Prepare the yuca by peeling it very well, making sure to remove the whole peel and the outer veins. It should be completely white. Quarter it and cut it into chunks.

Add the yuca and garlic to a large pot with boiling water. Make sure the yuca is fully immersed, adding water if needed. Boil for about 30 minutes, until the yuca becomes very tender and starts to flake.

Drain the yuca and garlic, reserving 1 cup of the yuca water. Using an immersion blender or large fork, mash the yuca and garlic while slowly drizzling in the oil. Add ½ to 1 cup of the yuca water as you are blending to get the right consistency.

Garnish with fresh herbs and a kefir sauce (recipe follows) or herb-lemon mojo (see page 340).

Kefir Sauce

1 to 2 cups kefir
½ cup fresh herbs of your choice (cilantro, mint, dill, or parsley)
2 garlic cloves, mashed
Optional: ½ teaspoon cayenne pepper
Optional: Sea salt to taste

Mix together the kefir with the herbs and garlic. Season with a little cayenne pepper or salt if needed.

Tahini Cookies

SERVES 2 TO 4

1 large pastured egg
½ cup xylitol or erythritol
1 teaspoon vanilla
A pinch of salt
½ cup 100% pure ground tahini (sesame paste)
¼ cup sesame seeds

Preheat the oven to 350°F and line a baking tray with parchment paper.

Beat the egg together with the sweetener. Add the vanilla and salt. Stir in the tahini until a solid batter has formed. It will be sticky.

Place sesame seeds onto a small plate. Form small balls of batter and tightly press them into the sesame seeds until fully coated.

Place the cookies on the baking tray 1 inch apart. Bake for 10 to 15 minutes or until golden. Let cool and store in an airtight container.

Almond Coconut Macaroons

SERVES 6 TO 12

1 cup almond flour
2 cups unsweetened shredded or flaked coconut
2 large pastured eggs
½ teaspoon salt

½ teaspoon vanilla extract
½ teaspoon cinnamon
Optional: 1 teaspoon cocoa powder

In a large bowl, mix together the almond flour and coconut. Add the cocoa powder, if desired. In a separate bowl, beat together the eggs.

Pour the eggs into the flour mixture. Add salt, vanilla, and cinnamon.

Wet your hands and form little balls of batter. Pat them tightly together. Place the macaroons at least 1 inch apart on a baking tray lined with parchment paper.

Bake at 300°F for about 15 to 20 minutes or until cookies are golden.

Chocolate-Avocado Ice Cream

SERVES 2 TO 4

1 avocado, peeled and pitted
1 can (13½ ounces) full-fat coconut milk (BPA-free)
½ cup unsweetened cocoa powder
½ cup xylitol
½ cup water
2 teaspoons vanilla extract
½ teaspoon sea salt

Place the avocado and coconut milk into a food processor or blender to combine. Add the remaining ingredients and blend for about 2 minutes, until smooth. You may need to scrape the sides.

Ice cream machine method: Place into a freezer-safe container in the refrigerator for 2 hours to set up before freezing. Prepare and freeze the ice cream according to the manufacturer's instructions.

Hand method: Place into a freezer-safe container and freeze for 1 hour. Over the next 3 to 4 hours, remove the mixture from the freezer and whisk the mixture slightly every 20 minutes to prevent it from getting too icy. It should thicken after each whisking until it's firm enough to scoop.

Prior to serving, let the ice cream thaw for 5 to 10 minutes.

Avocado Lime Sorbet

SERVES 2 TO 4

2 ripe avocados, peeled and pitted
2 cups unsweetened almond milk (or water, if you prefer a lighter taste and icier texture)
½ cup xylitol or erythritol
2 tablespoons fresh lime juice
1 tablespoon lime zest
½ teaspoon sea salt

Place the ingredients in a food processor or blender and combine.

Ice cream machine method: Transfer the mixture to the chilled container of your ice cream machine. Prepare and freeze according to the manufacturer's instructions.

Hand method: Place the mixture into a freezer-safe container and freeze for 1 hour. Over the next 3 to 4 hours, remove the mixture from the freezer and whisk it slightly every 20 minutes to prevent it from getting too icy. It should thicken after each whisking until it's firm enough to scoop.

Best if eaten within 24 hours.

Acknowledgments

Many people helped me complete this book. I'll narrow it down to the few who really made a difference, but I am grateful to all who contributed and made this book better, especially to the women who are represented here as case studies, although most of their names and details have been changed to protect their identities.

Warmest thanks to my digital team, editors, publishing team, readers, friends, and colleagues, especially Nathalie Hadi, Laura Friedlander, Kevin Plottner, Caroline de Lasa, Yoni Wiseman, Christina Wilson, Celeste Fine, Gideon Weil, Laina Adler, Melinda Mullin, Sydney Rogers, Andrea Vinley Converse, Elaine Hooker, Becca Edwards, Amy Mansfield Weinberg, Leslie Murphy, Leslye Robbins, Allison Post, Anne Zolfghari, Chris Kresser, Kevin Gianni, Nick Polizzi, Brent Eck, Katie Ferran, Todd Crane, Lisa Contreras, Nilima Desai, Roda Cisco, Alan Christianson, NMD, Bethany Hays, MD, Eric Hassid, MD, David Perlmutter, MD, and Martin Rossman, MD.

Special thanks to my dear friend Johanna Ilfeld, PhD, who cheerfully debated with me about how to make protocols doable for most people. Jo kept me laughing and going to yoga despite the many drafts and deadlines.

Above all, thanks to my family for enduring my years of left-hemisphere domination leading up to the fall that led to the epiphany behind this book, including Maya, Gemma, Juneau, Albert and Mary Lil Szal, Anna Esterline, and Justina Phillips. My husband, David Gottfried, continues to be my greatest sounding board, reader, and teacher—and the love of my life!

Thank you all for upgrading my social genomics and making my brain body better!

Appendix A

Cast of Characters

In order to get the most out of this book and your Brain Body Diet, it's worthwhile to become familiar with the various chemical messengers—neurotransmitters, growth factors, and hormones—that shuttle through the brain, affecting your thoughts and behavior. They are all regulatory proteins and may overlap, i.e., some hormones act like neurotransmitters and growth factors. Neurotransmitters relay signals from one nerve to another across a synapse, such as nerve to nerve, nerve to muscle, or nerve to gland. Growth factors are substances capable of stimulating cellular growth, proliferation, differentiation, and healing. Hormones are created in the endocrine glands and control most bodily functions, including metabolism, reproduction, and mood. Many of the brain messengers "crosstalk"; for instance, as serotonin levels rise, norepinephrine levels fall.

Here are the most important chemical messengers produced in the brain, their jobs, and what it feels like when they're off. You may have an aha moment when you read the list of symptoms if a part of your brain is not functioning properly.

Brain Messenger	Job	Conditions or Symptoms When Out of Balance
Brain-derived neurotrophic factor (BDNF)	Involved in neurogenesis and brain plasticity by promoting survival of nerve cells, especially the neurons that produce dopamine. Also supports long-term memory.	You feel like you cannot heal or rewire your brain. Depression, schizophrenia, obsessive compulsive disorder; Alzheimer's and other dementias; anorexia, bulimia; addiction to opiates.
Dopamine	Controls brain's reward circuit; regulates motivation, movement, and emotional responses.	Bored, apathetic, a loss of satisfaction and pleasure; impulsivity, reward deficiency, vulnerability to addiction; depression, fatigue, attention deficit; poor motor skills (extreme: Parkinson's disease).
Gamma-aminobutyric acid (GABA)	Calming or "downer" (inhibitory) neurotransmitter that counters the effect of glutamate and creates calmness, like nature's Xanax. GABA and glutamate act in a complementary fashion.	Too low: you feel overstimulated; panic, depression, anxiety, insomnia, PTSD, premenstrual syndrome (PMS), addiction (especially alcohol cravings).
Glutamate	"Upper" or excitatory neurotransmitter that may be the most important messenger for normal brain function. One type of glutamate receptor is the target of the drug MDMA (3,4-methylenedioxy methamphetamine, known as Ecstasy or Molly), a "party" drug that alters mood and perception. (Other targets of Ecstasy are the dopamine and the serotonin transporter.)	Too high: overexcitement, restlessness, inability to focus, anxiety, pain amplification (hyperalgesia). When extreme, neurodegeneration like amyotrophic lateral sclerosis (ALS) or Parkinson's disease. An example of a dietary glutamate that can excite the brain is monosodium glutamate, or MSG, which may cause headache, flushing, sweating, nausea, and palpitations.

Brain Messenger	Job	Conditions or Symptoms When Out of Balance
Neurosteroids	The brain has its own endocrine system and can produce sex hormones, known as *neurosteroids*, that act on the central nervous system. Examples: • pregnenolone • progesterone • allopregnanolone • 17ß-estradiol • dehydroepiandrosterone (DHEA, DHEAS) • testosterone • deoxycorticosterone • allotetrahydrodeoxy-corticosterone	Problems with neuron health, excess neuron excitability, seizure susceptibility including menstrual-cycle-related seizure disorder, alcohol abuse, anxiety, depression, negative moods especially in women, neurodegenerative disease, PMS.
Norepinephrine	Stress hormone involved in the brain's ability to pay attention and respond to action, cognitive function, motivation, and energy, all of which we need for healthy social relationships. Plays a key role in fight-flight-freeze by increasing arousal, alertness, and vigilance.	Too high: you feel stuck in fight-flight-freeze. High blood pressure, headache, profuse sweating, palpitations, nervousness, or worry. Too low: you feel a lack of focus and attention, depression, poor sleep, reluctance to socialize.
Oxytocin	The "cuddle" or "trust" hormone involved in love, bonding, and connection. Released in social interaction, orgasm, labor and delivery, and breastfeeding.	You feel like you're missing your cashmere hoodie: chronic stress, low libido, autism, poor connections with others.
Serotonin	Controls mood, sleep, thought flow, and appetite; regulates bowel function. (Many of the brain messengers crosstalk. For instance, as serotonin levels rise, norepinephrine levels fall.)	Life feels blah. Depression, osteoporosis, sugar cravings. Serotonin syndrome (agitation, restlessness, high blood pressure and heart rate, diarrhea, muscle rigidity).

Appendix B

Laboratory Testing

NEUROINFLAMMATION TESTS

1. **8-OHdG**

   Urinary 8-hydroxy-2′-deoxyguanosine (8-OHdG) is an excellent biomarker of oxidative stress and a risk factor for a variety of conditions (including oxidative stress and oxidative DNA damage) and diseases (including metabolic syndrome, cancer, Alzheimer's disease, and environmental exposures).

   www.doctorsdata.com/dna-oxidative-damage-assay

2. **Cyrex Arrays 2, 3, 4, 7X, 20**

   Cyrex is an immunology lab that assesses the crosstalk between the brain and body, especially the gut and hormones. I commonly test my patients for array 2, intestinal antigenic permeability; array 3, wheat/gluten proteome reactivity and autoimmunity; sometimes array 4, gluten-associated cross-reactive foods and food sensitivity; array 7X, expanded neurological autoimmune reactivity screen; and array 20, blood-brain barrier permeability.

   www.cyrexlabs.com

3. **Diffusion Tensor Imaging (DTI)**

   DTI is an emerging brain imaging technology that measures the flow of water through networks of the nervous system, thereby measuring the flow of energy in the brain. It's an MRI technique that helps us see the synaptic map and is better able to show brain damage when traditional brain imaging is less sensitive.

TOXICITY TESTS

1. **Quicksilver Scientific**

   This is the lab that I use for measuring heavy metals. I use its Mercury Tri-Test because it's the only current test that measures mercury speciation, which means it separates methyl mercury from inorganic mercury by measuring each directly. This avoids the need for a urine challenge test, which measures total mercury. Additionally, I use Quicksilver's Blood Metals Panel, which assesses other potentially toxic elements: arsenic, cadmium, cobalt, lead, mercury, silver, and strontium.

   www.quicksilverscientific.com

2. **Genova Toxic Effects CORE**

   Toxic body burden is at the root of brain/body dysfunction. This test from Genova assesses levels of bisphenol A (BPA), chlorinated pesticides, organophosphates, PCBs, phthalates and parabens, and volatile solvents (i.e., the toxins that are related to chronic, neurodegenerative, and autoimmune conditions, as well as diabetes and weight gain). Signs of exposure include but are not limited to allergies, asthma, autoimmune conditions, brain fog, heart disease, cancer, fatigue, frequent infections, hypertension, learning challenges, mood disorders, and obesity.

   www.gdx.net/product/toxic-effects-core-test-urine-blood

3. **Genova NutrEval**

   This test documents micronutrient deficiencies and heavy metals in the blood and urine and provides information about personalized supplementation need for antioxidants, amino acids, B vitamins, digestive support, essential fatty acids, and minerals.

   www.gdx.net/product/nutreval-fmv-nutritional-test-blood-urine

4. **Great Plains Toxic Non-Metal Chemical Profile (GPL-Tox)**

This test screens for 172 different toxic chemicals including organophosphate pesticides, phthalates, benzene, xylene, vinyl chloride, pyrethroid insecticides, acrylamide, perchlorate, diphenyl phosphate, ethylene oxide, acrylonitrile, and more. This profile also includes tiglylglycine (TG), a marker for mitochondrial disorders resulting from mutations of mitochondrial DNA. These mutations can be caused by exposure to toxic chemicals, infections, inflammation, and nutritional deficiencies.

www.greatplainslaboratory.com/gpl-tox

5. **Visual Contrast Sensitivity Test**

This test is administered online and involves a short questionnaire followed by a visual test (your computer screen will need to be eighteen inches from your eyes). It is a screening test for neurotoxins and biotoxins. You need 20/20 vision to perform the test accurately.

www.survivingmold.com/diagnosis/visual-contrast-sensitivity -vcs or www.vcstest.com

Genetic Testing

DNA LIFE

I use the DNA Life assays together with biomarker testing so that we can assess a patient's genotype and phenotype. I use **DNA Mind, DNA Diet, DNA Health, DNA Oestrogen, DNA Sport,** and **DNA Skin.** You will need to run the test with your health care practitioner.

http://www.dnalife.healthcare

GENOMIND

I use the **Mindful DNA** and **Genecept** assays frequently to personalize brain/body recommendations. Mindful DNA is a direct-to-consumer test available on Amazon and its website. For the best results, I'd recommend running the test with your health care practitioner so that you can simultaneously test biomarkers with genomics.

https://genomind.com

GENOVA

I recommend the following tests to review the genomics of detoxification. They need to be ordered through a licensed practitioner. Additionally, I use the EstroGenomic Profile before prescribing bioidentical estrogen therapy for a woman.

- **DetoxiGenomic Profile:** www.gdx.net/core/sample-reports /Detoxi-Genomics-Sample-Report.pdf
- **EstroGenomic Profile:** www.gdx.net/core/support-guides /Estro-Genomic-Support-Guide.pdf
- **NeuroGenomic Profile:** www.gdx.net/product/neurogenomic -test-saliva

PATHWAY

I commonly order the **PathwayFit** test because it provides actionable data on metabolism, optimal food plan, exercise, and supplements. The report is intuitive and easy to understand.

www.pathway.com/fit-products

SMARTDNA

SmartDNA provides genomic testing through registered practitioners.

www.smartdna.com.au

23ANDME

23andme.com is still the most affordable option, although you end up having to do much of the interpretation yourself or use additional interpretations systems for a nominal fee, such as MTHFR Support (https:// mthfrsupport.com) or Promethease (https://promethease.com).

www.23andme.com

Other Laboratory Testing

Additional tests that I use routinely in my lifestyle medicine practice are listed below for sex hormones, blood sugar, gut function, and telomeres. Measure your urine for four-point cortisol, estrogen, and steroid hormone metabolism with DUTCH. You can also measure your anabolic-to-catabolic ratio and estrogen and steroid hormone metabolism with Genova's Complete Hormones test. Review results with a functional medicine clinician.

- Sex hormones
  — **Dried Urine Test for Comprehensive Hormones (DUTCH)** by Precision Analytical will provide information about adrenal hormone metabolism, including estrogens: https://dutchtest.com
  — **Complete Hormones** test by Genova: www.gdx.net/product/complete-hormones-test-urine
  — **Essential Estrogens** by Genova: www.gdx.net/product/essential-estrogens-hormone-test-urine

- Blood sugar
  — Two home glucose meters that I like are the **Precision Xtra Blood Glucose and Ketone Monitoring System** and **Contour next EZ.** Both require that you prick your finger for a drop of blood, and the meters plus supplies are available at drugstores and online. I prefer the Precision because you can also check your blood ketones, and both glucose and ketones may be helpful to monitor while on the Brain Body Protocol.
  — Often your clinician will be willing to test your fasting blood sugar and hemoglobin A1C, a three-month average of your blood glucose. For direct-to-consumer testing of blood sugar, including fasting glucose and insulin, and hemoglobin A1C, I recommend **WellnessFx:** www.wellnessfx.com.

- Gut, microbiota, and microbiome testing (review results with a functional medicine clinician)
  — **American Gut Project:** http://humanfoodproject.com/americangut
  — **Gastrointestinal Microbial Assay Plus (GI-MAP)** by Diagnostic Solutions Lab
  — **Great Plains Organic Acids Test**
  — **Doctor's Data Comprehensive Stool Analysis**
  — **uBiome:** https://ubiome.com
  — **Viome:** www.viome.com

—Small intestinal bacterial overgrowth (SIBO) testing with the **lactulose breath test:** https://sibocenter.com/

- Telomeres
  —**SpectraCell:** www.spectracell.com/clinicians/products/telomere-testing
  —**TeloYears:** www.teloyears.com

Heart Rate Variability (HRV) Testing

My husband and I use HRV testing daily to assess our capacity for exercise. When my HRV is ≥ 50, I can walk, practice yoga or Pilates, or go to barre. When my HRV is ≥ 70 is when I feel best running or spinning. When I'm < 50, I use a foam roll and take a day off. We use the combination of a heart rate chest strap (from **Polar** or **Wahoo**) together with the **SweetBeat** app. If my HRV is < 50, I use **HeartMath** for HRV training. Learn more at Heartmath.org. Throughout the day, I measure my HRV using a wearable called **The WellBe,** available on Amazon or https://thewellbe.com.

Recovery

FOOD AND HUNGER

http://beyondhunger.org
www.foodaddicts.org

ALCOHOL AND OTHER SUBSTANCES

www.hipsobriety.com
http://moderation.org
www.aa.org
www.smartrecovery.org
http://womenforsobriety.org

Food and Drink Recommendations

Nondairy yogurt, cashew yogurt:
  http://livingculturessuperfoods.com
Prebiotic foods are indigestible fibers that fertilize the probiotics,
  but you may need to avoid them if you have dysbiosis or small
  intestinal bacterial overgrowth. If you don't have these gut issues,
  good sources include raw asparagus, cabbage, chicory root,
  dandelion greens, fennel, Jerusalem artichoke, jicama, garlic,
  onion, potatoes, radicchio, cooked onions, unripe bananas,
  watermelon, chickpeas, lentils, and pistachios.
Yucan Crackers are made by Mission Heirloom in Berkeley and are
  available on Amazon.com
Sleep Welle Calming Tea by Welleco: www.welleco.com
Super Elixir Greens by Welleco: www.welleco.com

Kitchenware

GreenPan. Ceramic nonstick, toxin-free cookware featuring the
  Thermolon coating, free of PFOA, PFAS, lead, and cadmium.
  Dishwasher- and metal utensil–safe.
Scanpan. Environmentally progressive nonstick pans made in
  Denmark and free from PFOA and PFOS, the toxins in Teflon, yet
  provide a durable nonstick surface. The Classic Fry Pan is the most
  versatile pan in my collection (9.5 inch/24 cm). www.scanpan.com
  and Amazon.com

Wearables

Fitbit Ionic is good for athletes (i.e., my husband).
Fitbit Surge is more appropriate for recreational exercisers like me.
Muse Headband is being used at 120 research institutions. I use it for
  ten to thirty minutes per day.

Oura Ring is a "smart ring" worn on a finger that tracks sleep, activity, body temperature, heart rate, and heart rate variability.

The WellBe provides continuous heart rate variability testing and offers visualizations if you need to calm down.

Saunas

https://infraredsauna.com
www.sunlighten.com

Other Resources

KUNDALINI YOGA

Guru Jagat, *Invincible Living* (San Francisco: HarperOne, 2017). Her website is https://ramayogainstitute.com/guru-jagat/, and her course called "Kundalini Yoga 101" on MindBodyGreen.com is one of the best courses out there (use code gottfried20 for 20 percent off): www.mindbodygreen.com/classes/kundalini-yoga-101.

Guru Gayatri (Gobinday Mukanday) is the Kundalini mantra recommended in chapter 5 and by Yogi Bhajan, master of Kundalini yoga, to clear deep-seated blocks. You repeatedly chant the eight names of the Divine in Sanskrit. I was introduced to it by one of my yoga teachers, Liya Garber of Berkeley (www.liyagarber.com). I like the version by Snatam Kaur at https://youtu.be/n8WFN-fzcko. You can listen and chant along while you sit quietly. Here's another by Tera Naam: https://youtu.be/JRun1qQEXkE. Here is the mantra:

Gobinday, Mukunday, Udaray, Apaaray, Hariang, Kariang, Nirnamay, Akaamay

Sustainer, Liberator, Enlightener, Infinite, Destroyer, Creator, Nameless, Desireless

GUIDED MEDITATION AND VISUALIZATION

Martin Rossman, MD, *The Worry Solution* (New York: Harmony, 2010), and *Anxiety Relief* (Louisville, CO: Sounds True, 2010); his website: https://thehealingmind.org

Tara Brach provides guided meditations and online classes through her website at www.tarabrach.com/guided-meditations

Index

Page numbers in *italics* refer to illustrations.

About the Author

Sara Gottfried, MD, is a world-renowned health expert, board-certified physician, and three-time *New York Times* bestselling author. After graduating from Harvard Medical School and MIT, Dr. Gottfried completed her residency at the University of California at San Francisco. She lives in Northern California with her husband and children.